AF555953

CHILDBIRTH AND POSTNATAL CARE

Management of Critical Care, Miscarriages and Diseases

CHILDBIRTH AND POSTNATAL CARE

Management of Critical Care, Miscarriages and Diseases

Encyclopaedia of Women Health and Empowerment—6

DR. R. KUMAR
MBBS, MS Ex PGI
Eye Specialist, Health Columnist, and
Advisor, Healthcare Medical Tourism,
Chandigarh

and

DR. MEENAL KUMAR
MBBS, MD, DGO
Senior Gynecologist and Menopause Consultant,
Chandigarh

Foreword by

PROF. N.K. GANGULY
MD, D.Sc (*hc*), FRC (Path.) London,
FAMS, FNA, FASc, FNASc, FTWAS (Italy)
FIACS (Canada), FIAMSA
Director General (Ex)
Distinguished Bio-Tech
Fellow, Dept. of Biotech, GOI
Visiting Professor, Universities of Boston, Minnesota, JNU

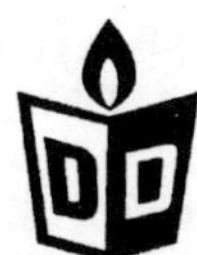

DEEP & DEEP PUBLICATIONS PVT. LTD.
F-159, Rajouri Garden, New Delhi-110027

CHILDBIRTH AND POSTNATAL CARE
Encyclopaedia of Women Health and Empowerment—6

ISBN 978-81-8450-128-5 (Vol. 6)
ISBN 978-81-8450-135-3 (Set)

Typeset by S.S. COMPOSERS,
3190, Mohindra Park, Shakur Basti, Delhi-110034.

Printed in India at MAYUR ENTERPRISES,
WZ Plot No. 3, Gujjar Market, Tihar Village, New Delhi-110018.

Published by DEEP & DEEP PUBLICATIONS PVT. LTD.,
F-159, Rajouri Garden, New Delhi-110027.
Phones: 25435369, 25440916
E-mail: ddpbooks@yahoo.co.in • ddpubs@gmail.com
Showroom:
2/13, Ansari Road, Daryaganj, New Delhi-110002 • Telefax: 23245122

Contents

	Foreword	vii
	Preface	ix
1.	The Normal Childbirth and Caesarean Delivery	1
2.	Mother Needs Critical Care after Childbirth	23
3.	Abortions and Miscarriages	85
4.	Infertility can make Life Fruitless	120
5.	Diseases and Medical Conditions in Women's Prime of Life	164
	Appendices	219
	Bibliography	338
	Index	377

आचार्य एन.के. गांगुली
महानिदेशक
Prof. N.K. GANGULY
MD, D.Sc (hc), FRC Path. (London), FAMS, FNA, FASc, FNASc
FTWAS (Italy), FIACS (Canada), FIMSA
Director General (Ex)
Distinguished Bio-Tech
Fellow, Dept. of Biotech, GOI
Visiting Professor, Universities of Boston,
Minnesota, JNU

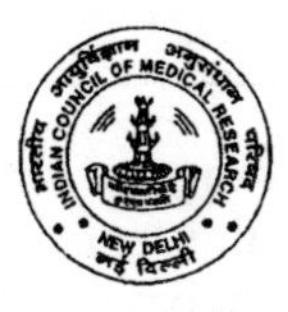

भारतीय आयुर्विज्ञान अनुसंधान परिषद
वी. रामलिंगस्वामी भवन, अंसारी नगर,
पोस्ट बॉक्स 4911, नई दिल्ली - 110 029
Indian Council of Medical Research
V. Ramalingaswami Bhawan, Ansari Nagar,
Post Box 4911, New Delhi - 110 029

Foreword

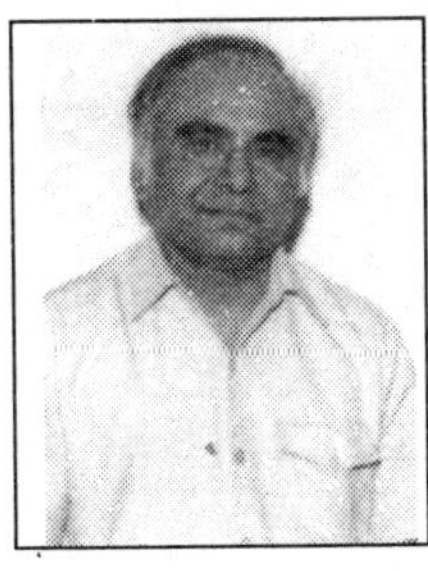

'Encyclopaedia of Women Health and Empowerment' contains a wealth of information in its 12 volumes for women across ethnic, racial, religious and geographic boundaries with tools to enable them to take charge of their health and lives. This is the first book of this magnitude on women's health, I have come across to support women and to work to create a just society in which good health is not a privilege but a human right.

Conventional medical care, with its heavy emphasis on drugs, surgery, and crisis intervention, helps us when we are sick, but it does not always keep us healthy. To a great extent, what makes us healthy or unhealthy is how we are able to live our daily lives: the quality of the food we eat and the air we breathe; access to healthcare; how we exercise; how much rest we get; how much stress we live with; how much we use alcohol, tobacco, or other drugs; how safe or hazardous our workplaces are; whether we experience the threat or reality of sexual violence. Some of these things are under our control as individuals. Many, however, are not; we can influence them only by working with others to bring changes: pressuring an employer to remove hazards, forming a co-op for cheaper high-quality food, protesting the pollution from a nearby chemical plant, starting a network of "safe houses" for women who may be experiencing domestic abuse. These books offer basic information to all women, who need to take care of their health at home and in the workplace.

This series of 12 books gives women the power and the knowledge to take charge of their own health, development and empowerment. It remains a valuable resource for women of all ages and backgrounds. It reflects that vital health concerns of women of diverse ages, racial backgrounds, and sexual orientations. In these pages, women will find new information, resources, and personal support for the decisions that will shape their health—and their lives—from living a healthy life, to relationships and sexuality, to childbearing, growing older, dealing with the medical system, and organizing for change. These volumes are for women of all generations to use, to rely on, and to share with others. This book is also for the governments, societies, communities and groups that are interested in women, in one way or the other.

The society must explore a range of strategies and tactics to reach a variety of women nationwide. At the level of Central and State level, we should work to promote healthful behaviours and practices by all women across all stages of their lives. We also need to work with NGOs and business organizations. I send this message of good wishes to the authors of this series of books and hope that these books would be of use to governmental and non-governmental organizations.

Within these pages, you will find the voice of a women's health movement that is based on shared experience. Listen to it—and add your own.

Nirmal Kumar Ganguly

New Delhi (N.K. GANGULY)

Preface

Just as there is no one type of woman, there is no single strategy for promoting good health among all women in India or other Asian countries, at all stages of their lives. Whether it's researching how to increase the survival of girl child, promote breastfeeding, immunization, mammogram usage among certain populations, increasing cardiovascular disease preventive behaviors, or promoting safer sex practices among at-risk women, you have to constantly look for new and innovative ways to have access to all the women from newborn babe to extreme old age. To truly have an impact on women's health, we must ask questions that address every aspect of a woman's life and at all the stages from birth to sunset. Does a young girl play sports? If she does, she's more likely to have good physical and psychological health. Does a young adult woman get regular screenings for cervical cancer? If so, cervical cancer can be prevented from developing almost 100% of the time. The lifelong interaction between a woman and her environment, cultural and social influences, personal and familial responsibilities, psychological and physical characteristics and lifestyle choices—these are true indicators of how healthy a woman's life can be. A life-cycle approach has been followed in this series of books.

Women's health is best explored not as a series of isolated medical conditions but in terms of all the factors that affect a woman's health and quality of life throughout her lifespan. On the one hand we see a new age woman whose life is changing on every level. She's living in a different family structure than her mother did; she's marrying later, if at all; she's more likely to be the sole head of a household; she's working; she's getting older; and she's living longer. On the other hand, there is a woman living in traditional society, who is fully subjugated and powerless even to survive or thrive. We consider women's health as encompassing all functions that relate to women's mental and physical wellness from conception, neonatal period, infancy, childhood, puberty through old age, the factors that affect wellness, and the activities and behaviors that promote it. Although lives are a continual process of learning and adapting and growing, women's lives involve several stages viz. newborn and neonatal period, infancy, childhood, puberty, adolescence, youthhood, marriage and pregnancy, antenatal period, childbirth and postnatal care, pre-menopausal stage, post-menopausal health problems, old age and so on. Each stage has to be studied in some detail to bring wellness, development and empowerment in her life.

We must explore a range of strategies and tactics to reach a variety of women nationwide. At the level of ministry of women and child in the central government and as well as at the state level, we should work to promote healthful behaviors and practices by all women, across all the stages of their lives. Among other things, for all ages we want to encourage routine and appropriate immunization, physical activity, good nutritional habits, safe sexual choices, no tobacco use, and healthy development and ageing. We also need to work with NGOs, non-profit and business organizations, and state and local health departments, among others. America's office of women's health (OWH) can be used as a model to set-up a nodal agency to supervise all aspects of women's health, at all stages of their lives.

The series of books under the umbrella of 'Encyclopaedia of Women Health and Empowerment' in 12 volumes highlights our approach to women's health development in India and other Asian countries. It discusses the key issues that affect women at each stage of life, from birth through the end of life. As you will see, much of the work focuses on promoting longevity coupled with better quality of life besides preventing disease, injury, and disability. Our main message is that just by changing the mindset towards the girl child and women, over time—many of the diseases, injuries, and disabilities experienced by women can be prevented and thus women of the nation can be empowered. The first volume entitled 'Newborn Girl Child' dealt with various issues concerning the hostility, neglect and discrimination towards girls from pre-birth times to the stages of neonatal period, infancy and subsequent stages of her life. The emphasis has been laid on the psyche of traditional Indian and other Asian families, while focusing on the aspects of female feticide, infanticide and the consequent unfavorable male to female ratio in our societies. It further dealt with the aspects of prematurity, birth defects and other aspects of parenting during neonatal period and infancy. The second volume dealt with the growth and development of girl children from 5-12 years of age. It highlights the feeding and nutrition, immunization, basics of different foods, common medical conditions, pre-pubertal zone and rapid growth, specific problems of girl children and the forms of violence unleashed on them. Similarly, the health and development aspects of teenager girls and the female youth has been dealt with in subsequent volumes (3-4).

The preceding volume (5) dealt with the aspects of pregnancy and antenatal care. Complications during early pregnancy can include a miscarriage, which is the natural termination of the pregnancy by the body, or an ectopic pregnancy, where the fetus develops outside the uterus, in the fallopian tubes. During mid-pregnancy, complications sometimes include an incompetent cervix, in which the cervix opens and expels the fetus prematurely. Other complications during mid-pregnancy include urinary tract infections, excessive weight gain, insufficient weight gain, and premature labor. During late pregnancy, the most common complication is high blood pressure. Polyhydramnios can occur during late pregnancy when extra amniotic fluid develops around the fetus. Intrauterine growth retardation occurs, when the fetus doesn't get the nutrition it needs from the placenta. Other late pregnancy complications include bleeding, premature labor, and overdue delivery. It's important to be aware of signals that could indicate something is wrong. Call your doctor immediately if you experience any of the following symptoms viz. vaginal bleeding, swelling of the face or feet or hands, abdominal pain, loss of fluids from the vagina, prolonged vomiting, blurred vision, painful urination, severe headache, or a fever over 100 degrees. Also, contact a physician if you have regular contractions three to four weeks prior to your due date, if you're injured, or if you notice a significant decrease in the movement of the baby. Discrimination in the area of health care during antenatal period, esp. among the poor and uneducated communities is well known.

Anemia is one of the primary contributors to maternal mortality (20-25%). Most mothers have a lower body mass index (BMI) . A low BMI status, indicative of chronic energy deficiency, is a particularly important aspect of the nutritional risks of women, during reproductive years. The birth weights of newborns appear to be linearly correlated with both maternal body weight and height. The proportion of low birth weight infants increases among mothers with low BMI. Significant incidence of prolonged/obstructed labor and hypotonic uterine contractions in such pregnancies have been reported. Infant Mortality Rate (IMR) for malnourished mothers is 40% higher than for well nourished mothers. As many as 55% are illiterate in this age group and only 17% have completed primary schooling. Low levels of literacy adversely affect reproductive and sexual health awareness and thus quality of life. It was observed that 52% of illiterate mothers gave birth to low birth weight babies suggesting that education plays a considerable role in preventing LBW. The lower socio-economic status of the mother is also associated with low birth weight babies. Domestic responsibilities, working for livelihood, inadequate rest along with malnutrition especially when the energy demands are increased, contribute to a large number of women delivering low birth weight infants.

This book (6) has described the aspects of childbirth and the care during postnatal period. In an attempt to provide a comprehensive picture of women's health and development during reproductive years of life, a variety of sources of information were used—both quantitative and qualitative, national and sub-national or local, including reports, research and studies, and the like. The burgeoning literature on modern and complementary medicine is critically evaluated. Written by primary care physicians, this will be useful for not only the pregnant and lactating women themselves, but also their family practitioners, nurses, paramedics, health planners and administrators, care givers, parents, husbands and other family members. Besides it will also work as reference book for the planners, trainers, health professionals and researchers alike.

Chandigarh

DR. R. KUMAR
DR. MEENAL KUMAR

[illegible] from the [illegible] is both [illegible] It is important to be aware [illegible] of the [illegible] fever over 100 degrees. After [illegible] [illegible] the abnormal [illegible]

Anemia is one of the [illegible] birth weights of newborns appear to be [illegible] [illegible] lack of [illegible] breeding [illegible] along with malnutrition [illegible] contribute to a large number of women [illegible]

This book has described these aspects of [illegible] of women's health and development [illegible] quantitative, national and international [illegible] and studies and [illegible] physicians [illegible] women themselves, but also their family members, nurses [illegible] Health [illegible] other family members [illegible]

Chandigarh [illegible] Dr [illegible] KUMAR

1

The Normal Childbirth and Caesarean Delivery

No one will tell you that giving birth is pain-free or easy, but if you know what to expect, you're much less likely to panic and more likely to feel confident about any choices you are asked to make. Labor is commonly divided into three stages. In the first stage, you will experience shorter, less painful contractions as your cervix begins to dilate and thin out (called effacement of the cervix). Later in the first stage, your contractions will be more frequent and painful as you reach transition, when your cervix will be fully dilated. The second stage involves actually delivering your baby, and the third stage refers to the delivery of the placenta.

Most women dread the pain of labor more than they dread the series of sleepless nights that will follow. Every woman experiences pain during labor differently, and it is very difficult to describe the pain of contractions. In early labor they can feel like menstrual cramps, or can be confined to your back and feel like a lower backache. Some describe contractions as waves of tightening of the stomach and accompanying discomfort. You can often see your stomach harden with the contraction. You can't control your contractions, but your state of mind can greatly affect the amount of pain you feel. If you are having a hospital birth, you should thoroughly discuss your pain relief options in advance when you choose your hospital. Remember, the medical staff is there to help you, and there is no "right" or "wrong" way to give birth. There's nothing wrong with asking for pain relief if you want it. It is important to know what all the options are, and to be fully aware of the implications that your choice will have.

Labor is usually longest with the first child, lasting 12-14 hours or more in most cases. Typically if you have light contractions, your labor will be longer. During the first stage of labor, your cervix will dilate and thin out to allow the baby to pass through the birth canal. Dilatation is measured in centimeters, so when your midwife or doctor says that you have reached ten centimeters dilatation, you know that your baby is ready to be born. The so-called transitional stage at the end of the first stage of labor can be difficult, as you may be quite uncomfortable and yet not be allowed to push. You may shiver or tremble; some women experience nausea or vomiting. Try to employ the breathing techniques you have learned, and try varying your position to make things a little easier. If you have asked for an epidural, the anesthetist will visit you shortly after your admission to hospital. Your baby's heart rate will be monitored by fetoscope, sonicaid, or by a machine. You will have a number of internal examinations to determine how dilated you are. If a long period of time has gone by, or you are experiencing particularly strong contractions, or you are feeling discouraged, ask for an examination so you'll know what progress you've made.

The average duration of the second stage of labor for first-time mothers is about an hour, although it can be as long as two hours or as short as 15 minutes for some. You will feel an overwhelming urge to bear down. When the midwife or doctor tells you, take a deep breath, bend your knees and push. Pushing is very hard work, so don't despair if you're feeling a bit exhausted. It is much easier if you are in a sitting or squatting position, or on your knees or all fours. Take your time with pushing in order to give your tissues and muscles a chance to stretch and thereby avoid the need for an episiotomy. Be sure to push during contractions, not between them. Try to relax your pelvic floor (although this sounds impossible, it can be done). Don't worry if you pass a little urine or stool during pushing. Your midwives and doctors have seen it all before, and it will be whisked away before anyone notices. Try to relax gradually after each push so that the baby maintains some momentum. When the baby is about to be born, your perineum and anus will begin to bulge. Your baby's head will appear more with each contraction, although it may slip back a little in between contractions. After the top of the baby's head appears (called "crowning"), the head will be delivered in the next couple of contractions. As the baby's head stretches the end of the birth canal, you will usually feel a burning or stinging sensation. This lasts only a short time and is followed by numbness as the baby's head stretches your tissues so thin that the nerves are blocked. This creates a natural anesthetic. When you feel this burning sensation, stop pushing and allow your uterus to push the baby out. This can help prevent tearing and avoid the need for an episiotomy. If your doctor or midwife feels that you will need an episiotomy, it will be performed now.

Once the baby's head has emerged, the midwife will ensure that the cord is not around the baby's neck. She will then wipe the baby's eyes, nose and mouth and remove any fluid from the baby's nose and airway. The contractions may stop for a few moments and then restart for the delivery of the baby's shoulders and body. Sometimes the entire baby is delivered in just one contraction! The midwife will probably help with the last part of the delivery by pulling the baby out and lifting him up towards you. Your new arrival will be quite a sight. He will be bluish in color, slippery and covered with blood, amniotic fluid, and vernix, the white greasy substance that protected his skin from amniotic fluid in the womb. His head may be pointy or misshapen from the delivery. He may cry after the delivery and continue to cry for a short while. If your baby is breathing normally, you should be able to hold him and put him to your breast immediately. Both of you should be kept warm. The midwife or nurse will assess your baby and check to make sure breathing is normal. Newborns are assessed by a series of five tests called the Apgar score, administered at one minute and five minutes. Each test is scored with 2, 1, or 0. A breakdown of the tests and their scores is shown below.

Heart rate

- Above 100 beats per minute—2
- Below 100 beats per minute—1
- Absent—0

Breathing

- Regular—2
- Irregular—1
- Absent—0

Movements

- Active—2
- Some—1
- Limp—0

Skin Color

- Pink—2
- Bluish extremities only—1
- Blue—0

Reflexes

- Cries—2
- Whimpers—1
- Absent—0

After your baby is born, the uterus will probably stop contracting for a few minutes. Eventually it will start up again, perhaps helped along by an injection in your thigh of syntometrine or ergometrine, synthetic hormones, which speed up the delivery of the placenta. The third stage of labor is basically nothing more than the delivery of the placenta. The placenta will detach from the uterine wall and be expelled painlessly by the contractions of the uterus. The large blood vessels attached to the placenta will be torn apart and then clamped together by the tightening of the uterine muscles, nature's way of stanching the flow of blood. It is absolutely essential that the entire placenta be delivered, otherwise there is a risk of prolonged bleeding and infection. The midwife will inspect the placenta after it is delivered to ensure that it is intact. You can look at it as well if you're interested. Don't be alarmed if you shake like a leaf after the delivery of the placenta. The shivering and shaking should stop after a half an hour or so. Get your birthing partner to fetch your jumper or cover you with blankets. The umbilical cord will be clamped and cut, and you can put your baby to the breast or simply cuddle up get to know one another. Newborns are usually quite alert in that first hour after birth. You will be washed, stitched if you had an episiotomy, and asked to urinate to ensure that your plumbing is functional. Your baby will be wiped down and weighed, and placed in a cot beside your bed or in a nursery. Labor may occur prior to 36 weeks of pregnancy and is then called preterm labor.

The labor is divided into 3 stages—first, second and third.

Management of First Stage

It starts from the beginning of true labor pains and ends with full dilatation (opening) of cervix. The average duration is approximately 12 hours in first pregnancy and 6 hours in 2nd or more pregnancies. Initially pains are not strong and come at intervals of 15 to 30 minutes and last for 30 seconds. Gradually the interval shortens and intensity and duration increases. In late first stage the pains come at every 3-5 minutes and last for 45 seconds. Pains are usually felt shortly after uterine contraction begins and pass off before complete relaxation of uterus. Maternal and fetal condition remains unaffected except during contraction. Non-interference with watchful expectancy so as to prepare the woman for a smooth delivery in 2nd stage.

- The progress of labor, maternal condition and fetal behavior is monitored so that any deviation from the normal is detected at the earliest possible moment.
- Woman is admitted in hospital, allowed to be in a comfortable position, walk, sit or lie down, enema is given, asked to empty her bladder frequently, adequate fluid intake is advised but should avoid solid food.
- Relief of pain—Various painkillers can be given to help the woman tolerate the pain. Epidural injection can be given if required or opted by the patient.

- Regular monitoring of blood pressure, fetal heart rate and progress of labor is done by the doctor.

Management of Second Stage

Starts from full dilatation (opening) of cervix and ends with expulsion of the fetus. Its average duration is 2 hours in the first delivery and 30 minutes in 2nd or more deliveries. This stage concerns with coming down of fetus and delivery of the fetus through the birth canal. The intensity of pain increases. It comes at interval of 2-3 minutes and lasts for 1-1½ minutes. It becomes successive and unbearable in terminal stage. The patient feels like pushing the baby down and out called "bearing down." The head comes out first followed by shoulders and rest of the body. Patient shows signs of exhaustion.

- Is to assist expulsion of fetus.
- To prevent injury to perineum
- Patient is better lying down under constant supervision of the doctor.
- Nothing has to be taken by mouth except water or ice.
- Patient is shifted to the labor table and given the position for delivery.
- With the help of the doctor the head of fetus slowly passes out of the vagina then the shoulder and rest of the body slips out.
- The slow process prevents injuries to the perineum of the patient.
- The umbilical cord is clamped (tied) and cut.
- If the pediatrician is present, baby is handed over to him.

Management of Third Stage

It begins after the expulsion of fetus and ends with expulsion of placenta and membranes. Its average duration is 15 minutes. The pain stops for a short time. However, intermittent discomfort in the lower abdomen re-appears, corresponding with the uterine contractions. Placenta is expelled by "bearing down" efforts or manual manipulation. Slight bleeding may be present. The patient may have chills and shivering. This is a very crucial stage of labor. This can be done by watchful expectancy or Active management. The placental descent into vagina is allowed to occur spontaneously. If this does not happen spontaneously it can be manually removed by the doctor.

What is Puerperium?

Puerperium is the period following childbirth during, which the body and the organs involved in pregnancy and childbirth, revert back to approximately the pre-pregnant state both anatomically and physiologically. It starts with the expelling of placenta and lasts 6 weeks. It can be divided into—

- Immediate within 24 hours.
- Early—up to seven days.
- Remote—up to 6 weeks.

Lochia is the vaginal discharge for the first fortnight during puerparuim. It comes from uterus, cervix and vagina. It has a fishy smell. Depending up the color its divided into—

- Lochia rubra-red and lasts for 1-4 days.
- Lochia serosa yellowish or pink and lasts for 4-10 days.
- Lochia alba-pale white and lasts for 10-15 days.
- It may be seen up to 3 weeks.

It's smell, color, amount and duration give an idea of infection, retained bits, subinvolution or other lesions. If the woman is not breastfeeding menstruation starts by 6 weeks. If breastfeeding it may be delayed. But usually comes before stoppage of breastfeeding.

Caesarean Section

Caesarean section (C-section) is the delivery of a baby through a cut in the mother's lower abdomen and the uterus, after the end of 28th week. Caesarean births are more common than most surgeries (such as gallbladder removal, hysterectomy or tonsillectomy) because a caesarean section may be life saving for the baby, or mother (or both). Caesarean birth is also much safer today than it was a few decades ago. Hence, 'caesarean' is not something that should scare you, as the ultimate goal is a healthy mother and healthy baby, regardless of the method of delivery. About 10% of all deliveries these days are conducted through caesarian section.

It is important to know a few things about caesarean section in order to be prepared for a caesarean birth if it does happen to you. Types of operations: There are two types of caesarean sections. Lower Segment Caesarean Section (L.S.C.S): Here the extraction of the baby is done through an incision made in the lower segment of uterus. It is the only method practiced in present day obstetrics. Classical or upper segment. Here, the baby is extracted through an incision made in the upper segment of the uterus. Its indications in present day obstetrics are very much limited.

Indications for L.S.C.S. are divided into two categories:

Absolute indications

Previous two caesarean sections, Vaginal atresia (narrowing of the vaginal opening), Advanced carcinoma of the cervix, Placenta Praevia type IV.

Relative indications

These indications are more common:

- Contracted pelvis and cephalo-pelvic disproportion is the commonest indication.
- Previous caesarean section associated with other risk factors.
- Fetal distress during first stage of labor.
- Abnormal uterine contractions leading to non-progress of labor.
- Ante-partum hemorrhage—due to placenta praevia or abruptio placenta.
- Mal-presentations like breech, transverse lie, and brow and mentoposterior position of face.
- Bad obstetric history.
- Failed induction.
- Primigravidae with associated other risk factors.
- Uncontrolled diabetes with previous history of fetal wastage.
- Pelvic tumors such as cervical/broad ligament fibroid, impacted ovarian tumor.

Contraindications of caesarean section in the absence of maternal interest are:

(a) Dead fetus.
(b) Baby is too premature to survive.
(c) Presence of blood coagulation disorders.

Timing of operation can be:

(a) Elective

When the operation is done at a pre-arranged time during pregnancy to ensure best surgical conditions. It is done between 36-38 weeks to deliver a mature baby.

(b) Emergency

When operation is performed in emergency due to unforeseen maternal and fetal complications either during frequency or labor.

There is no doubt that caesarean section is a safe operation, but it is not without problems, and this is why many doctors and midwives feel strongly that there is still a place for normal breech births. A caesarean section means a stay in hospital of around 4-5 days, a more prolonged recovery, and implications for future pregnancies or operations. Overall the risk of dying following caesarean section is 5 times higher than after a normal child-birth. Death is, of course, extremely rare, but infections and above average blood loss are very common. Scar tissue formed during the healing can lead to pain and make future operations more difficult.

For elective surgery you normally come into hospital either the night before the operation or the same morning if it is to be done in the afternoon. Most often an epidural or spinal anesthetic is advised. This involves a very small needle in the back which numbs everything below the navel so you feel no pain. Most women feel a bit of tugging and pulling, but it should not be uncomfortable. This type of pain-relief is safer for you than a general anesthetic. It also means that you can see your baby immediately, and usually hold him before the operation is finished. You will need to have a drip in your hand and a catheter in the bladder to ensure it is empty. Both of these will be removed the day after the operation.

Procedure

- Caesarean section may be an emergency procedure or an elective and hence planned procedure.
- Preparation for the surgery may be done in the labor room or in the theatre itself. This includes putting a catheter into your bladder to drain urine, and an intravenous line (needle) into a vein in your hand or arm to give your body fluids and medications as required.
- You may be given an antacid orally, or injections like Perinorm or Ranitidine to reduce the level of acid in your stomach and prevent vomiting.
- Your abdomen and pubic hair will be shaved, and the area washed with an antibacterial solution.
- Suitable anesthesia is given to you so that you are pain-free during the procedure.

The doctor makes the skin incision first. This is either a vertical incision in the middle from below the navel up to the pubic bone. A transverse or 'bikini cut' incision from side to side just above your pubic hairline. This incision is most common as it heals better and has a shorter recovery time, besides being more cosmetically acceptable. After going through the various layers of the abdominal wall, and opening the bladder fold of peritoneum, the lower segment of the uterus is exposed. The incision is now made on the uterine wall, usually horizontal (side to side) this is preferred as it heals better and bleeds less. However, due to certain circumstances it may be necessary for your doctor to make a vertical incision on the uterus.

Incision on the uterus

- The amniotic sac (bag of water) is broken and your baby is delivered either by hand or using forceps. At this point if you are under regional anesthesia, you may feel some tugging, pulling or some pressure on the upper abdomen.
- The umbilical cord is clamped and cut, and your baby is handed to the neonatologist or nurse for evaluation.
- The placenta is detached from the uterine wall and removed.
- The uterine incision is closed using sutures (usually) or staples, and bleeding is controlled.

- The abdomen is now closed, and the skin sutured. Depending on the initial skin incision, the skin may be closed with removable sutures, staples, or sub-cuticular (under the skin surface) dissolvable sutures.
- You may be given your baby to hold if you are feeling upto it, after observing your vital parameters (pulse, blood pressure, etc.) for some time you may be shifted to your room.
- The complete procedure takes about 45 minutes to one hour in an uncomplicated case. From the initial incision to delivery of the baby takes about 5 minutes, and the remaining time is taken for repairing your uterus and abdominal wall.

Anesthesia and Pain Relief

Different measures may be used for pain relief before, during and after your caesarean. If you had been in labor, you may have been taking medications for pain relief. If an epidural is already in place, for example, when you have been in labor for a while before you needed a caesarean section, it is usually continued for the surgery.

During the surgery, regional anesthesia, which acts to block the pain only at the operative area (and below), is usually preferred. This may be an epidural, typically being continued from labor analgesia. Another type of regional anesthesia is spinal anesthesia, which can be given more quickly, provides better pain relief and is usually preferred if an anesthetic is not already given. The advantages of regional anesthesia include the fact that you are not unconscious, only the lower half of your body is numb. Hence, you are aware of when your baby is delivered and may even see/hold the baby before he/she is shifted out of the operating room. More than that, some risks of general anesthesia like aspiration, respiratory complications and delayed breastfeeding are also avoided. It may be possible that a regional anesthetic cannot be given to you for medical reasons. Another possibility is that, in an emergency caesarean there may not be enough time to give a regional block. In such cases general anesthesia is given, where you will be completely unconscious during the surgery. Some women, who are apprehensive about the surgery may infact opt for general anesthesia as a personal choice. Your doctor, in conjunction with the anesthesiologist (doctor giving the pain relief) will be the right person to help you decide what is best for you.

Common indications for emergency caesarean sections are:

- Fetal distress.
- Dystocia or non-progress of labor.
- Bleeding from your placenta.

An emergency surgery is always more risky than a planned procedure. This may be because you are not on empty stomach, or there are life threatening problems like severe bleeding or rise in your blood pressure, or complete facilities like experienced anesthetist/neonatologist/operative team/blood may not be immediately available.

This is one reason why your doctor may suggest a planned or elective caesarean section to you. If there are certain pre-existing conditions, which make it nearly certain that you will not be able to deliver safely vaginally, it may be better to do a planned procedure. This could be for reasons like—

- Previous 2 or more caesareans.
- Placenta praevia.
- Mal-presentations of your baby, etc.

Let us now understand some of the reasons for which caesarean births may be required.

Dystocia (difficult or abnormal labor patterns)

The causes of dystocia are many, but basically the end result is that labor fails to progress, is prolonged excessively, or gets arrested. Your doctor may try measures like augmenting contractions with oxytocin, or rupturing the amniotic sac to improve the labor pattern. If these fail, however Caesarean section may be the only option.

Fetal distress

Your baby may not be tolerating the forces of labor well, and may show problems like irregularity or slowing of the heart rate, or acid in the blood. Sometimes greenish discoloration of the amniotic fluid (passage of meconium or fetal stools in utero) may be a sign of distress. If vaginal delivery cannot be completed quickly, a caesarean may be the best way to save your baby.

Mal-presentations

Unfavorable positions of the fetus in utero can make vaginal delivery difficult, dangerous or impossible. These include:

- Transverse lie,
- Shoulder presentation,
- Oblique lie,
- Breech presentation (buttocks first),
- Posterior face presentation,
- Face presentation, and
- Brow presentation.

Some of these conditions may be corrected before the onset of pains by a procedure called 'external cephalic version', by which your doctor attempts to turn the baby to the correct position. This may not be feasible or safe in all cases. Though, for breech, particularly if you have had a normal delivery earlier, it may be possible in some cases to deliver the baby vaginally. However, even without difficulties in delivery, breech babies have a less favorable outcome. Hence many doctors opt for planned caesarean. This is a problem which needs prior discussion with your doctor.

Placental or cord problem

The placenta is the main connection between the mother and the fetus providing nutrition, oxygen and other essentials to the baby via the umbilical cord. Bleeding occurring from the placenta before delivery can be risky. It may be due to an abnormal location of the placenta 'placenta praevia'. It may be due to early separation of a normally located placenta called 'abruption placenta'. These can endanger your life or your baby's health. Hence a Caesarean section may be done.

The umbilical cord may prolapse (come out) into the vagina before the baby's birth. This is more common with malpresentations. Pressure on the prolapsed cord can lead to baby's death. Hence an emergency caesarean section is usually required.

Cephalo-pelvic Disproportion or mismatch between the size of the baby and the birth passage. This may be due to abnormalities in the bony pelvis such as:

- A small or contracted pelvis.
- Resulting from previous pelvic injury or fracture.
- A large sized baby where the baby is too big to deliver through the pelvis.

Proper evaluation of fetal and pelvic relative sizes is best done after 38 weeks or ideally at the onset of labor. Even if mild disproportion is suspected, your doctor may suggest a 'trial of labor' where a wait and watch policy is followed to see what the forces of labor can achieve. This may avoid unnecessary caesareans.

Sometimes, other conditions may be present which may be the reasons for your doctor suggesting caesarean section:

- A stenosed cervix.
- A thickly cervix, which does not open up.
- Previous pelvic repair of a urinary or rectal fistula.
- Active herpes lesions of the genital tract.

Maternal medical conditions

- Pre-eclampsia or Pregnancy Induced Hypertension (PIH) is a leading cause of maternal and fetal problem, even today. Due to uncontrolled blood pressure or impending complication likes eclampsia, HELP syndrome it may be necessary to opt for caesarean birth.

- Maternal diabetes in pregnancy is also associated with problems, which may make caesarean birth a safer option.
- Other medical illness like severe asthma, certain types of cardiac diseases, etc. may also preclude labor as mother, baby or both may not be able to tolerate labor well.
- *Previous Caesarean Delivery*: This is now becoming a very common indication for repeat caesarean section. Most patients with one prior caesarean delivery may deliver safely vaginally in the later pregnancies. This is more likely if the prior caesarean section was for a non-recurrent or temporary condition of that pregnancy, such as: Malpresentation, Fetal distress, Bleeding from the placenta.

The options should be discussed by you and your doctor prior to onset of labor. If a vaginal birth trial is opted for, certain guidelines need to be followed. In some cases, you and your doctor may opt for an elective or planned repeat caesarean. This is more commonly done if you have had:

- More than one caesarean previously.
- Your baby is now larger.
- Not in a favorable presentation.

The type of prior caesarean is also important, as with an incision. Other uterine surgeries done in the past such as myomectomy or septum resection may also influence the decision for type of delivery.

Risks Involved

Caesarean births are much safer now than they were a few decades ago. In fact, hardly a century ago, having a caesarean was like a death sentence for the mothers. Today, the procedure carries a 'risk' of less than 1 in 2500. Yet, this risk is 4 times more than the risk of death after a normal vaginal delivery. However, when talking about risks, one must keep in mind that statistics show that most people die at home or in bed. That doesn't mean that by not staying home or not sleeping you can escape the inevitable! While talking of risks what needs to be seen in the risk-benefit ratio. The ultimate aim is to have a healthy mother and healthy baby. In a given situation, if the benefits offered by caesarean birth to the mother, the baby or both are more than the risks; the procedure needs to be done regardless. Individual medical conditions like uncontrolled blood pressure or profuse bleeding from the placenta may make a vaginal birth more dangerous for the mother.

Risk for Mother

- *Infection*: Post-operative infection of the uterus, or nearby organs like the bladder may occur. Use of antibiotics has reduced this risk.

- *Increased bleeding*: Some blood loss is inevitable at birth, but it is twice as much at caesarean as compared to a vaginal delivery.
- Complications of the anesthesia.
- *Urinary tract*: Difficulty in passing urine, urinary retention, infection may occur. Rarely, surgical damage to the bladder or ureters may occur, particularly in cases of repeated surgery.
- *Bowel function*: Post-operatively, the bowel movements may become sluggish or slow down completely. This leads to distension, bloating and abdominal discomfort.
- *Respiratory tract*: Occasionally, due to aspiration of stomach contents, pneumonia may result. This is more common with general anesthesia.
- *Wound problems*: There may be a blood clot or pocket of pus in one or more stitches. In more severe cases there may be infection of the whole abdominal wound, and partial or complete dehiscence (splitting open) of the wound.
- *Blood clots*: They may form in the leg veins, or collect in the uterus. Clots in the pelvis organs or veins may travel to the lungs causing embolism, a serious complication. This is reduced by early ambulation.
- *Delayed recovery*: The hospital stay after a caesarean birth is usually twice as long as after a vaginal birth. In case of a 'bikini' incision, the average stay is 5 days, with a vertical midline incision, it may be 7 days or more. Full recovery of daily activities may take 4 weeks or more.
- *Long-term*: Increased chance of repeat Caesarean section.

Risk for Fetus

Prematurity

The baby may have been delivered too early if there was miscalculation of the due date. Sometimes, despite knowing that the baby will be premature, an emergency caesarean may be needed, such as, for bleeding from the placenta, uncontrolled hypertension, etc. in the mother's best interest.

Low Apgar Score

The baby may have depressed activity at birth, as measured by the Apgar score. This could be due to the anesthesia, other medications, or pre-existing factors. This need not indicate any long-term problem, however.

Breathing difficulty

Transient tachypnoea of the newborn (rapid or irregular breathing) is more common with caesarean birth. This is thought to be due to lack of the 'squeezing out' of lung fluid, which occurs in vaginal births. This usually settles in a few days.

Fetal injury

Although this is rare, the baby may be accidentally nicked while the surgeon is opening the uterus. With malpresentations, or deeply engaged head (as in caesareans after a long and difficult labor) there may be some trouble delivering the baby, a minor fetal bruising or injury.

Basic Rules

- Wear loose comfortable clothing, a support bra and proper flat or low-heeled shoes.
- Include warm-up and cool-down exercises.
- Start slowly and gradually increase the intensity of exercises.
- Stop exercising when fatigued and don't exercise to exhaustion.
- Stop if you feel any pain, light headed, breathless, or faint.
- Don't exercise in supine position (flat on your back), after the 1st trimester because pressure from your heavy uterus on the major blood vessels can diminish blood flow to your heart and to the placenta.
- A sudden change in position can also make you feel giddy, so be careful.
- Because of the enlargement of your uterus and breasts, your physical center of gravity changes. So don't do exercises, which require balancing, especially in the third trimester. Also wear low-heeled or flat footwear.
- During pregnancy both basal metabolic rate and heat production increase. Avoid hot tubs, steam rooms and saunas as these cause overheating.
- Do mild to moderate exercise routines three days a week.
- Drink enough water (at least 8 glasses).
- You need an extra 300 calories over pre-pregnant requirement. While exercising, be sure to eat enough.

It is desirable to take an insurance policy, where even available to get cover against maternity-related problems and the expenditure thereon. See Appendix I.

Cesarean section (C-SECTION)

If natural birth is not possible, C section may be done to take out the newborn surgically, from the womb, confirm fetal heartbeat indicators with fetal scalp blood oxygen readings. Anesthesia: As little as possible depending on circumstances. No general anesthesia unless absolutely necessary. Participation: Screen lowered at the time of delivery. Events explained as they occur. Contact with baby: Held by father immediately after birth, where mother can touch and see. Breastfeeding as soon as possible. Discharge of mother and baby: As soon as possible.If the infant is sick, parents visit and care for baby as much as possible. If baby must be transferred to another hospital, mother goes, too; if that's not possible, father goes with baby. Feeding: Mother nurses baby. If that's not possible, parents feed mother's expressed milk to baby.

A cesarean section is major abdominal surgery. When a cesarean is necessary, it can be a life saving technique for both mother and infant. The World Health Organization states that no region in the world is justified in having a cesarean rate greater than 10 to 15 percent. However, in the past twenty years, the cesarean section rates have nearly quintupled in the US to 23.8% in 1989 and nearly quadrupled in Canada to 18.3% in 1987-8. A cesarean section poses documented medical risks to the mother's health, including infections, hemorrhage, transfusion, injury to other organs, anesthesia complications, psychological complications, and a maternal mortality two to four times greater than that for a vaginal birth. An elective cesarean section increases the risk to the infant of premature birth and respiratory distress syndrome, both of which are associated with multiple complications, intensive care and burdensome financial costs. Even mature babies, the absences of labor increases the risk of breathing problems and other complications.

After the skin is thoroughly cleansed with an aseptic solution and sterile drapes spread over the surgical field, the abdomen is entered by making an incision through all layers of the abdominal wall: the skin, the fat, and then several muscle layers and muscle sheaths (fascia). This incision can be made either vertically below the umbilicus like a zipper, or horizontally right above the pubic bone, a "bikini cut." Usually all the intestines have been pushed up into the upper abdomen by the enlarged uterus and the uterus lies directly against the abdominal wall. Next, the incision through the muscle wall of the uterus is made and stopped just short of the amniotic sac that contains the baby. At this point, everybody gets ready for the arrival of the baby. The amniotic sac is ruptured carefully, so as not to hurt the baby, and the baby is delivered much as if she were coming out through the vagina. After the baby is dried and wrapped in soft cloths, the mom can often hold her baby, or at least touch while nurse holds the baby. The time from the incision of the skin to the delivery of the baby can be less than three minutes if an emergency requires it, but usually takes about 10 minutes. If the incision into the uterus is made horizontally in the lower part of the uterus (low transverse incision), the woman is eligible for a trial of labor in a later pregnancy. Rarely, the incision has to be made, or extended, vertically into the upper part of the uterus ("classical" incision) in order to get the baby out. After a classical incision, future labor is too much of a stress for the uterine scar—it will burst and all subsequent pregnancies will have to be delivered by cesarean section. Rupture of the uterus during labor can occur even without a previous cesarean section but it is rare. It is life threatening to both mom and baby. Immediate surgery, however, can save both their lives (another reason not to have a home birth!). After the baby is delivered, the placenta is removed through the same uterine incision as the baby, and the uterus and abdomen are closed layer by layer in reverse order. This takes about 15 to 20 minutes.

Do I Need a Cesarean Section?

A cesarean delivery should be performed when it is safer for the mother or the baby than a vaginal delivery. That can sometimes be determined before labor and a cesarean section will be scheduled. In this case, it is important to be very sure how far along the pregnancy is, so as not to deliver a baby prematurely.

Listed below are some of the more common reasons that a cesarean section needs to be performed:

- Previous surgery on the uterus, such as removal of fibroids from deep in the muscle wall of the upper part of the uterus or cesarean section with a high (classical) incision.
- Infectious conditions, such as HIV, large vaginal warts or acute herpes outbreak at the onset of labor; these could otherwise transmit to the baby once he enters the birth canal.
- Medical conditions that make labor too great a risk for the mother, such as extremely high blood pressure or severe diabetes.
- The baby is too big for the size of the mother's pelvis ("cephalopelvic disproportion"). Sometimes this is so obvious that a cesarean delivery is scheduled from the outset; sometimes the decision is made to do a "trial of labor" and see what happens, only resorting to cesarean delivery when the baby appears to be stuck ("failure to progress in labor").
- Having more than one baby; risks are greatly elevated, especially for the second or third baby, as the placenta may detach from the wall of the uterus before all the babies are out.
- The exit is blocked; if a large tumor is located in the lower part of the uterus, it may block passage of the baby through the birth canal. The placenta can cover the cervix and block the exit. This is called placenta praevia.
- Malpresentation, such as a breech presentation. Even though many babies can be delivered in the breech position (bottom first), the risk of complications is greatly increased because the head and shoulders are the largest parts of the newborn. Once they've stretched the birth canal, the rest follows automatically. When the smaller bottom end comes out first, the head may get trapped and the umbilical cord can be compressed between the baby's skull and the mother's pelvic bones. The baby then does not get any oxygen because the placental blood is cut-off and the head isn't yet in the air. The American College of Obstetricians and Gynecologists now recommends that an attempt should be made to turn breech babies in late pregnancy and only deliver them by cesarean section if turning them fails.

- If the mother wants a c-section, she can opt to have one. She may choose this because she had one before and feels as she already has a scar, she doesn't want to subject her pelvis and vagina to the trauma of labor. The mother may just decide that labor is not for her, in which case she'll have problems getting her insurance company to pay. Even with a previous cesarean, women and their doctors have been pressured by insurance companies to do a "trial of labor" (see section on VBAC).

Reasons for Cesarean Section

Often the need for a cesarean section becomes apparent only during labor on a more or less emergency basis—

- *Fetal distress.* During labor, the baby's heart rate, including how it responds to contractions, is followed either with a monitor or by auscultation. A non-reassuring fetal heart rate pattern can be a sign that the baby is not receiving enough oxygen. This can occur because the cord is tightly wrapped around the baby's neck or shoulder, the placenta is separating from the uterine wall or the baby is at risk for a host of other reasons.
- *Placental problems.* This usually involves the placenta beginning to separate from the uterine wall (placenta abruption). Signs of this are excessive bleeding and fetal distress.
- *Labor problems or "failure to progress."* About 30% of cesarean deliveries are performed for this reason. The most common reason the baby stops advancing down the birth canal is that the baby does not fit ("cephalo-pelvic disproportion"). If labor is allowed to continue indefinitely, something will eventually give—either the baby will develop fetal distress or the uterus will rupture.
- Rarely, the laboring woman will develop medical problems, such as seizures, that make it unsafe for her to continue with labor.

Use all the help you can get, be that a supportive side-kick to help you breathe through all your contractions or an epidural when the pain gets to be more than you are willing to endure.

If a general anesthesia was used during the delivery, you may not wake up for a few hours. When you do, you may feel groggy and confused. Don't be surprised if your baby is still being affected by the anesthesia for six to 12 hours after delivery and appears a little sleepy. If you're going to breastfeed, try to nurse her as soon as you feel well enough. Even if she's drowsy, her first feeding will provide a reason for her to wake up and meet her new world and you. You'll probably experience some pain where the incision was made. But you'll soon be able to hold your baby, and you'll quickly make up for the lost time. You may need to stay in bed for a while.

A hospital stay after cesarean birth is usually four days. The length of your stay depends on the reason for the cesarean birth. It will take a few weeks for your abdomen to heal. It's important to help yourself heal. For a few weeks after the cesarean birth, you should not place anything in your vagina or do any strenuous activity. Many maternity centers have childbirth classes and support groups for couples who may need cesarean birth. If you have questions or concerns about cesarean birth, ask your doctor or nurse.

Cesarean Section Complications

When a cesarean is done, the risks and benefits of the procedure need to be weighed. This includes looking at the added benefits and risks of doing a cesarean or of birthing the child vaginally. Sometimes the benefits of the cesarean will outweigh the risks, and sometime the vaginal birth benefits will outweigh the risks of the cesarean. Cesarean birth is major surgery, and, as with other surgical procedures, risks are involved. The estimated risk of a woman dying after a cesarean birth is less than one in 2,500 (the risk of death after a vaginal birth is less than one in 10,000). These are estimated risks for a large population of women. Individual medical conditions such as some heart problems may make the risk of vaginal birth higher than cesarean birth.

Risks for the Baby

Premature birth. If the due date was not accurately calculated, the baby could be delivered too early.

Breathing problems. Babies born by cesarean are more likely to develop breathing problems such as transient tachypnea (abnormally fast breathing during the first few days after birth).

Low Apgar scores. Babies born by cesarean sometimes have low Apgar scores. The low score can be an effect of the anesthesia and cesarean birth, or the baby may have been in distress to begin with. Or perhaps the baby was not stimulated as he or she would have been by vaginal birth.

Fetal injury. Although rare, the surgeon can accidentally nick the baby while making the uterine incision.

Risks for the Mother

Infection. The uterus or nearby pelvic organs, such as the bladder or kidneys, can become infected.

Increased blood loss. Blood loss on the average is about twice as much with cesarean birth as with vaginal birth. However, blood transfusions are rarely needed during a cesarean.

Decreased bowel function. The bowel sometimes slows down for several days after surgery, resulting in distention, bloating and discomfort.

Respiratory complications. General anesthesia can sometimes lead to pneumonia.

Longer hospital stay and recovery time. Three to five days in the hospital is the common length of stay, whereas it is less than one to three days for a vaginal birth.

Reactions to anesthesia. The mother's health could be endangered by unexpected responses (such as blood pressure that drops quickly) to anesthesia or other medications during the surgery.

Risk of additional surgeries. For example, hysterectomy, bladder repair, etc.

You can get blood clots in the legs, pelvic organs or lungs.

Your bowel or bladder can be injured.

Vaginal Birth after a Cesarean

Vaginal Birth After Cesarean is what VBAC stands for. It is a vaginal birth after one or more cesareans. More than 80% of women will be able to have a VBAC. VBAC is safer than repeat cesarean and VBAC with more than one previous cesarean does not pose any increased risk.

Tips for a healthy vaginal birth

Get in training. Labor is the hardest work you'll ever do, but it's worth it! Focus on good nutrition and exercise.

Make a daily checklist to ensure you are getting essential nutrients.

Daily exercise: swim, walk, yoga, prenatal fitness class—whatever feels good.

Prenatal classes. Be sure to register early for VBAC, refresher or any other quality prenatal program Even though you may have taken classes in a previous pregnancy, an evening out together with your partner will help to prepare you both, promote discussion, give you ideas on coping with labor and focusing on this baby and its birth.

Supportive care provider. Find someone who believes in VBACs, has a VBAC success rate over 75% and a cesarean rate that is lower than community average. If you are unsure about anything, get a second opinion. Read "Working with Your Birth Attendant."

Information. Get as much of it as you can. Obtain a copy of your medical records from the previous birth(s) for yourself. Ask your current care provider to explain anything that you don't understand. Talk to your care provider, make plans with them. Talk to other people who have been there. Read a lot of books and journals.

Physically you need to prepare your body. Being in good physical condition can help your labor move more quickly as well as speed healing. Regular exercise and special birth exercises are good ways of doing this.

Establish a safe supportive birth environment to facilitate labor.

Try a variety of positions. Standing or walking instead of lying down facilitates labor and squatting to push can be most effective. Try sitting on the toilet.

Continue calorie and fluid intake. Labor is hard work and takes a lot of energy. Far from eliminating the risk of aspiration with general anesthesia, total fasting (NPO) may increase the risk by raising the acidity of the stomach contents. Fasting may also make it harder for the uterus to work.

Believe in yourself, your body, and the process of birth. Say affirmations silently to yourself or write them down or work through fears. Accept the pain of birth as a sign of how strong and well your body is.

Learn to trust, cooperate with and listen to your body and your own unique labor pattern.

Feel good about yourself and your relationship as a couple and keep a positive outlook.

Reassure family and friends. Remember that according to medical studies VBAC is usually safer for both you and your baby than a repeat cesarean. Read and make available to your friends and relatives, "Yes, I'm Having a VBAC."

Why a VBAC?

There are many reasons that you may want a vaginal birth after a cesarean. Some may be medical and some may be emotional. Others may be financial or in terms of recovery. Here are some brief lists of the benefits of a vaginal birth.

Benefits for the mother:

- Prevention of Death from surgery.
- Prevention of lesser complications from surgery.
- Prevention of blood loss.
- Prevention of infection.
- Prevention of injury (bowel, urinary tract, etc.).
- Prevention of blood clots in the legs.
- Prevention of feelings of guilt or inadequacy that surgery sometimes causes.
- Breastfeeding is generally easier after a vaginal birth.
- The cost of a vaginal birth is about $3,000 less.

Benefits for the baby

Prevention of Iatrogenic Prematurity (meaning surgery was done, because of an error in guessing a due date).

Reduction in the cases of Persistent Pulmonary Hypertension.

Labor prepares the baby for extrauterine life.

Prevention of surgery related fetal injuries (lacerations, broken bones).

VBAC results in fewer fetal deaths than elective repeat cesareans.

Risks of VBAC

A common fear among women who have had a previous cesarean is rupture of the uterus. Most of this fear dates back to when the incisions of the original cesarean were of the classical variety (vertical incisions), nowadays most incisions are the low transverse type. There are two types of uterine ruptures: complete and incomplete. Complete uterine rupture is very unlikely today, for a variety of reasons. One is that when we use Pitocin, if needed, during a labor, we regulate the amount that goes in. In other times it was given IV to a woman and allowed to flow freely. These have also decreased due to some obstetrical practices being abandoned, like high forceps, internal version, etc. And the final reason is because of the rarity of the classical incision. A complete rupture occurs in much less than 1% of women attempting VBAC.

Am I a candidate for VBAC?

Whether or not you will be able to try VBAC will depend on several things. These include: Low transverse incisions on both the abdomen and uterus from previous cesarean. If you had a low-transverse uterine incision (which means the incision was across the lower part of the uterus), as 95 percent of women do today, your chances of having a VBAC are good. However, if you had a classic vertical incision down the middle of your uterus, you will probably not be allowed to attempt a vaginal delivery because of the possible risk of rupture of your uterus. If the reason that you had the previous cesarean was something that is not likely to repeat during this pregnancy, such as infection, drug or alcohol abuse, pre-eclampsia, etc., you are a good candidate for VBAC. If however, the reason for your cesarean was a chronic illness that is likely to impact your current pregnancy such as high blood pressure or diabetes, you will probably require a repeat cesarean.

Willingness to prepare for VBAC

Typically, there is no limit as to the number of cesareans you can undergo. Having repeat cesareans is much safer than it used to be, thanks to new procedures and growing technology in the world of obstetrics. However, certain things will affect how safe repeat cesareans will be. These include the type of incisions made and the status of the scars from your previous cesarean(s). One of the risks associated with repeat cesareans is uterine rupture due to the scar tissue on the uterus from your past procedure. Thus, you should always notify your doctor and go to the hospital immediately if you experience unexplained vaginal bleeding or persistent abdominal pain during your pregnancy.

Must mother have a repeat C-Section?

The common opinion among many health professionals for a long time was "Once a cesarean, always a cesarean." However, many women nowadays are choosing to deliver babies vaginally after having a c-section in a previous pregnancy. But some women still continue to have repeat cesareans, either by choice or because of medical necessity.

Is it safe for mother?

There has been some controversy over whether or not it is safe for a woman to have repeat c-sections. Should there be a limit to the number of cesareans a woman can have? Research on this topic has found that repeat cesareans do not necessarily put the mother at an increased risk of complications. However, it is important to remember that a cesarean is considered to be major surgery and therefore will always carry a certain amount of risk, as well as a longer recovery period than a vaginal birth. For women who have had four or more cesareans, the surgery may be a bit harder to perform, as there are often quite thick adhesions to deal with. See Appendix I for provision of an insurance policy to cover the expenditure of childbirth.

2

Mother Needs Critical Care after Childbirth

Child birth is not a disease situation to be feared. Most of the child births occur in a normal manner and without much assistance. However, it is an important life situation, where the life of mother and her infant may be threatened, if not managed properly and adequately. A large number of deaths and many more moribund conditions arise, during delivery of the child and thereafter, i.e. during puerperium. Safe Motherhood programmes are designed to reduce the high number of deaths and illnesses resulting from complications of pregnancy and childbirth. In many Asian countries, maternal care mismanagement is the leading cause of death for women of reproductive age. Most maternal deaths result from haemorrhages, complications of unsafe abortions, pregnancy-induced hypertension, sepsis and obstructed labour. Safe Motherhood programme seeks to address these direct medical causes and undertake related activities to ensure women have access to comprehensive reproductive health services. The activities related to Safe Motherhood help prevent excess neonatal and maternal morbidity and mortality by: providing clean delivery kits for use by mothers or birth attendants to promote, clean home deliveries, providing midwife delivery kits (UNICEF or equivalent) to facilitate clean and safe deliveries at the health facility; and by initiating the establishment of a referral system to manage obstetric emergencies. See Appendices II, III and IV for post-delivery care and stabilization of mother and newborn, 1996. Appendix V firther outlines the criteria for discharge, within 24-36 hours of delivery.

Causes of Maternal Mortality Globally

- Severe bleeding 25%
- Indirect causes 20%

- Infection 15%
- Unsafe abortions 13%
- Eclampsia 12%
- Obstructed labour 8%
- Other direct causes 8% (WHO: World Health Day—Safe Motherhood—1998)

Comprehensive services for antenatal care, delivery of the child and look after in the postpartum period must be well organised to prevent morbidity and loss of life. Planning for such services should take into account existing facilities for the population. Services should be able to deal with obstetric and other medical emergencies. Approximately 15 per cent of pregnant women will develop complications that require essential obstetric care, and up to five per cent of pregnant women will require some type of surgery. The minimum needs are: (a) one health clinic with trained community health workers and traditional birth attendants (TBAs) to be able to identify problems and refer (to health centre/hospital) for every 5,000 people; (b) one equipped health centre providing basic essential obstetric care for every 30,000-40,000 people; (c) one operating theatre and staff, capable of performing 24 hour comprehensive essential obstetric care, for every 150,000 to 200,000 people. To make sure that the services provided are appropriate and of the highest quality and will be fully used, it is essential to identify skilled care providers involved in childbirth, viz. physicians, midwives, experienced nurses, trained TBAs. Be aware of and discuss community beliefs and practices and health-seeking behaviour related to delivery, such as position for delivery, presence of relatives for support and traditional practices both positive (breastfeeding) and harmful (female genital mutilation); and ensure that all women and their families know where to obtain assistance for antenatal care and delivery.

Appropriate antenatal care

This includes not only determining the pregnant woman's overall health status, but also identifying factors that may adversely affect pregnancy outcome. These factors include: age (younger than 17 or older than 40), grand multipara, short stature, and obstetric history of any previous complications, including surgery. While this screening may help identify some women who will develop postnatal complications, it will not identify all of them. Thus, it is critically important to identify and manage complications as they arise among all pregnant women. Female genital mutilation is a particular risk in some countries. Women who have been subjected to this procedure, especially to infibulation, should be identified during the antenatal period.

Detection and management of complications

This includes Special emphasis on identifying the acute complications of unsafe abortions or ante-partum haemorrhages. Other complications, such as hypertensive disease, anaemia, diabetes, malaria or an STD, are less obvious and require more detailed physical examination. Treatment for existing health conditions should be undertaken. Syphilis testing is recommended at least once during pregnancy, preferably before the third trimester. Systematic testing for syphilis in pregnancy is cost-effective if the prevalence of syphilis is one per cent or more in the general population.

Observation and recording of clinical data

Height, blood pressure, search for oedemas, proteinuria and haemoglobin, uterine growth, fetal heart rate and presentation should be recorded.

Maintenance of maternal nutrition

The recommended minimum nutritional requirements for a pregnant woman have been set at 2,300 kcal per day of a balanced and culturally acceptable diet. Supplementary food may be required if the basic food ration available is inadequate. The offer of supplemental food can be a good incentive to get women to attend for antenatal care. Doctors should be alert to signs of iron-deficiency anaemia and iodine deficiency disorder (IDD). Either due to ignorance or poverty, the incidence of malnourishment among young mothers is very high. A malnourished mother is bound to produce a Low Birth Weight (LBW) baby, who will lead the life of a retarded and sick child.

Health education

The following topics should be part of the educational activity related to antenatal care:

- choosing the safest place for delivery;
- clean delivery; the major symptoms of complications (bleeding, severe abdominal pain, headache);
- where and when to seek care for complications;
- exclusive breastfeeding;
- maternal nutrition;
- STD/HIV/AIDS prevention;
- immunisation; and
- family planning.

Prevention of major diseases

Preventive measures should include: iron folate prophylaxis (anaemia occurs in over 60 per cent of pregnant women in Asian countries); tetanus toxoid immunisation; Vitamin A supplements; antimalarials and antihelminthics (hookworms) in endemic areas. Iodized oil/salt may be given in areas of moderate or severe IDD and following national protocols.

Childbirth/Delivery Care

Even with the best possible antenatal screening, any delivery can become a complicated one, requiring emergency intervention. Therefore, skilled assistance is essential to delivery care. In the absence of midwives or doctors, TBAs (who usually perform home deliveries) should be trained to identify complications, provide immediate first aid, and know when and where to refer women for additional care. It should also be remembered that: the first priority for a delivery is to be safe, atraumatic and clean; and most maternal deaths are due to a failure to get skilled help in time for delivery complications. It is critical to have a well-coordinated system to identify complications and ensure their management with immediate first aid and/or referral. As a rule, the further away the referral facility, the earlier you intervene. Delays in obtaining help may be at the community level (in identifying and referring women with difficulties); en route to the referral facility (inability to get transport, poor road conditions); or on arrival at the referral facility (absence of staff, lack of drugs or other materials). All three possibilities for delay must be minimised. Midwives and TBAs should also take care of the newborn by: clearing the airway, keeping the baby warm, providing eye and cord care, helping mothers begin breastfeeding (and not giving any other foods or liquids to the baby), and identifying complications, which require referral. Birth weights should also be measured.

TBAs or family members will often assist deliveries. Therefore, early identification of midwives or TBAs within the community, their training and supervision on the proper use of clean delivery kits (clean place, clean hands, proper cord care) and identification and management of complications, are essential to prevent excess maternal morbidity and mortality. These health facilities, whether temporary or permanent, should be equipped with the appropriate human and material resources to take care of all but surgical cases. The following basic essential obstetric care should be provided and standard protocols used to monitor and manage labour. These include:

- initial assessment of mother;
- assessment of fetal well-being;
- episiotomy;
- special care for women who have undergone genital mutilation;
- use of vacuum extractor;
- management of haemorrhage;
- management of eclampsia;
- multiple births;
- breech delivery; and
- and procedures for referral to next level of care, if necessary.

Protocols must be taught to health staff, publicly displayed and made available in all health centres. Basic essential obstetric care should be performed at the health-centre level to address, or stabilise before referral, the main complications of delivery, such as ante-partum haemorrhage, eclampsia, prolonged labour, uterine rupture, postpartum haemorrhage, repair of vaginal and cervical tears, and retained placenta. These facilities should therefore be equipped with broad spectrum injectable and oral antibiotics (ampicillin, penicillin, doxycycline, gentamicin, metronidazole), plasma expanders, anti-convulsants, oxytocics, ergometrine, analgesics, magnesium sulphate, suturing kits, "high" sterilisation techniques, gloves, syringes and needles, delivery equipment, and materials for universal precautions. These facilities should also be able to provide for resuscitation and basic care of the newborn (e.g., management of hypothermia and hypoglycemia), including measurement of birth weight. A readily available prophylactic to prevent neonatal ophthalmia, ideally tetracycline eye ointment, should be given to all newborns.

However, very often, severe complications will be managed at the nearest major health facility. In this case, try to avoid swamping the facility with the demands of the normal population to the detriment of the people in real distress. The referral hospital should be able to perform safely comprehensive essential obstetric care, such as Caesarean sections, laparotomy, hysterectomy, repair of cervical and severe (third degree) vaginal tears, care for complications due to unsafe abortions, and safe blood transfusion. An appropriate referral system requires referral protocols specifying when and where to refer and an adequate record of referred cases. This implies coordination, communication, confidence and understanding between the TBAs and their supervisors and between the health centre and the hospital with surgical facilities. An effective referral system will also have to take into account security, geographical and transport constraints.

Postpartum Care, after birth supervision

Since up to 50 per cent of maternal deaths occurs after delivery, a doctor and midwife should visit all mothers as soon as possible within the first 24-48 hours after birth. The doctor should assess the mother's general condition and recovery after childbirth and identify any special needs. This attention is particularly important when the woman is alone in the family. The postpartum visit provides an occasion for assessing and discussing issues of cleanliness, care of the newborn, breastfeeding and appropriate methods and timing of family planning. Health providers should support early and exclusive breastfeeding, and discuss proper nutrition with the mother. Iron folate tablets should be continued and Vitamin A and iodised oil/salt should be provided when necessary. During the postpartum visit, the health and well-being of the newborn should also be assessed and its birth weight measured. Newborns should be referred to the under-five clinic to start immunisations, growth monitoring and other well-child services. Community Health Workers (CHW) and TBAs should be trained for appropriate referral of postpartum complications, such as haemorrhage, sepsis, perineal trauma, breastfeeding problems, and newborn complications, such as prematurity or failure to thrive, that may require additional surveillance and/or treatment.

Integrating Services

Some situations may benefit from a "women's house", which offers peer support, counselling and health promotion in a non-threatening environment. This resource is especially important for adolescent and new mothers. Such a place might also provide a suitable venue for small-scale income-generation or female literacy activities. Effective dissemination of information is vital if women are to enjoy access to available services. The community's knowledge and attitudes regarding medical care during pregnancy and childbirth must be assessed. If there is suspicion and fear of medical interventions, such as hospital delivery, Caesarean section or blood transfusion, appropriate IEC activities may be necessary. New procedures, such as screening blood for syphilis, should be preceded by educational activities that explain and dispel misconceptions about the procedures. Health workers should consider inviting a companion who will be present at the time of delivery to attend antenatal clinics with the pregnant woman. Through TBAs and/or CHWs, the population as a whole, should be made aware of the warning signs of impending complications in pregnancy and labour and encouraged to plan how to reach the equipped medical facility, if necessary. Given that men and older family members often make the decisions within the family, it is particularly important that educational activities target these groups.

A midwife or an experienced doctor is best suited to organise and supervise the Safe Motherhood programme. A midwife can effectively supervise 10 to 15 TBAs for an estimated population of 20,000-30,000. In many societies, TBAs are usually the key people at the community level who will influence maternal and newborn care, although their influence and skills may vary from culture to culture. In general, one TBA can look after 2,000 to 3,000 population. With a crude birth rate of three per cent per year, this means roughly five to eight deliveries per month per TBA. With adequate training and supervision, some experienced TBAs can: identify complications; refer women with delivery complications to appropriate medical facilities;provide care for normal pregnancy through labour, delivery and the postpartum period; and offer family planning information and services.

TBAs, however, are no substitute for a more skilled attendant at birth. Training and supervision of health workers in Safe Motherhood practices should be evaluated and planned in coordination with the community, NGOs and UN agencies. The nature of the training will vary depending on the services the health worker provides and the skills required for those services. Services should be continuously reviewed. Efforts should be made to collect reliable information on maternal deaths. Every maternal death should be investigated to determine the cause and action taken and to ensure that the referral system is responding appropriately to obstetric emergencies.

Record keeping is essential for appropriate surveillance. Home-based maternal records, kept by the mother, have proven advantageous.

Safe Motherhood Indicators

Indicators to be collected from the health-facility level

- Crude birth rate,
- Neonatal mortality rate,
- Stillbirth ratio,
- Coverage of antenatal care,
- Coverage of syphilis screening,
- Coverage of trained delivery services,
- Coverage of postpartum care, and
- Incidence of obstetric complications.

Supervisors should periodically assess the skills of doctors to ensure quality of care of Safe Motherhood interventions.

India and other Asian countries

Complications of pregnancy and childbirth are a leading cause of death and disability among women of reproductive age (ages 15 to 44) in India and other Asian countries. About half of the nearly 120 million women, who give birth each year experience some kind of complication during their pregnancies, and between 15 million and 20 million develop disabilities such as severe anemia, incontinence, damage to the reproductive organs or nervous system, chronic pain, and infertility, according to Lori Ashford, Elizabeth Ransom and Nancy Yinger of PRB, in their thought provoking article entitled, "Hidden Suffering: Disabilities From Pregnancy and Childbirth in Asian Countries" (August 2002). These disabilities are tragic on two counts: They occur in the process of giving life, and they are almost entirely preventable. Disabilities from maternal causes affect the health and productivity of women who are in the prime of their lives. These disabilities are also strongly associated with infant deaths and poor health and development in children and adversely affect family income and well-being. Reducing women's disabilities, therefore, is as important for alleviating poverty as it is for reducing needless suffering. The interventions for preventing and treating complications of pregnancy and childbirth are well-documented, but greater commitments and investments are needed to make such interventions widely available and effective. See Appendix VII for ICPD Programme of Action.

A Giant Problem Indeed

Each year, more than 500,000 women, predominantly in Asian countries, die of causes related to pregnancy and childbirth. Yet the deaths are only the tip of the iceberg: For every death, at least another 30 women suffer serious illness or debilitating injuries. Though these women are fortunate to survive, their injuries can have devastating social and physical consequences. Maternal disabilities have received relatively little attention, because they are often hidden from view. In Asian countries, many women receive no medical care before, during, or after childbirth, so there are few medical records available for analysis. Numerous studies have documented the incidence of pregnancy-related complications, but few large-scale studies have included medical verification of women's conditions after childbirth. Much of the available data is derived from women's self-reported symptoms on surveys, which experts consider unspecific and not clinically valid. Nevertheless, case studies in a number of countries reveal an enormous but unaddressed problem, shrouded in a "culture of silence and endurance" because of cultural values that encourage women to give lower priority to their health than to other family matters. See Appendices VIII and IX for aspects of 'Women's Health in India'.

Causes of Maternal morbidity

Maternal morbidity can be defined as any illness or injury caused or aggravated by pregnancy or childbirth. The disability can be acute, affecting a woman during or immediately after childbirth, or chronic, lasting for months, years, or a lifetime. The vast majority of maternal disabilities stem from health complications that are a direct result of pregnancy or childbirth. These "direct causes" include severe bleeding, infection, obstructed or prolonged labor, pregnancy-induced hypertension (high blood pressure), and unsafe abortions.

Morbidity can also be caused by illnesses that are aggravated by pregnancy, such as anemia, malaria, cardiac disease, hepatitis, tuberculosis, sexually transmitted infections, and diabetes. Interactions between illnesses and complications can also cause a disability, making this a particularly difficult problem to quantify. No matter what the cause, pregnancy complications can pose a serious health risk to the fetus or newborn, as well as for the mother's subsequent pregnancies. Maternal disabilities are strongly associated with poor or non-existent medical care during labor and delivery and immediately after the birth. Only about half of all births in Asian countries are attended by a doctor, nurse, or trained midwife. In many cases, women who experience complications do not receive adequate medical attention in time to avert serious illness or injury. Women and their families may not recognize the warning signs of complications or may fear poor treatment or high fees at health facilities. Even deliveries in health facilities can be risky, because the quality of obstetric care may be inadequate. In some cases, the delay between arriving at a health facility and receiving care results in the death of the mother or child. Unsafe abortions, those that are self-induced or carried out by unskilled providers, are also a major cause of maternal death and disability. In contrast, complications of abortions conducted by skilled providers in medical

Complications of Pregnancy and Childbirth: Asian and other less Developed Countries

Complication	*Incidence as a Percent of Live Births*	*Maternal Disabilities that may Result*
Severe bleeding (hemorrhage)	11	Severe anemia Pituitary gland failure and other hormonal imbalances Infertility
Infection during or after labor (sepsis)	10	Pelvic inflammatory disease* Chronic pelvic pain Damage to reproductive organs Infertility
Obstructed or prolonged labor	6	Incontinence Fistula* Genital prolapse* Uterine rupture, vaginal tears Nerve damage
Pregnancy-induced hypertension (pre-eclampsia and eclampsia)	6	Chronic hypertension Kidney failure Nervous system disorders
Unsafe abortion	16	Reproductive tract infection Damage to uterus Infertility Pelvic inflammatory disease* Chronic pelvic pain

Source: C. Murray and A. Lopez, eds., Health Dimensions of Sex and Reproduction (1998).

settings are rare. The World Health Organization (WHO) estimates that 18 million unsafe abortions occur each year in less developed countries, i.e. about one in 10 pregnancies, or one abortion for every seven live births.

The deliveries in case of adolescent mothers are more risky, entailing greater morbidity and mortality. See Appendix VI for a Singapore report on the subject.

Major Maternal Problems

Maternal disabilities can severely affect women's quality of life, fertility, and productivity long after pregnancy and delivery.

The following sections describe some of the major disabilities that may result from pregnancy and childbirth-related complications.

Consequences of Severe Bleeding

About 11 percent of women who give birth, or 13 million women per year, experience postpartum hemorrhage, defined as loss of more than 500 milliliters of blood following the delivery of a baby (the exact amount is difficult to monitor without trained assistance). Without prompt and effective treatment, women who bleed profusely can die in a matter of hours, making postpartum hemorrhage as a leading cause of maternal death. Women who survive may develop severe anemia or, in rare but serious cases, permanent hormonal imbalances due to failure of the pituitary or adrenal glands. Pituitary failure can lead to inability to breastfeed, loss of menstruation, chronic weakness, premature ageing, and confusion or apathy.

Anemia, or low levels of iron in the blood, deserves special mention because it is so common, affecting about half of all pregnant women worldwide. Anemia is both an indirect cause of death and a consequence of pregnancy complications, such as severe bleeding. The main cause of anemia is insufficient iron in the diet, but other causes include malaria, intestinal worms, folate deficiency, and HIV/AIDS. Because pregnancy and severe postpartum bleeding can aggravate existing anemia; anemic women are exposed to increased risk of death and disability with each subsequent pregnancy. Women with moderate to severe anemia suffer from fatigue and lack of energy that dramatically reduce their productivity and quality of life. A recent analysis using WHO data estimated that anemia associated with maternal causes in Asian countries in 2000 alone resulted in a loss of women's productivity valued at more than US $ 5 billion.

Consequences of Infection

About 10 percent of women who give birth suffer from sepsis, or blood poisoning caused by an untreated infection during or immediately after childbirth. Sepsis can result from prolonged labor, inappropriate care, or unclean practices during a delivery or induced abortion. Women who survive the initial infection may develop pelvic inflammatory disease (PID), in which the infection spreads to the fallopian tubes and ovaries. If left untreated, PID can cause chronic pelvic pain, which affects women's lives continuously. PID can also permanently damage the reproductive organs, putting women at future risk of ectopic pregnancy—a life-threatening condition in which a fertilized egg develops in the fallopian tube. Apart from suffering the physical pain associated with these conditions, women who become infertile experience emotional pain and, in some cases, abandonment or abuse by their husbands.

Obstructed or Prolonged Labor

Affecting about 6 percent of live births, obstructed labor occurs when the fetus will not pass through the mother's pelvis. Very young mothers who have not attained their adult stature are particularly at risk. Lacking the option of a Caesarean section delivery, a woman can suffer the agony of obstructed labor for days or even a week. As a consequence, she may experience chronic incontinence or, in severe cases, a ruptured uterus or the formation of fistula, with likely loss of her child. Some women suffer genital prolapse after bearing several children. The prolapse occurs when the vagina or the uterus drop below their normal positions because of repeated stretching and damage to the muscles that support these organs. The condition is extremely uncomfortable, especially for women who do their chores in a squatting position. Genital prolapse can also lead to chronic backache, urinary problems, pain during sexual intercourse, and complications in future pregnancies. Women with this condition rarely report it because they consider it a normal consequence of childbearing. Obstructed or prolonged labor can also lead to severe postpartum infections and increased risk of PID, infertility, and neurological injuries (damage to the nervous system), including a condition called "foot drop" that makes walking difficult.

Pregnancy-induced Hypertension

About 6 percent of women who give birth, develop pregnancy-induced hypertension which includes a dangerous condition called pre-eclampsia (previously known as toxemia) that is characterized by high blood pressure, swelling over the body and the presence of protein in the urine. If pre-eclampsia is not detected and treated, it can result in seizures or convulsions, at which point it is defined as eclampsia. Management of eclampsia requires a trained health practitioner, who can provide timely care such as anticonvulsant drugs and expedited delivery of the infant. Pregnancy-induced hypertension is a leading cause of maternal mortality and it can also lead to long-term health problems such as chronic hypertension, kidney failure, or nervous system disorders.

The Impact on Infant

The same pregnancy-related complications that threaten women's survival can also cause death and disability in newborns. The vast majority of the estimated 8 million perinatal deaths (late miscarriages, stillbirths, and deaths in the first week of life) that occur each year in Asian countries are associated with maternal health problems or poor management of labor and delivery. For example, obstructed and prolonged labor asphyxiates an estimated 3 percent of newborns, resulting in death for nearly 25 percent of these infants and brain damage for another 25 percent. In addition, women suffering from poor nutrition and infections during pregnancy are more likely to have low birth-weight infants (weighing less than 2,500 grams). Low birth-weight infants are 20 times to 30 times more likely to die in the first week of life than infants of normal weight, and those who survive are more likely to suffer disabilities such as cerebral palsy, seizures, and severe learning disorders.

A mother's disability can have profound consequences for her family and the broader community, due to changes in household responsibilities, earnings and expenses.

- The cost of the mother's medical treatment can change patterns of household consumption and reduce savings and investments.
- The mother's reduced productivity can reduce family output and earnings, compelling children to enter the labor force.
- Children whose mother is ill may have inferior nutrition, hygiene and health.
- Older children may drop-out of school to assume some of the mother's responsibilities.
- Family members may suffer from psychological problems, including depression and feelings of isolation.

Interventions to Improve Maternal Health

All pregnant women, even healthy ones, face some risk of complications that can result in death or serious disabilities if not successfully treated. The same assistance that would save women's lives could also prevent suffering on the part of the women who survive, as well as their newborn babies.

The following sections will describe some of these issues.

Ensure Access to Essential Obstetric Care (EOC)

EOC includes the ability to perform surgery, anesthesia, and blood transfusions; management of problems such as anemia or hypertension; and special care for at-risk newborns. Providing such care requires trained professional staff, a good logistics system for medical supplies, a functioning referral system, and good supervision. Wherever possible, families and communities should have specific plans for transporting women who suffer from serious complications to facilities that can provide essential care.

Provide Postpartum Care and Post-abortion Care

Postpartum and post-abortion care can detect and manage problems, such as hemorrhage, infection, and damage to the reproductive organs, that arise immediately after delivery, miscarriage, or unsafe abortion. Increased funds for training and equipment would also increase the availability of surgical repair of obstetric fistula.

Promote Family Planning

Making low-cost contraceptives and information on family planning available can prevent unintended pregnancies and reduce women's exposure to the health risks associated with pregnancy and childbirth. Family planning allows women to delay motherhood, space births, prevent unsafe abortions, and stop bearing children when they have reached their desired family size.

Provide Adequate Antenatal Care

WHO recommends that women have at least four antenatal visits, starting in the first three months of pregnancy. Timely antenatal visits allow for screening and treatment of STIs, malaria, hookworm, and anemia; immunization against tetanus; and detection and treatment of pregnancy-induced hypertension. The visits also give health workers the chance to educate women about diet and healthy behaviors and to give women nutritional supplements. Antenatal care providers should inform women about the importance of safe delivery with a skilled birth attendant, the warning signs of complications, and how to plan for emergency care.

Improve Girls' Nutrition and Increase Women's Age at First Birth

These earliest preventive measures can help ensure adequate growth of the pelvis, reducing the chances of obstructed labor and its debilitating consequences. Addressing chronic undernutrition and micronutrient deficiencies can also increase women's resistance to infections, hypertension, and other illnesses during pregnancy. Taken together, these interventions could have substantial benefits, given that poor maternal health is a major drain on women's productivity. An analysis conducted in Uganda showed that the implementation of a "mother-baby package" for the 1.2 million Ugandan women who give birth every year would, over 10 years, save more than 12,000 women's lives and 60,000 children's lives, and spare more than 250,000 women from disability. The resulting gain in productivity was valued at US $ 90 million. In low-income settings, therefore, promoting safe motherhood is as important for moving families out of poverty as it is for alleviating human suffering. While the interventions to improve maternal health are well-documented, a lack of commitment and funding has prevented them from being effectively implemented. Given the evidence available on maternal disabilities, the payoffs in reduced suffering and increased productivity may be well worth the investment.

Obstetric Fistula sums up the lack of antenatal care

An obstetric fistula is a devastating injury. It is an abnormal opening between the vagina and the bladder or rectum (or both), results from extreme pressure and tissue damage during prolonged or obstructed labor, as the baby attempts to pass through the mother's birth canal. If a Caesarean section delivery is not available to end the ordeal, the baby is usually stillborn and a fistula forms, permitting the uncontrollable passage of urine and feces into the vagina. Women who suffer fistula have not only lost their babies (in most cases), they also constantly leak urine and feces, producing a foul odor. Women with fistula usually feel ashamed or disgraced, and are often deserted by their husbands and cut off from family, friends, and daily activities, resulting in a life of destitution. The women most at risk include very young women and women having their first birth; women whose growth has been stunted because of poor nutrition or childhood illness; women in rural areas; and those who use traditional care and home delivery. It is estimated that some 2 million women, predominantly in Africa and the Indian sub-continent, suffer from fistula. Each year, another 50,000 to 100,000 women are affected, mostly under age 20.

Fistula can be surgically repaired but only where trained surgeons and good postoperative care are available. Only two centers in Africa specialize in fistula care: one in Addis Ababa, Ethiopia, and the other in Jos, in northern Nigeria. The operation costs about US $ 150, beyond the means of most affected women (United Nations Population Fund).

Given a clinical scenario, the midwife should be able to prevent many of the unfortunate situations mentioned above. She should be able to assess pregnancy and its signs and symptoms on the following lines:

- Recognize the number one cause of secondary amenorrhea in childbearing years.
- Establish the diagnosis of pregnancy and recognise the signs and symptoms of impending child birth and the possibility of its being normal.
- Determine the estimated gestational age of the fetus.
- Define the health status of the mother and the fetus.
- Establish the plan for ongoing care.
- Determine when to consult and/or refer to High Risk Obstertric Clinic.

On getting the referral, the physician has the opportunity to offer advice, guidance, and intervention when indicated. The possible effects of treatment on the patient, the developing fetus, and involved others must be considered. Of primary importance is an awareness on the part of every physician, who assumes responsibility for the medical care of any woman in her reproductive years, irrespective of the physician's type of practice or special interest, must always raise the question, "Is she pregnant?" Failure to do so may lead to incorrect diagnoses, inappropriate therapy, and, at times, to medicolegal problems.

Positive Signs

- identification of fetal heart action separate from the mother's (normal: 120-160 BPM),
- perception of active fetal movements by the examiner (by palpation of the abdomen),
- recognition of the embryo or fetus sonographically (may be detected after only 5 weeks of amenorrhea),
- enlargement of the abdomen (by 12 weeks gestation, the uterus can be felt through the abdominal wall just above the symphysis),
- changes in the size, shape, and consistency of the uterus (uterus becomes softened or "doughy"), softening of the isthmus

between the still firm cervix and the softened uterus (Hegar's Sign),
- changes in the cervix (softening of the cervix at 6-8 weeks gestation can also occur),
- Braxton Hicks contractions (palpable but ordinarily painless contractions at irregular intervals from early stages of gestation),
- ballottement (near midpregnancy, pressure on the uterus will cause the fetus to sink in the amniotic fluid, and with release of pressure, the rebound to its original position will be felt as a tap),
- outlining the fetus (in the second half of pregnancy), and
- results of endocrine tests (presence of hCG in matemal plasma and its excretion in urine).

Presumptive signs

- cessation of the menses (especially after predictable menstruation),
- changes in breasts (tenderness, tingling, increase in size),
- discoloration of vaginal mucosa (dark bluish or purplish-red and congested- Chadwick's Sign),
- increased skin pigmentation and the appearance of abdominal striae (can be absent during pregnancy or present with the use of OCPs),
- nausea with or without vomiting (appears usually at 6 weeks, lasting 6 to 12 weeks),
- frequent micturation,
- easy fatigueability, and
- sensation of fetal movement (16-20 weeks).

Initial Obstetric Visit

Major goals are identification of risk factors, determination of the estimated gestational age of the fetus, patient education, and initiation of a plan for ongoing obstetric care. This also entails management of the women and child after the child birth.

History and Physical Examination

- Assess general health and risk factors.
- Attempt dating of pregnancy: Last menstrual period (LMP)—accurate if verified by calendar or coincident with holiday, etc.; reliable if no interfering factors present (i.e., prior menstrual irregularity, oral contraception).
- Bimanual examination for uterine size and pelvic adequacy (esp. diagonal conjugate).

- Auscultation or doppler examination for foetal heart.
- General examination of all other systems.

Prematurity Risk Factors

- Age <18, low socio-economic status, sexual promiscuity, DES exposure, prior premature delivery, 2 or more spontaneous abortions, uterine anomalies or fibroids, thin patient or poor weight gain, multiple gestation, polyhydramnios, UTI/renal disease, acute infections.

Placental Insufficiency Risk Factors

- Post-dates, previous stillbirth, intrauterine growth retardation, anemia/hemoglobinopathies, medical illness (DM, HTN, thyroid disease, renal disease, cardiac disease, collagen or vascular disease).

Congenital Anomalies/Disease Risk Factors

- Race (Asian, Jewish, Mediterranean, Black), mother >34 years of age, advanced paternal age, family history of congenital anomaly, previous delivery of child with anomalies, teratogen exposure, infection exposure, diabetes.

Clinical Criteria

- LMP, bimanual examination in first trimester, doptone FHTs at 10-12 weeks, fetoscopic FHTs at 20 weeks, quickening (primiparous at 18-20 weeks and multiparous at 17-19 weeks), fundus reaches umbilicus at 20 weeks, after 20 weeks fundal height in cm = weeks gestation.

Laboratory Measures

Ultrasound

- Approximate accuracy: <10 weeks—3-7 days, <20 weeks—10 days, <30 weeks—2 weeks, 30-40 weeks—3 weeks. Urine pregnancy test can give the diagnosis of pregnancy in the 7-14 days of missing the date.
- Best single scan for dates and anomalies is at 16-18 weeks.

Routine Screening Tests

- CBC (r/o anemia).

- Sickle cell prep (Black or Hispanic patients).
- Urinalysis (r/o bacteriuria, proteinuria, glycosuria).
- VDRL/RPR (r/o syphilis).
- Type, Rh, and antibody (r/o potential hemolytic disease of the newborn. If Rh- and neg antibody screen, repeat antibody screen at 28 weeks and administer Rhogam if still neg. Administer Rhogam for threatened abortions. If antibody screen is positive, consult HR OB immediately. If positive for any other antibodies except Anti I, Anti Lewis A, and Anti Lewis B, refer to HR OB).
- Rubella titer (r/o need for postpartum vaccination).
- PAP smear (inflammation—repeat PAP in 6-8 weeks and treat possible etiology; other abnormalities—refer for colposcopy).
- Glucose screening (Patients at risk, i.e., age >25, family history of DM, previous stillbirth, previous anomalous child, previous child >4000 gm, obesity, HTN, glycosuria. O'Sullivan abn if 1 hour glucose >140. Do at first prenatal visit if very high risk; follow up at 26-28 weeks if normal.)
- Triple Screen (should be done at 15-19 weeks.)
- Hepatitis screening (r/o chronic hepatitis carriers).

Patient Education

- Avoidance of possible teratogens, i.e., cigarettes, alcohol, medication, illicit drugs, radiation, work hazards.
- Healthy diet and appropriate weight gain (ideally 20#-28# total), prenatal vitamins.
- Physiologic changes in pregnancy—quickening should occur at 17-20 weeks.
- Sexuality during pregnancy.
- Warn of potential hazards that may require immediate attention.
- Schedule prenatal classes.

Follow-up Prenatal Care

- Frequency—monthly until 30-32 weeks (weekly from 17-20 weeks if necessary for dating), then biweekly until 36 weeks, then weekly.
- Brief history.

Parameters to Follow each Visit

- Weight (ideal—20-28 pounds; think PIH for rapid weight gain).
- Blood pressure (Think PIH if B/P >140/90 or if systolic increases >30 or diastolic increases >15 from first trimester B/Ps).

- Urine protein (if >1+, think PIH; if no signs of PIH, think UTI).
- Fundal height (ultrasound if EGA <36 weeks and size > or < dates by 3 cm, fundal height not increasing over a 2-week period, or fundal height increases by more than 3 cm in 1 week).
- Fetal heart tones (120-160).
- Fetal presentation: FHT (after 32 weeks).
- New problems/patient complaints.
- Repeat Rh antibody screen and titer on Rh negative mothers following any episode of supracervical vaginal bleeding or abdominal trauma, and at least once during second trimester and twice during third trimester. Rh negative mothers should receive Rhogam at 28-32 weeks.
- Repeat pelvic examination at 36-38 weeks and as indicated.
- Encourage preparation for breast feeding of infant.
- Explain false labor and onset of labor (i.e., when to come to the hospital).
- Schedule parenting classes.

Previous Cesarean Section (C/S)

1. Eligible for vaginal trial (Vaginal Birth After Cesarean—VBAC): Candidates with two or fewer low transverse C/S or undocumented scar in a patient who underwent an uncomplicated term vertex C/S for failure to progress.
2. Ineligible for vaginal trial: Refer to maternity centre at 35 weeks for evaluation.

Post-dates

- Non-Stress Test at 41 weeks with referral to Obstetrician, Arrange at 40 weeks.
- Family History of Congenital Anomaly, Genetic Disease, or Advanced Maternal Age.
- Less than 16 weeks EGA (schedule appointment with genetic counselor).
- Greater than 16, less than 22 weeks EGA (refer immediately to genetic counselor).
- Greater than 22 weeks EGA (make certain dates are correct and encourage genetic counseling).

Herpes

- Culture prenatally only if patient complains of symptoms near term and/or confirmation of the diagnosis has not been previously established.

Hypertension

- *1st or 2nd trimester*: Consider chronic HTN and obtain obstetric (OB) evaluation.
- *3rd trimester*: Consider pre-eclampsia. Refer to OB ER if B/P >140/90 and/or if symptoms of scotomata, headache, or abdominal pain. Consult HR OB for mild disease after obtaining CBC, BUN, creatinine, and LFTs.

Vaginal Bleeding (more than bloody show)

- *1st trimester*: THINK ECTOPIC PREGNANCY. Check cervical os with ring forceps to assess for inevitable abortion, check Hct and quantitative B-Hcg, check for doptones if >10 weeks, ultrasound only if patient is having evidence of abdominal cramping/pain, consult with GYN resident, and if agreeable, obtain serial B-Hcgs every other day x 3.
- *2nd trimester*: Assess for fetal cardiac activity; refer for ultrasound examination.
- *3rd trimester*: THINK PLACENTA PREVIA. Refer to Hospital immediately. Do not perform cervical examination unless the placenta has already been evaluated by ultrasound and is not a placenta previa

Premature Labor

- OB ER evaluation for abnormal cervical examination or complaints of possible uterine activity.

Premature Rupture of Membranes

- Confirm PROM by sterile speculum examination (pooling in vaginal vault, nitrazine positive, ferning).
- No digital examinations.
- Refer to maternity centre.

Six Week Postpartum Check-up

- Inquire in general about delivery, i.e., "difficult time," long, painful bleeding, etc.
- General state of mother and family:
  - o How is she coping with the baby? mood, appetite, exercise activities, rest and sleep.
  - o Involvement and interest of father.
  - o Reactions of siblings to new baby.
- Problems with baby at birth or now.

High Risk Critiera

Prior OB Complications	Maternal Medical Problems
Previous stillborn	Diabetes
> 2 miscarriages	High blood pressure
History of preterm delivery	Asthma (COPD)
Prior C/S (VBAC eval)	Thyroid disease
Present OB Complications	Liver disease
Age <14 or> 34	Chronic renal disease
Preterm labor this pregnancy	Acute pyelonephritis
Premature rupture of membranes	Cardiac disease (not murmur)
Third trimester bleeding	Hematologic disorders
Fetal anomaly	• severe anemias
Post-term>41 weeks	• sickle cell
Pre-eclampsia	• hemoglobinopathies
Incompetent cervix	• thrombocytopenia
Polyhydramnios	• Rh sensitization
Poor weight gain	Seizure disorders
Fetal growth retardation	Lupus
Mutiple gestation	Actibe tuberculosis
Fetal demise/missed abortion	Active hepatitis
	Active mumps, rubella

- Specifically ask the mother about:
  - o Fever, vaginal bleeding, cramping, discharge, episiotomy pain, breast soreness or discharge, swelling, headaches, urinary symptoms, and bowel movement.
  - o Medications currently taking (particularly if breast feeding).
  - o Contraception (consider BCPs, diaphragm, IUD, etc.).
- Menses should start 6-8 weeks after birth (longer if breast feeding).

Physical Examination

- Vital signs (particularly BP and WT).
- *General*: breast, chest, abdomen, and extremities.
  - o Brief HEENT, chest, abd. and ext.
  - o Breast examination for infection or masses.
- *Pelvic examination*: including rectal examination.
  - o State of perineum (episiotomy, if done).
  - o Character of discharge (should be scant blood or normal menses).
  - o *Cervix*: laceration, uterine size and tenderness, adnexa for tenderness or masses.
  - o *Rectal*: sphincter tone, fistula.
  - o *Uterine size*: should be normal size and non-tender in 6 weeks.

Laboratory tests

- Pap and GC culture.
- CBC if indicated by history.
- Recheck rubella titer from prenatal lab (will need immunization if titer < 1:8), if will not become pregnant within the two months following

STAGES OF NORMAL LABOR

Labour is divided into three stages—the dilation of the cervix, the delivery of the baby, and the delivery of the placenta. For first-time mothers, labour takes around 12 to 24 hours. Women who have undergone childbirth before, can expect about seven hours of labour.

Braxton-Hicks contractions are sometimes mistaken for labour. These 'false' contractions usually start halfway through the pregnancy and continue for the entire duration. You may find these contractions visibly harden and lift your pregnant belly. It is not known what triggers the onset of labour, but it is thought to be influenced by the hormone oxytocin, which is responsible for causing uterine contractions. Some of the signs and symptoms of going into labour may include:

- Period-like cramps.
- Backache.
- Diarrhoea.
- A small bloodstained discharge as your cervix thins and the mucus plug drops out.
- A gush or trickle of water as the membranes break.
- Contractions.

The first stage of labour

The first stage of labour is concerned with the thinning of the cervix and its dilation to around 10 cm. The different phases include:

- *The latent phase*—generally, this stage is the longest and the least painful part of labour. The cervix can thin out over weeks, days or hours and be accompanied by mild contractions. The contractions may be regularly or irregularly spaced, or else you might not even notice them at all.
- *The active phase*—the next phase is marked by strong, painful contractions that tend to occur around three or four minutes apart and last up to a minute or so. The cervix dilates to around 7 cm.
- *The transition phase*—the contractions become more intense, painful and frequent. It may feel like the contractions are no longer separate but running into each other. The cervix may take

around an hour or so to dilate the final 3 cm. It is not unusual to feel a strong urge to go to the toilet as the baby's head pushes against the rectum.

The second stage of labour

Once the cervix is dilated to around 10 cm, the second stage of labour can begin. The contractions should now be regular and spaced apart, so that you can relax between them (as best as you can). As each contraction builds to a peak, you may feel the urge to bear down and push. The sensation of the baby moving through the vagina is described as a stretching or burning, particularly as the baby's head crowns (appears at the vaginal entrance). Once the head has emerged, the delivery staff will turn the body to deliver the shoulders. The rest of the baby will then slip out. The second stage of labour typically lasts around 15 minutes to one hour.

The third stage of labour

The placenta is then delivered, usually five to 30 minutes later. Your uterus gently contracts to loosen and push out the placenta, although you may not be able to feel these contractions.

Be guided by your doctor or midwife, but general suggestions for a woman approaching early labour include:

- Once you go into early labour, take the opportunity to rest and relax at home. There is no need to be in hospital until the contractions are regular and painful.
- Once the contractions are around seven to 10 minutes apart, you might like to start timing them. You do this by noting how many minutes elapse between the start of one contraction and the start of the next.
- If you are unsure whether to stay home or head to the hospital, ring and speak to one of the midwives. They will ask you a number of questions and help you decide what to do.
- Once your contractions are five minutes apart, or if you no longer feel comfortable being at home, go to the hospital.
- If your waters break or if you start bleeding from the vagina, go immediately to hospital.

Once in hospital the suggestions include:

- Resist any urge to push until your cervix is fully dilated.
- The pressure of your baby's head helps to widen your cervix, so use gravity and walk around, stand or sit upright.
- Don't feel embarrassed or inhibited by your appearance or behaviour—the medical team have seen it all before. If you want to grunt, yell or swear—go ahead. Remember that passing a

bowel motion during labour is normal and nothing to be concerned about.

Where to get help

- Your doctor
- Obstetrician
- Midwife

Labour is divided into three stages—the dilation of the cervix, the delivery of the baby, and the delivery of the placenta. For first-time mothers, labour takes around 12 to 24 hours. Women who have undergone childbirth before can expect about seven hours of labour.

Suggestions for the early stages of labour

Be guided by your doctor or midwife, but general suggestions for a woman approaching labour include:

- Once you go into early labour, take the opportunity to rest and relax at home. There is no need to be in hospital until the contractions are regular and painful.
- Once the contractions are around seven to 10 minutes apart, you might like to start timing them. You do this by noting how many minutes elapse between the start of one contraction and the start of the next.
- If you are unsure whether to stay home or go to the hospital, ring and speak to doctor. She will ask you a number of questions and help you decide what to do.
- Once your contractions are five minutes apart, or if you no longer feel comfortable being at home, go to the hospital.
- If your waters break or if you start bleeding from the vagina, go immediately to hospital.

Once in hospital, suggestions include:

- Resist any urge to push until your cervix is fully dilated.
- The pressure of your baby's head helps to widen your cervix, so use gravity and walk around, stand or sit upright.
- Don't feel embarrassed or inhibited by your appearance or behaviour—the medical team have seen it all before. If you want to grunt, yell or swear—go ahead. Remember that passing a bowel motion during labour is normal and nothing to be concerned about.

Many women in India are vulnerable to complications in the postpartum period because they lack effective care. Although 60 percent of all maternal deaths occur after delivery, only 1 in 6 women receive care during the postpartum period. More women in India access maternal health services during pregnancy than during delivery or after childbirth. NFHS data indicate that among the births that took place in non-institutional settings in India, where postpartum care is particularly important, only 17 percent were followed by a checkup within two months of delivery. Shockingly, among those who deliver at home only 2% receive postpartum care within 2 days of delivery and only 5% receive care within the first 7 critical days. Often the entire range of information and services is not provided to women during a postpartum visit. According to NFHS figures, only 38 percent of the women who did not deliver at a facility but received postpartum care had an abdominal examination and a mere 27 percent were given family planning advice. Information on breastfeeding and care was more routinely provided, with around 4 out of 10 postpartum women receiving this advice. This was in spite of the fact that a significant number of women reported health problems in the first months after delivery. The same NFHS data show that 23 percent of women reported problems six weeks after delivery, of which the most frequently reported were lower abdominal pain (4.4 percent), high fever (5.3 percent) and foul discharge (0.5 percent). Massive vaginal bleeding and very high fever during the two months after delivery—symptoms of possible postpartum complications—were reported for 11 percent and 12.6 percent of births, respectively. However we must remind ourselves that these data were collected from the survivors.

Postpartum Best Practices

Most important is planning Interventions to the First 24 hours and First 7 Days to Reduce Maternal and Neonatal Deaths. From the recent evidence, it has become clear that the first 24 hours is perhaps the most critical period for postpartum and newborn care. Women regardless of where they deliver—at home or in an institution—and their newborns need to be closely monitored for the first 24 hours. Those who deliver in an institution should remain for observation for the first 24 hour period while those who deliver at home need to ensure that the birth attendant provides close monitoring for the first 24 hours for signs of an emergency. During this critical 24-hour period, the birth attendant needs to monitor for signs of any serious complications in the mother and newborns such as:

- Hemorrhage
- Atonic uterus
- Retained placenta
- Shock/fainting—cool/clammy
- Convulsions—may be preceded by severe headache/visual disturbance
- Tears/lacerations
- Urine output decrease

- Decreased blood pressure
- Neonatal complications—birth asphyxia or labored breathing, convulsions, signs of jaundice

All of these require immediate medical attention and referral to a hospital.The following 6 days are next in importance for postpartum care. It is in this period that health providers must look for signs of infection in mother—foul smelling discharge, high fever/chills, hemorrhage—and in the newborn—hypothermia/skin blue, fever/chills, redness of cord, signs of tetanus-stops sucking/rigidity. The postpartum period is also very important for providing advice to the mother and family on preventing unplanned pregnancies, on effective breastfeeding practices, importance of fully immunizing the newborn, and care of mother and baby during this period. Thus, when we design a postpartum intervention, it is essential that we include the following components for effective postpartum care: prevention and early detection and treatment of complications and disease, a system of blood donation/system for hemorrhage, a referral system and transport for emergencies, and the provision of advice and services on breastfeeding, birth spacing, prevention of infection (mother and the newborn), immunization and maternal nutrition.

Care and service provision should Identify the community's perceptions of events in the postpartum and of the health system before designing services. Explore the community's resources and involve the community itself in planning and evaluating services. Establish the incidence and prevalence of postpartum conditions in the community. Ensure culturally acceptable services for women and newborns. Develop/provide home-based maternal record for all women and newborns. Ensure care at all levels: in the community, health centre (including domiciliary services), and at the referral level. Develop, together with the community, a complete functional chain of referral from community to the district hospital and back. Strengthen district hospitals and health centres as appropriate to their levels to cope with emergencies, including blood transfusion services.

Obstetric Emergency

1. Postpartum hemorrhage (PPH)

The first few hours postpartum are especially critical in the diagnosis and management of abnormal bleeding. During the first hours after birth, the caregiver has to make sure that the uterus remains well-contracted and that there is no heavy loss of blood. In cases where bleeding is particularly severe, blood transfusion may be the only way of saving a woman's life. Signs of PPH include: Heavy bleeding, e.g. soaking one pad/cloth every hour in the first 8 hours, soaking 1 pad/cloth every 2 hours in second 8 hours. Shock (e.g. sweating, cool clammy, sweating, fainting, rapid weak pulse). Atonic or soft/boggy uterus, Tears/lacerations.

2. Retained Placenta

Retained placenta, defined as when the placenta is not delivered within 30 minutes after delivery. Retained placenta—either full or partial—can lead to hemorrhage or infection. There are many indigenous practices associated with removing the placenta. Some of these—pressing hard on the fundus, pulling on the cord, hanging heavy objects on the cord—can be dangerous and lead to complications. A retained placenta needs to be removed by a skilled birth attendant in a setting that has blood transfusion facilities. Signs of Retained Placenta include: No signs of placental separation (lengthening of the cord, gush of blood) within 15 minutes after delivery. The placenta is not delivered within 30 minutes after birth of the baby.

3. Sepsis

Puerperal infection (such as sepsis) continues to be a major cause of maternal mortality in many developing countries. Fever is the main symptom of puerperal infection and antibiotics are the main treatment. Prevention by ensuring cleanliness and hygiene at delivery is the best course of action. Signs of Sepsis include: Fever with or without chills (3-5 days postpartum usually), Foul smelling/discharge from uterus, Uterus tenderness/atonic uterus, Convulsions/rigidity.

4. Eclampsia

Eclampsia is a most important cause of maternal mortality worldwide. A woman suffering from eclampsia or severe pre-eclampsia in the first days postpartum should be hospitalized. The treatment recommended by WHO is Magnesium Sulphate. Signs of Eclampsia include:

Facial and/or hand edema (not swelling of ankles), Headache, visual disturbances, Delirium convulsions, Decreased urine output.

Counseling for Breastfeeding and Contraception

1. Immediate and Exclusive Breastfeeding

The establishment and maintenance of breastfeeding should be one of the major goals of postpartum care. Although the Government of India recommends that breastfeeding should begin immediately after childbirth and that infants should be exclusively breastfed in the first four months of life, very few children begin breastfeeding immediately after birth—only 16 percent in the first hour and 37 percent on the first day. Moreover, only 55 percent of children under four months of age are exclusively breastfed. Immediate breastfeeding is important for both mother and newborn. It helps to stimulate uterine contractions and can prevent postpartum hemorrhage. The colostrum—or first yellow milk—provides life-protecting immunities and nutrients needed by the newborn. Breast milk provides optimal nutrition for newborn infants, protects them against infections and allergies, and promotes mother-infant bonding. The baby should be given to the mother to hold immediately after delivery, to provide skin-to-skin contact and for the baby to start suckling as soon as it shows signs of readiness—normally within ½-1 hour of birth. In institutions, babies should be kept with their mothers and unrestricted breastfeeding should be allowed. Mothers need help and advice on how to breastfeed. Supplementary feeds and fluids should be avoided.

2. Birth spacing and Postpartum Contraception and counseling services

In India, data indicate that infant mortality is nearly three times higher among children born less than 24 months after a previous birth as among children born after a gap of 48 months or more (110 deaths compared to 39 per 1,000 live births). The use of temporary contraceptive methods to delay and space births would help reduce maternal and infant mortality as well as fertility. During the postpartum period women need counseling on postpartum contraception. For mothers who do not breastfeed exclusively, fertility can return as soon as 6 weeks after delivery. For mothers who breastfeed exclusively with day and night feeds, fertility can return anytime after supplemental feeding begins.

Postpartum Contraceptive Methods include the following:

(a) Lactational Amenorrhea Method (LAM) is an effective and reliable method of birth control. The method is well adapted to cultures where breastfeeding is practiced for long periods, and for women and couples who wish to avoid or postpone a subsequent pregnancy without using other family planning methods. There are three conditions for effective LAM:
   1. The mother must be fully or nearly fully breastfeeding—at least 6 times a day, with day and night feeds.
   2. Menstruation has not returned since delivery.
   3. Less than six months postpartum.

   If these three conditions are met, the mother can rely on the contraceptive effect of lactation amenorrhea (LAM). After six weeks an alternative contraceptive will be required.

(b) Combined oral contraceptives (OC) Pills can be used by postpartum women who are not breastfeeding after 6 weeks postpartum and by breastfeeding women after the first 6 months postpartum. If women do not want to rely on lactation amenorrhea or another form of contraception, low-dose combined OCs may be started earlier, but after the first six weeks postpartum.

(c) Progestogen—only contraceptives pills, injectables and more recently implants have been extensively investigated during the postpartum period. The conclusion of the study was, that the progestogen—only contraceptives used from 6 weeks postpartum during lactation did not adversely affect growth and development of the infants, compared with the infants of mothers who used non-hormonal methods. Progestogen—only pills and DMPA (Depo-Provera) injections are safe for use by postpartum women anytime after delivery and by breastfeeding women after 6 weeks.

(d) Intra-uterine devices: Intra-uterine devices (IUDs) are reliable contraceptives with lower rates of pregnancy specially for the copper-medicated IUDs: The lowest pregnancy rate is achieved by the progesterone (levonorgestrel)—releasing IUD: 0.2. It can normally be introduced from 4 to 6 weeks postpartum; in the case of the progestogen-releasing IUD it is advised to introduce it from 6 weeks. It is possible to introduce an IUD within 48 hours postpartum, but there is an increased risk of expulsion and/infection in developing countries.

(e) Female sterilization: Female sterilization in the postpartum situation is usually accomplished by minilaparotomy and surgical ligation of the fallopian tubes. Tubal ligation is a minor operation, which can be performed under general or local anesthesia, on one of the first days postpartum. It is very effective and safer. However, it is important that the woman and her husband are thoroughly counseled preferably during pregnancy. Method and the permanent nature should be explained to people who are certain that they do not want any more children.

Similarly, Male sterilization (vasectomy) can be performed when the couple are sure they do not want additional children as this is a permanent method of contraception. The operation is simple and can be performed under local anesthesia as an outpatient procedure. Complications are rare, and there are no proven long-term health effects. The postpartum period may be suitable for a vasectomy, because generally after the operation a period of some weeks is necessary as waiting time until a test shows that there are no sperms in the ejaculate. Good counseling is as important here as in the case of female sterilization, particularly given that male acceptance of sterilization is far less than that of tubal ligation by females.

The care of newborn

The provider should also Recognize complications in the newborn and postpartum woman and provide appropriate management. It also includes promoting health and preventing disease in newborn, including:

- Thermal protection
- Promotion of breastfeeding
- Eye care
- Cord care
- Immunization
- Provide Vitamin A and iodine in areas of deficiency

- Inform the woman and family of the existence of emergency funds
- Refer to higher levels of care, when appropriate
- Support and value the use of a skilled provider during the postpartum period
- Ensure that the woman is not alone in the postpartum period
- Recognize the danger signs and support implementation of the complication readiness plan (see section on Complication Readiness)
- Support mother- and baby-friendly decision-making in case of newborn emergencies
- Support timely transportation of woman and the newborn to the referral site, if necessary
- Have a functional blood donor system
- Have access to facility and community emergency funds
- Educate community members about complication readiness.

The family should:

- Ensure the mother and newborn are able to recuperate in a clean room with limited visits from outsiders to reduce the risk of infection, are provided clean clothes and clean change of sanitary pad/cloth
- Support the woman's use of postpartum and newborn care, and adjust responsibilities to allow for her attendance
- Recognize complication signs and facilitate implementing the complication readiness plan
- Agree with the woman on the decision-making process in case of postpartum or newborn emergency
- Know transportation systems, where to go in case of emergency, and support persons to stay with in the family
- Support provider, woman and newborn in reaching referral site, if necessary
- Know how to access community and family emergency funds
- Have personal savings for costs associated with postpartum and newborn care
- Purchase drugs or supplies needed for normal or emergency postpartum and newborn care
- Know-how and when to access a community blood donor system
- Identify blood donor.

The woman should Seek postpartum and newborn care at least twice in the first week of delivery—within 24 hours and within the next six days (calls a skilled provider to provide a home visit or obtains money and transport to seek care in a health facility):

- Recognize danger signs and implements the complication readiness plan
- Speak out and act on behalf of her and her child's health, safety and survival
- Know transportation systems, where to go in case of emergency, and support persons to stay with the family
- Have access to community and facility emergency funds
- Have personal savings and access these in case of need.

Key Behavior Change Messages

- The first 24 hours and the first week is when most postpartum and newborn deaths occur
- Ensure the mother and newborn are kept in a clean room with clean clothes and clean sanitary pad, and few outside visitors to prevent infection
- Families need to ensure that postpartum care by a skilled provider is provided during the first 24 hours after delivery and during the first week
- Ensure that the postpartum woman is not left alone during the first 24 hours
- Know the signs of postpartum emergency—bleeding, fever/ chills, convulsions, retained placenta after 30 minutes—and have a plan for responding without delay to an emergency
- Ensure the newborn is kept warm at all times, is breathing well, is put to the breast within one hour of birth, and is not given any other fluids besides breastmilk
- Never put any substance on the cut umbilicus—keep it dry and clean
- Seek care at a medical facility immediately if the newborn is not well—is blue/cold, has difficulty breathing, has fever, is very small and cannot suck, stops sucking or has convulsions or rigidity
- Ensure the newborn is given immunization as per schedule.

After delivery

The first month after a delivery (the postpartum period) is a time of major changes for women. Their hormones and weight are rapidly readjusting. There may be new and stressful changes in relationships with other children, the father of the baby, parents and in-laws, colleagues at work, and friends. Of course, the new baby needs almost constant attention and feeding every two hours, resulting in sleep deprivation. All of these factors can contribute to postpartum mood swings. If the moodiness only lasts 2-3 weeks and then goes away, it's commonly called the "baby blues." This natural reaction to stress is experienced by more than half of new mothers. However, if the feelings of depression or anxiety continue more than three weeks, a more serious condition called postpartum depression may exist. About 10% of women experience significant depression after a pregnancy.

Postpartum Depressioon (PPD)

You have a higher chance of postpartum depression if:

- You had mood or anxiety disorders prior to pregnancy, including depression with a previous pregnancy
- You have a close family member who has had depression or anxiety
- Anything particularly stressful happened to you during the pregnancy, including illness, death or illness of a loved one, a difficult or emergency delivery, premature delivery, or illness or abnormality in the baby
- You are in your teens or over age 40
- The pregnancy is unwanted or unplanned
- You currently abuse alcohol, take illegal substances, or smoke—these are also serious medical health risks for the baby.

Symptoms and Signs

Most of the symptoms are the same as in major depression. In addition to mood fluctuations, the woman becomes preoccupied with the infant's well-being. The intensity of this varies—the preoccupation may become delusional. Women who are depressed may feel withdrawn and unconnected to their baby, and can even feel as if they might harm the baby. The presence of severe or delusional thoughts about the infant are symptoms that need immediate attention. These can be accompanied by psychotic "command hallucinations" to kill the infant or delusions that the infant is possessed.

Having good social support from family, friends, and co-workers probably helps to reduce the seriousness of postpartum depression, but may not prevent it. Those at high risk should be screened both before and after delivery and followed closely with repeated screening, depending on symptoms, for at least four months after the delivery.

Diagnosis and Tests

There is no single test to diagnose postpartum depression. Sometimes depression following pregnancy can be related to other medical conditions. Hypothyroidism, for example, causes symptoms such as fatigue, irritability, and depression. Women with postpartum depression should have a blood test to screen for low thyroid hormones. This condition is easily treated with supplemental hormone. Another clue to this condition can be weight gain or failure to lose weight after pregnancy, despite breastfeeding the baby. Since postpartum depression is so common, questionnaire screening tests are available. Women with any of the risk factors, or with symptoms of depression, should consider taking such a test to determine if they need treatment.

Treatment

The treatment for depression after birth often includes medication, therapy, or a combination of both. Fortunately, several anti-depressant medications may be given to breastfeeding mothers. Once depression is diagnosed, the woman will need to be followed closely for at least six months.

The Puerperium

- The interval from the birth of the baby until the reproductive tract returns to its pre-pregnant condition.
- Usually time for this is 4 to 6 weeks.
- 'Involution' is the term referring to the return of the uterus to its pre-pregnant state.

Normal Body Changes

- Reproductive System has the most significant changes.
- The Uterus
- Involution
- Lochial flow and return of menses
- Cervix/vagina
- The breasts
- Breastfeeding mothers
- Non-breast feeding mothers

Other Body Changes

- Vital signs
- Cardiovascular changes
- Urinary effects
- G-I effects
- Muscular changes
- Integumentary effects

Nursing Care and Assessment

- Mental observations
- Alertness
- Bonding
- Mood changes
- Vital signs
- Temperature

- Blood pressure
- Pulse rates

Assessment-"Bubble"

- B-Breasts
- U-Uterus
- B-Bladder
- B-Bowel
- L-Lochia
- E-Epistomy/Extremities

Teaching Points

- Breasts care
- Good support bra
- Use only water
- Lubrication and air dry
- Prevention of cracks or fissures
- Lochial flow
- Normal pattern should not reverse
- Should not have an offensive odor
- Should not contain large clots
- Perineal Care
- Cleanse after each elimination
- Wipe from front to back
- Change peri pads often
- Good handwashing
- Episiotomy care
- Bladder care
- Increase fluids
- Heed the urge and void frequently
- Avoid a distended bladder
- Bowel care
- Increase fluids, fiber and activity
- Stool softeners
- Rest and activity
- No heavy lifting
- Rest when infant sleeps
- Exercises according to MD's recommendations

Emotional Care

- Single, unwed mothers
- Unwanted child
- Infant with illness or anomalies
- Sorrowing mothers

Complications of the Puerperium

(a) Bleeding complications are the leading causes of mortality/ morbidity: Uterine Atony, Acreta, Retained placental fragments, Cervical lacerations. Normal blood loss is 250-350 mls with delivery. More than 500 mls in 24 hours is excessive. Greatest danger is within the first 24 hours
(b) Infections; Endometritis, Mastitis, Cystitis
(c) Others Complications; Thrombophlebitis, Pulmonary Embolus, DIC

PPH

Postpartum haemorrhage (PPH) remains an important complication. Primary PPH is classically defined as blood loss from the genital tract, exceeding 500 mls within 24 hours of delivery. This definition is of limited practical use as accurate quantification of blood loss is seldom possible, and the average blood loss at delivery is 500 to 600 mls. Blood loss of >1000 mls is a more useful definition of PPH as this corresponds to the 95th centile for blood loss associated with spontaneous vaginal delivery. Secondary PPH is defined as excessive blood loss from the genital tract after 24 hours following delivery, until six weeks post-delivery. Incidence varies: 4%-22%. The reported incidence of PPH in the UK varies from 4% to 11%. National figures for New Zealand are not available. National Women's Hospital reports a high incidence of PPH with 18% of all women suffering a primary PPH of 500 to 1000 mls and 4% suffering a primary blood loss of >1000 mls. These figures suggest that there is scope for improvement in the management of the third stage of labour amongst Indian doctors, as that of other countries.

Causes

Uterine Atony

Failure of sustained uterine contraction following partial or complete placental separation may result in massive haemorrhage from the placental vascular bed. Prolonged labour, uterine overdistension, grand multiparity, retained placental tissue or haematometria (abruption) may contribute to inadequate myometrial contraction. Uterine inversion is a rare but dramatic cause of uterine atony and haemorrhage.

Trauma

Haemorrhage may result from vulval, perineal, vaginal or cervical tears. Rupture into the clitoral venous plexus may cause remarkable loss. Occult bleeding into the para vaginal space, ischiorectal fossa and broad ligaments may follow vaginal laceration. Occasionally, uterine rupture presents as a PPH.

Coagulopathy

Clotting dysfunction and disturbance of platelet function are unusual but important causes of PPH. In the majority of cases, the clotting disorder is secondary to pre-eclampsia, abruption or massive blood loss. Almost all maternal mortalities attributable to PPH are associated with coagulopathy and, in most cases, the bleeding dysfunction is recognised late and inadequately treated. Failure to control PPH quickly with standard measures behoves exclusion of coagulopathy and full specialist support.

Risk Factors

Although the risk of severe PPH (>1000 mls) is low (<5%), many haemorrhages are predictable. The following are risk factors:

- previous PPH;
- uterine overdistension (multiple pregnancy/macrosomia/ polyhydramnios);
- prolonged labour (especially prolonged second stage);
- instrumental delivery;
- grand multiparity (>5);
- pre-eclampsia; and
- clotting/platelet dysfunction.

To reduce the risk of PPH, aspirin therapy (used in pre-eclampsia) should cease at least 3 days prior to delivery. The management of the third stage of labour in at-risk women should be active with:

- intravenous access;
- cross matched blood available for transfusion;
- ecbolic at delivery (Syntocinon 10 IU or Syntometrine 1 ampoule); and
- placental extraction (controlled cord traction).

Active *vs.* physiological management : There are two methods of management of the third stage of labour; either active management or physiological management. Active management of labour is practised routinely in western countries such as: the UK, Australia and New Zealand. Expectant or physiological management of the third stage is popular in Northern European countries, in parts of the USA and Canada and is the practice of choice for domiciliary practice. Active management entails interventions, which reduce the chances of PPH. It involves the administration of an oxytocic drug either intramuscularly or intravenously with, or immediately after, the birth of the baby. The cord is then clamped and cut, and once signs of placental separation have occurred the placenta is delivered by controlled cord traction. The fundus should be contracted and the uterus splinted by suprapubic pressure.

In most Asian countries, physiological management, i.e. "leave well alone" approach is practised. No oxytocic drug is given at delivery. The cord is not cut until pulsation ceases and no clamp is applied, other than the umbilical clamp. Controlled cord traction is not used. Once signs of separation have occurred, the placenta will deliver spontaneously either with the aid of gravity or nipple stimulation. This kind of management of the third stage should only be practised where there has been a normal progression through labour and delivery. In India both methods are used, depending upon the educational and economic status of the patient concerned.

PPH Risk and Active Management

Three randomised trials of active *versus* expectant management of the third stage of labour were reviewed by Prendiville, Elbourne and McDonald in the Pregnancy and Childbirth Module of the Cochrane Database Systematic Reviews. The outcomes measured were maternal and perinatal complications of the third stage of labour. Results demonstrated that active management of the third stage of labour is associated with a two-fold reduction in the risk of PPH, and a significant reduction in postpartum anaemia and the need for blood transfusions during the puerperium. Women did, however, experience some adverse affects. Nausea, vomiting, headaches and hypertension were more common. One trial in Dublin demonstrated that there were more retained placentas requiring manual removal. No differences in neonatal outcomes were observed. One trial (in Bristol) measured neonatal outcomes. There were no significant differences in Apgar scores, neonatal respiratory problems or breastfeeding rates. There were fewer admissions to the special care baby unit with active management. Active management with informed consent should be routine practice. Active management of third stage of labour has positive outcomes for women in terms of a reduction in the amount of blood loss in PPH, the need for blood transfusions and postpartum anaemia. For the woman, postpartum well-being is improved. Offsetting this is the higher risk of experiencing short-term adverse side effects such as nausea, vomiting and headache. In domiciliary practice where labour and delivery have been straightforward, and with full informed consent, there may be a place for physiological management of the third stage. However, in most hospital settings, active management of the third stage should be the routine practice.

Management of Postpartum Haemorrhage

Let us assume that the placenta has been delivered and routine initial measures for the management of heavy bleeding post-delivery have been taken, i.e. fundal massage to contract the uterus, the administration of an ecbolic, either Syntometrine or Syntocinon depending on the woman's blood pressure, and emptying of the bladder.

The treatment suggested is for the management of severe rapid onset primary postpartum haemorrhage, i.e. when blood loss is perceived to have exceeded 1000mls. This management protocol is not suggested for women with minor degrees of postpartum bleeding, or for the routine management of the third stage of labour.

Uterine massage

There has been considerable criticism that the management protocol suggests that uterine compression be applied after establishment of intravenous access. We agree that uterine massage is the first action if deemed appropriate to the situation. All elements of the initial measures and treatment should take place within 5 to 10 minutes, hence it is essential that immediate assistance is obtained. Intravenous access and vigorous replacement of intravascular volume remain the mainstay of treatment for severe acute haemorrhage of any origin. If heavy and persistent bleeding occurs with the placenta *in-situ,* it is important that an attempt be made to remove the placenta and if unsuccessful to proceed immediately to surgical removal. The authors believe that the process of intravenous access and fluid replacement, use of ecbolics and recourse to obstetric/anaesthetic help, would remain unchanged. An empty bladder is said to aid uterine contraction. Catheterisation with an indwelling cathether will maintain an empty bladder and is useful in assessing fluid balance. In cases of severe haemorrhage due to uterine atony, Syntometrine IV rapidly and effectively restores uterine tone in most cases and its use in these circumstances can be justified.

Dealing with HIV

HIV-positive women having either a managed caesarean delivery or a managed vaginal birth are more likely to experience a post-delivery complication than HIV-negative women. Elective caesarean section delivery reduces the risk of mother-to-baby transmission of HIV. However, there are risks of post-delivery complications following a caesarean section and it has been suggested that these risks might outweigh the benefits for HIV-positive women with low viral loads.

To gain a better understanding of the safety of elective caesarean delivery in HIV-positive women, investigators from the European Collaborative Study collected prospective data from 13 sites across Europe on the frequency of major and minor postpartum complications. Two case controlled studies were used (using matched HIV-positive women and HIV-negative controls), one looking at managed vaginal delivery, and one at elective caesarean delivery. Investigators compared the frequency of both major and minor postpartum complications in HIV-positive women giving birth naturally or by caesarean intervention. The investigators also compared the frequency of complications in HIV-positive and HIV-negative women. Overall, HIV-positive women were significantly more likely to have a postpartum complication than HIV-negative women (29% *versus* 19%, $p<0.001$). There were a total of five major postpartum complications in HIV infected women having a caesarean delivery and none in women having a managed vaginal delivery. However, the investigators found that the five-fold increased risk of complications after a caesarean was also present for HIV-negative women. There were no major complications in either HIV-positive or HIV-negative women having a managed vaginal delivery. HIV-positive women had, however, a significantly increased risk of postpartum fever than HIV-negative women (OR 4.5, p=0.001), and HIV-positive women undergoing episiotomy (an incision into the area of skin between the vagina and the anus) had an increased risk of puerperal fever (p=0.001). The use of antibiotics, iron supplementation and spinal anaesthetic, which is associated with reduced blood loss, would be good places to start, the investigators suggest.

A Type 2 Diabetes Prevention Initiative

Five years ago I was diagnosed with impaired glucose tolerance (IGT). This diagnosis was really no surprise knowing my strong family history of diabetes. Being a nurse and a diabetes educator, I realized it was only time before I was faced with the initial steps of this progressive disease. So when I was diagnosed with gestational diabetes (GDM), I realized this was going to be a more serious matter. I now had three major risk factors for the development of type 2 diabetes—family history of type 2 diabetes, impaired glucose tolerance and gestational diabetes. This was stated by a nurse-patient.

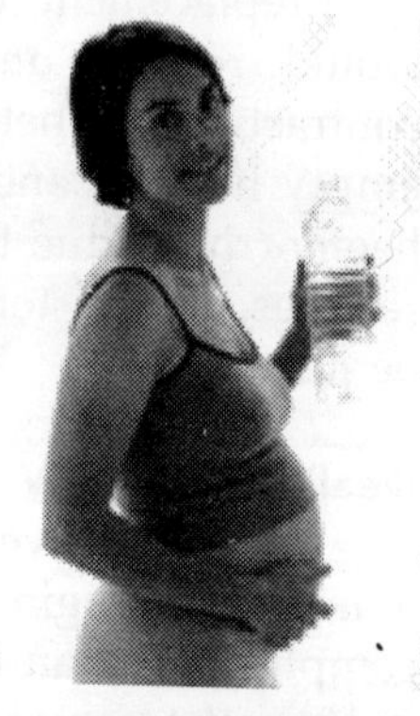

Gestational diabetes (GDM) is defined as carbohydrate intolerance, first recognized during pregnancy. GDM occurs in 2-4% of all pregnancies. It is usually diagnosed in the beginning of the third trimester when insulin resistance is high. Some women can control their blood sugars with diet and exercise. Others end up requiring insulin therapy in order to avoid the fetal and maternal complications that can arise from uncontrolled blood sugars during the pregnancy. For the most part, as the baby is delivered the insulin resistance stops and the woman returns to a non-diabetic state. However, in a clinical study, scientists found that more than 50 percent of women who had GDM, developed type 2 diabetes within 15 years after the pregnancy. Once the pregnancy is over, the implications of GDM for the future health of the mother consist of not only increased risk for the development of type 2 diabetes but also a potential recurrence of GDM in subsequent pregnancies, the development of impaired glucose tolerance, and an association with other cardiovascular risk factors. The cardiovascular risk factors that constitute the metabolic syndrome consist of dyslipidemia, hypertension and abdominal obesity. The patient has to struggle each and every day with the hardship of following a proper balanced diet, a daily exercise regimen and continued random monitoring of blood sugar. But what happens to these women after the delivery. The continuous educational support we provide during the pregnancy should not end with the delivery of the baby. We firmly believe in the need to provide education and teaching to women in a gestational postpartum program.

Primary diabetic prevention

Women with a history of GDM are an ideal group for primary diabetic prevention. They are mothers of young families, often responsible for the shopping and the preparation of the family meals. The risk factors include ethnicity, age, parity, family history of diabetes and degree of glucose intolerance in pregnancy and immediately postpartum. The modifiable risk factors are: obesity, future weight gain, level of activity, dietary fat and subsequent pregnancies. The information would then allow for the application of preventative strategies such as changes in nutrition and physical activity that might help minimize the progression to those significant diseases. Only through education will women with GDM understand the potential benefits to be gained by adopting and following positive lifestyle changes. It is imperative that the education does not stop after the delivery of the children—it must be an extension of the prenatal education these women already receive our gestational postpartum program should extend to identifying the modifiable and unmodifiable risk factors that our new mothers are faced with. We focus on making sure they understand the implications of these risk factors and stress the value of ongoing attention to nutrition and exercise. Our gestational postpartum program can assist women in changing their lifestyle routine sufficiently to reduce not only the reoccurrence of GDM in further pregnancies but in delaying and/or preventing the later development of diabetes, IGT and cardiovascular disease.

Child birth is special time

Pregnancy is one of the most exciting times in a woman's life. It can also be one of the most confusing! There are so many choices to make, to research, to learn about. Today, women have more choices than ever before, when it comes to where and how they give birth to their babies. In Indian conditions many choices are not available. Many women are rail-roaded into the OBE-GYN/hospitals, simply because they don't have other options out there! Other course, not safe at all is domicilliary child birth under supervision of a TBA. For the benefit of several other countries, below are given four options that each woman should at least consider when trying to make the best choice for herself and her baby.

(1) Assisted hospital birth

This is the option most people think of first. Giving birth in a hospital with a doctor or Certified Nurse Midwife (CNM) in attendance has become the standard most WELL TO DO women choose. Women generally see their chosen doctor at their office or at the hospital throughout pregnancy. Hospital procedures and requirements vary greatly from hospital to hospital, and it's very important to take a tour of the hospital you are considering delivering at to see if they will support you in the choices you wish to make. Your doctor will only have a limited amount of control over the type of care you receive at the hospital, so it's VERY important to determine the atmosphere where you will be giving birth.

Government Hospitals or private maternity centres provide the highest level of medical care available, and should be able to handle any crisis situation that may arise during labor and birth. Obstetricians are trained to handle high risk pregnancies and complications. The hospital birth scenario generally offers women the most technology available. Babies are monitored throughout labor and after birth with machines, mothers are generally given IV fluids instead of food or oral liquids, pain relief is immediately available, and mother's have the option of letting the nursery staff completely care for their new baby during their stay. The downside to this high level of medical management is that a lot of parents are left feeling out of the loop and without many choices. They are processed through the system instead of being treated like individuals with individual rights and needs.

(2) Certified Nurse Midwife (CNM) or Certified Professional Midwife; assisted Birthing Center Birth

In some areas Birthing Centers are becoming very popular (not in India). They offer an environment that is much closer to a home like setting, while still having some medical technology on hand. They are generally not as well equipped as hospitals and are unable to handle emergencies. They also may not be able to provide the same spectrum of pain relief during labor (such as epidurals). Patients generally see their doctor for prenatal visits at the Birthing Center. A much stronger emphasis on natural birth, breastfeeding, and family bonding is usually found at Birthing Centers as opposed to hospitals. Birthing centers may also offer special amenities not found at hospitals such as labor pools and equipment designed to help women cope with labor without drugs. Care is generally more relaxed, and women are allowed greater freedom to follow the needs of their bodies during labor and birth than at a hospital. Because there is a lower level of medical technology on hand. Birthing Centers generally require that their clientele be fairly low risk, which means, not all women will be accepted as clients.

(3) Certified Nurse Midwife (CNM); assisted Home Birth

There are many variables in the type of care offered by a midwife that provides services for home births. The amount of medical type prenatal and labor care provided will depend completely on the midwife you select. Some midwives are as medically oriented as doctors, others view pregnancy, labor and birth as completely natural and treat it as such. Enough emphasis cannot be placed on the value of researching the midwife you choose. Speak with her in detail about your views on birth, the type of care you wish to receive, and request references. Research her medical training and her credentials, and inquire about her amount of experience with various situations. Speaking to past clientele is a great way to get a true feel for how a midwife practices. Most midwives also practice with at least one assistant, or apprentice midwife. Be sure to meet all her assistants and see if you like them as well. Midwives are generally able to handle a wide range of complications, and will bring the medical equipment necessary to handle those complications to your home during the birth. Because not all complications can be handled at home, midwifes frequently work with a back-up obstetrician, whose care you will be transferred into if you have a complication that would prevent you from being able to give birth at home. Women generally choose a midwife assisted home birth because it offers them a great deal of freedom, but still affords them the security of having a medically trained professional on hand. Because midwives are unable to handle higher level of medical complications they may screen out women they consider to be high risk and refuse to provide care for them. It's also important to note that although midwives are generally assumed to be greater supporters of natural childbirth, they may not be as hands-off as some women expect.

(4) Unassisted Childbirth

Unassisted Childbirth offers a woman the ultimate freedom and control over their own pregnancies. Women either provide their own prenatal care, or seek limited care from outside medical sources (midwives). A great deal of emphasis is placed on trusting the natural process of pregnancy, labor and birth. All three are viewed as normal, safe, natural events that do not require medical care. Women have the innate ability to give birth to and care for their own babies without a trained medical assistant on hand. By choosing to give birth without medical assistance, women have complete freedom in all aspects of pregnancy and birth and follow the urgings of their own bodies instead of medical doctrine. Women generally labor and birth at home with their spouse, close family and friends, or alone. The choice is left up to the pregnant or laboring mother and what she feels is best. Intuition and instinct is used to handle any problems that may arise. Some women choose to have medical backup made available ahead of time in case there is a problem. Other women feel that nature will resolve all issues, and see no need for medical back up. Risk factors determined by the medical community are no longer an issue because women who choose to birth unassisted generally see these "risks" simply as variations of normal instead of inherent problems.

Support for Breastfeeding

Breastfeeding is important issue in Indian situations because of the increased risk of diarrhoea and other infections, and because the warmth and care, which breastfeeding provides is crucial to both mothers and children. In these situations, it may be the only sustainable source of food for infants and young children. The well-known risks associated with bottle feeding and breast milk substitutes are dramatically increased due to poor hygiene, crowding and limited water and fuel. Since breastfeeding is also an esteemed traditional activity for women, it can help uprooted women preserve a sense of their self-worth.

Optimal Feeding Practices

- Initiate breastfeeding within one hour of birth.
- Promote colostrum as a health benefit to newborns, while being sensitive to commonly held beliefs to the contrary.
- Implement the "Ten steps to successful breastfeeding" (1989 Joint WHO/UNICEF statement, protecting, promoting and supporting breastfeeding).
- Encourage frequent, on-demand feeding (including night feeds).
- Promote exclusive breastfeeding. On-demand breastfeeding during the first six months provides 98 per cent contraceptive protection, provided menses has not returned, and no other food is given to the baby.
- Surrogate feeding/wet nursing is an alternative for an orphaned child or if the mother is disabled or absent.
- Supplement breast milk with appropriate weaning foods starting at six months of age.
- Encourage breastfeeding well into the second year of life or beyond.
- HIV-positive mothers may need special support and counseling.
- During a child's illness, breastfeeding frequency should be increased, as it should after a child's illness so the child can catch up on its growth.
- 2,500 kcal per person per day of appropriate food is recommended as a minimum requirement for lactating women. The distribution of supplementary food to lactating women may be necessary when the diet available to the population is inadequate.

Counteracting Common Myths about Breastfeeding

MYTH: Women under stress cannot breastfeed.

TRUTH: Women under stress CAN successfully breastfeed. Milk production is stable; but milk release (let down) can be affected by stress. The treatment for poor milk release and for low production is increased suckling and social support. The most effective support for a breastfeeding woman comes from other breastfeeding women.

MYTH: Malnourished women don't produce enough milk.

TRUTH: Malnourished women DO produce enough milk. It is extremely important to distinguish between true cases of insufficient milk production (very rare) and mistaken perceptions. Milk production remains relatively unaffected in quantity and quality except in extremely malnourished women. Malnourished women and children are best served by feeding the mother and letting her breastfeed the infant. By doing so, you protect the health of both mother and child. Giving supplements to infants decreases suckling and so can reduce milk production. The treatment for insufficient milk production—real or perceived—is to increase suckling frequency and duration, ensure the mother has sufficient food and liquids, and offer reassurance from other breastfeeding women.

MYTH: Breast milk substitutes are always needed.

TRUTH: Usually, breast milk substitutes are NOT appropriate. There are good guidelines on the use of breast milk substitutes and other milk products in emergencies. They include the WHO International Code of Marketing of Breast Milk Substitutes (May 1981), the UNHCR guidelines on the use of milk substitutes (July 1989), and the World Health Assembly Resolution 47.5 (May 1994). Under the Code, donors must ensure that any child who receives a breast milk substitute is guaranteed a full, cost-free supply for at least six months. These guidelines include stipulations that breast milk substitutes are:

- not used as a sales inducement;
- used only for a limited target group of babies (i.e., for orphans in instances where wet nurses are not available);
- used under controlled conditions (i.e., for therapeutic feeding; never in general distribution); and
- accompanied by additional healthcare, diarrhoea treatment, water and fuel.

In addition, the guidelines assert that feeding bottles and teats should not be provided by government agencies except under strict supervision; and their use should otherwise be discouraged.

MYTH: General promotion of breastfeeding is enough.

TRUTH: Breastfeeding women NEED assistance; general promotion of breastfeeding is NOT enough. Most health doctors have little knowledge of breastfeeding and lactation management. Women who are displaced or are in emergency situations are at increased risk of breastfeeding problems. They need help, not just motivational messages. Health workers may need to be trained to give practical help to women who have difficulty breastfeeding because of incorrect positioning, cracked nipples or engorgement. A mother's fear that she "may not have enough milk" is often a cause of early termination of breastfeeding. Health workers should encourage optimal breastfeeding behaviours, even if they require selective feeding of lactating women. Policies and services, which undermine optimal feeding, such as giving food supplements to infants under six months and using bottles for Oral Rehydration Salts (ORS) delivery, should be avoided.

Nutshell for Safe Motherhood Services

- Provision of delivery kits: UNICEF midwifery kits for health centres and clean delivery kits for home use
- Identification of referral system for obstetric emergencies
- One health centre for every 30,000-40,000 people
- One operating theatre and staff for every 150,000 to 200,000 people
- Skilled doctors trained and functioning (one midwife for 20,000-30,000 people, one CHW/TBA for 2,000-3,000 people)
- Community beliefs and practices relating to delivery are known
- Women are aware of service availability.

Antenatal Services are in place:

- Record systems in place (clinic and home-based maternal records)
- Maternal health assessment routinely conducted
- Complications detected and managed
- Clinical signs observed and recorded
- Maternal nutrition maintained
- Syphilis screening in pregnancy undertaken routinely
- Educational activity related to antenatal care provision in place
- Preventive medication given during antenatal services: iron folate for anaemia, Vitamin A, tetanus toxoid, others as indicated (malaria)
- STD prevention and management undertaken
- Materials available to implement antenatal care services.

Delivery services are in place:

- Protocols for managing and referring complications in place and transport system functioning
- Training and supervision of TBAs and midwives undertaken
- Complications are detected and managed appropriately
- Awareness of warning signs of complications in pregnancy is widespread
- Standard protocols are used to manage deliveries
- Medical facilities are adequately equipped
- Breastfeeding is supported.

Postpartum services are in place:

- Educational activities undertaken (especially family planning and breastfeeding)
- Complications managed appropriately
- Iron folate and Vitamin A provided.

Newborn weighed and referred for under-five services (e.g., EPI, growth monitoring).

Emergency Child Birth Situation

As a general guideline, there are three cases in which you would not try to transport the mother to a hospital or doctor:

1. When you have no transportation available.
2. When the delivery of the baby can be expected within five minutes.
3. When the hospital or doctor cannot be reached.

Imminent delivery can best be determined by simply talking to the mother. Open lines of communication and good rapport with the mother are necessary for a successful delivery. The mother is naturally nervous and apprehensive, since she expected to have her baby in the well-controlled environment of a hospital delivery room—not in the street or at home. When you arrive at the scene and find a woman in labor, you will first need to determine whether you have adequate time to transport her to the hospital. To make this decision, ask the mother certain questions:

1. Has the mother had a baby before? Labor during the first pregnancy is usually slower than in later pregnancies, allowing more time for transport. If this is a first child, you will have time to transport unless the mother's vagina is bulging and you can see the crown of the baby's head in the birth canal. In women who have had several children, there may not be much time. Previous deliveries cause most of the structures used in the birth process to stretch, permitting easier delivery.
2. How frequent are contractions? Contractions more than five minutes apart generally allow enough time to get the mother to a nearby hospital. Contractions less than two minutes apart, especially in a woman who has had more than one pregnancy, signal impending delivery and do not allow enough time for transport. False contractions, or "false labor," may begin as early as three or four weeks before actual delivery. These contractions, part of the natural stretching process that begins early in pregnancy, allow the uterus to grow with the development of the fetus. As the fetus grows and the uterus enlarges, these contractions become more and more evident. They are usually confined to the lower part of the abdomen and groin but do not increase in intensity. True labor contractions are felt in the lower back and extend in a gird like fashion from the back to the front of the abdomen. There is a definite pattern to the rhythm and a gradual increase in intensity, frequency, and duration. False labor pains are irregular and are usually

relieved by walking. In true labor, the intervals between contractions are regular and do not cease with exercise. During labor, the interval between contractions gradually diminishes from ten minutes in early labor to two or three minutes in the second stage. The duration of the contractions is usually forty-five to ninety seconds. For the woman bearing her first child, the total length of labor can be up to eighteen hours. For women who have had several children, eight hours or less is not uncommon. However, remember that no two women are alike.

3. Has the mother's amniotic sac (bag of waters) ruptured, and if so, when? If rupture occurred many hours before, the likelihood of fetal infection is increased, and the hospital staff should be alerted.
4. Does the mother feel as though she has to move her bowels? This sensation is caused by the baby's head in the vagina pressing against the rectum and indicates that delivery is imminent. Under no circumstances should you allow the mother to sit on the toilet. Excessive bearing down by the mother will cause early delivery and may result in the death of the child.
5. Examine the mother to see whether the crown of the baby's head (or whichever part of the baby comes out first) is bulging out of the vagina. If so, the baby is about to be born, and you will not have time to go to the hospital before delivery. This can only be determined by direct examination. Communication with the mother is crucial at this point; you must have gained the mother's trust and confidence. A simple explanation about the necessity for examination should suffice for the mother and or father. Every step of the examination should be carefully explained in simple, easily understandable terms. If you think that you have plenty of time for a trip to the hospital, transport the mother:
    1. Keep her lying down, and remove any underclothing that might obstruct delivery.
    2. If possible, place a stretcher underneath the mother during transport.
    3. Place a folded blanket, sheet, or other clean object underneath her buttocks and lower back.
    4. Have the mother bend her knees and spread her thighs apart so that you can watch for the fetal crowning (appearance of the crown of the baby's head in the birth canal).
    5. If the father or someone else is present, ask that person to reassure the mother and to talk to her during this part of the examination, since it can be embarrassing for both parties.
    6. Do not allow the mother to go to the toilet.
    7. Never ask the mother to cross her legs or ankles, and never

tie or hold her legs together in an attempt to delay delivery. Never try to delay or restrain delivery in any way, since this causes undue pressure and may result in death or permanent injury to the infant.

8. In case of vomiting, turn the mother's head to one side and clean out her mouth, either manually or by suction.

Birth

Position: Squatting, or if that doesn't work, hands and knees. If neither of those two work, try whatever.

Expulsion techniques: Bearing down with contractions.

Speed up birth: Gravity-enhanced positions.

Bed for birth: Mother's choice of bed, or whatever else is available.

Cleanliness of perineum: Undraped, mother touches baby during birth.

Care of perineum: Try for intact perineum with massage, support, and hot compresses.

Presence of family: Coach (Dad) present at all times. Children and their adult friends present at parents' discretion.

Handling of baby: Mother gets to hold baby immediately, with father helping, so baby doesn't accidently get dropped. Suctioning or whatever done while baby is in mother's arms.

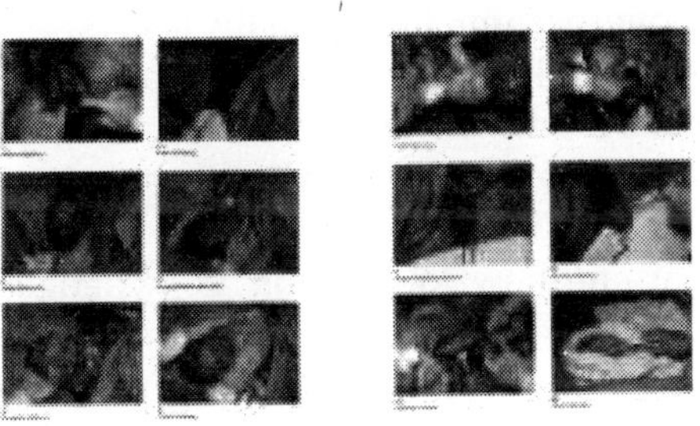

Crowning

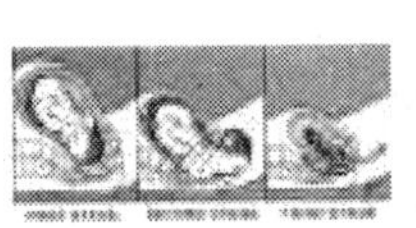

Baby Delivers

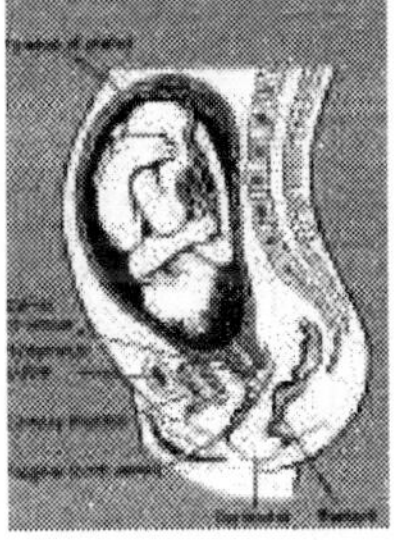

Fetus in Womb

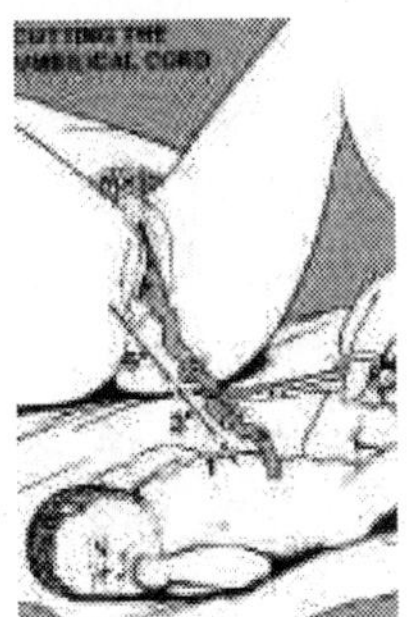

Cutting of Cord

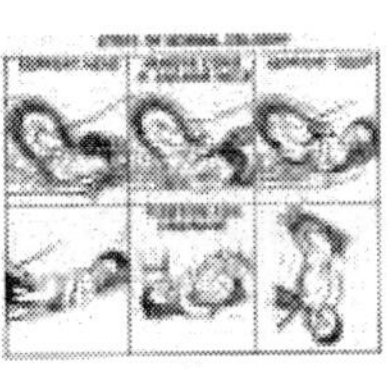

Steps of Normal Delivery

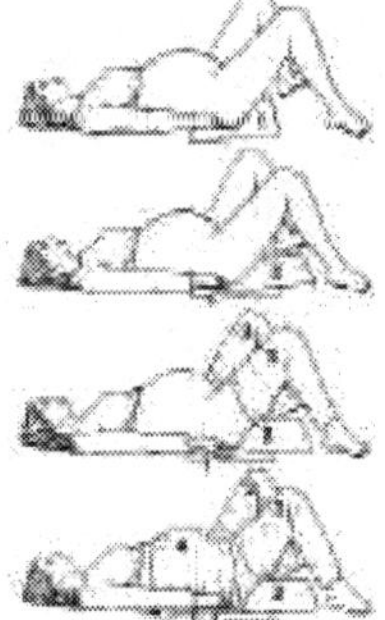

Turning of the Head, Positioning

After Birth

Delivery of placenta: Spontaneous or encouraged with breast stimulation and nursing the baby.

Cord cutting: Clamp and cut after it stops pulsating.

Discharge of mother and baby: As soon as possible. If medically feasible, within 24 hours of admission.

Baby Care

Airway: Baby coughs and expels own mucus. Suctioned only if necessary.

Warmth: Baby skin-to-skin with mother, with blanket covering both.

Immediate care: Baby held by parents and nursed by mother. Observed in parents' arms. If parents need a break, baby is kept nearby in bassinet.

Eye care: Non-irritating agent, such as erythromycin or tetracycline, as late as possible, so baby has a chance to look at her family.

First feedings: Breastfeeding on demand, start within one hour of delivery.

Contact with baby: 24-hour rooming in.

Taking care of yourself after birth

The postpartum period begins after the delivery of the baby and ends when the mother's body has returned as closely as possible to its pre-pregnant state. This period is called puerperium that usually lasts six to eight weeks. The postpartum period involves the mother progressing through many changes, both emotionally and physically, while learning how to deal with all the changes and adjustments required with becoming a new mother. The postpartum period also involves the parents learning how to care for their newborn and learning how to function as a changed family unit. A mother needs to take good care of herself to rebuild her strength. You will need plenty of rest, good nutrition and help during the first few weeks.

Rest

Every new parent soon learns that babies have different time clocks than adults. A typical newborn awakens about every three hours and needs to be fed, changed and comforted. Especially if this is their first baby, parents—especially the mother—can become overwhelmed by exhaustion. While a solid eight hours of sleep for you may not happen again for several months, the following suggestions may be helpful in finding ways to get more rest now:

- In the first few weeks, a mother needs to be relieved of all responsibilities other than feeding the baby and taking care of herself.
- Sleep when the baby sleeps. This may be only a few minutes rest several times a day, but these minutes can add up.

- Save steps and time. Have your baby's bed near yours for feedings at night.
- Many new parents enjoy visits from friends and family, but new mothers should not feel obligated to entertain. Feel free to excuse yourself for a nap or to feed your baby.
- Get outside for a few minutes each day. You can begin walking and postpartum exercises, as advised by your physician.
- After the first two to three weeks, introduce a bottle to breastfed babies for an occasional night-time feeding. This way, someone else can feed the baby, and you can have a longer period of uninterrupted sleep.

Nutrition

A mother's body has undergone many changes during pregnancy, as well as with the birth of her baby. She needs to heal and recover from pregnancy and childbirth. In addition to rest, all mothers need to maintain a healthy diet to promote healing and recovery. The weight gained in pregnancy helps build stores for your recovery and for breastfeeding. After delivery, all mothers need continued nutrition so that they can be healthy and active and able to care for their baby.

Whether they breastfeed or formula feed, all mothers need to eat a healthy and balanced diet. Most experts recommend that breastfeeding mothers should eat when they are hungry. But many mothers may be so tired or busy that food is forgotten. So, it is essential to plan simple and healthy meals that include choices from all of the recommended groups from the food pyramid. Vitamin A Supplementation in Pregnancy is a must. Where Vitamin A Deficiency is endemic among children and maternal diets are low in Vitamin A, health workers should provide: a daily supplement not exceeding 10,000 IU vitamin A during pregnancy or a weekly supplement not exceeding 25,000 IU Vitamin A after the first trimester. These supplements will benefit the mother and her developing fetus with little risk of harm to either after the mother gives birth, she should receive 200,000 IU Vitamin A.

Although most mothers want to lose their pregnancy weight, extreme dieting and rapid weight loss can be hazardous to your health and to your baby's if you are breastfeeding. It can take several months for a mother to lose the weight, she gained during pregnancy. This can be accomplished by cutting out high-fat snacks and concentrating on a diet with plenty of fresh vegetables and fruits, balanced with proteins and carbohydrates. Exercise also helps burn calories and tone muscles and limbs. Along with balanced meals, breastfeeding mothers should increase fluids. Many mothers find they become very thirsty while the baby is nursing. Water, milk and fruit juices are excellent choices. It is helpful to keep a pitcher of water and even some healthy snacks beside your bed or breastfeeding chair.

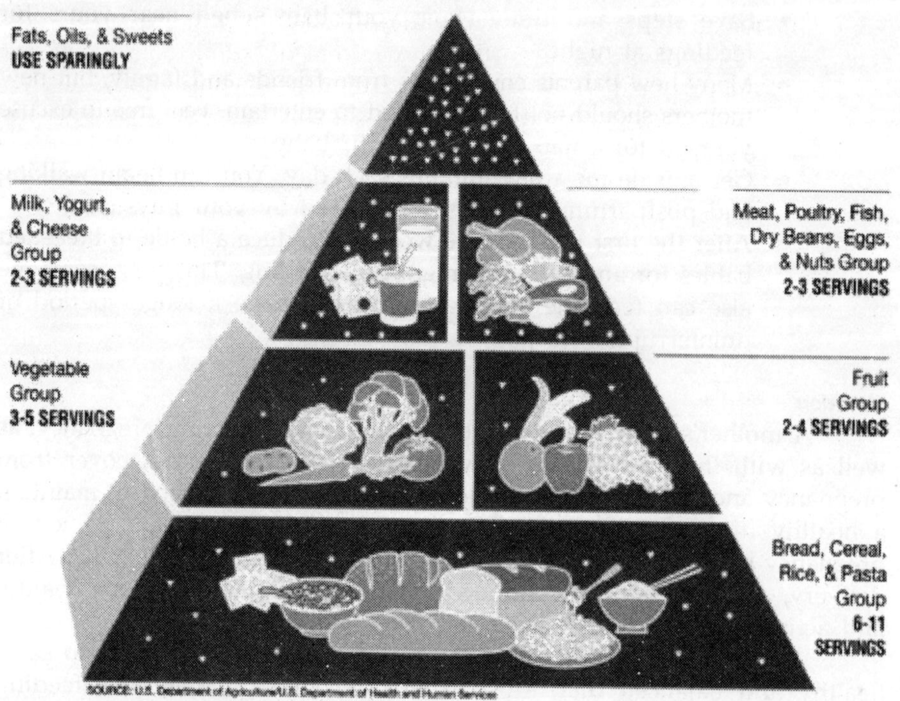

Help for new parents

New as well as experienced parents soon realize that babies require a lot of work. Meeting the constant needs of a newborn involves time and energy and often takes parents away from other responsibilities in the home. Although many parents do fine on their own, having someone else helping with the household responsibilities usually makes the adjustment to a new baby easier. Parents can concentrate on the needs of mother and baby, rather than the laundry or dirty dishes. Helpers can be family, friends or a paid home care provider. A family member such as the new baby's grandmother or aunt may be able to come for a few days or longer. Home care providers offer a variety of services, from nursing care of the new mother and baby to housekeeping and care of other children. Whoever you decide to have as helpers, be sure to make clear all the things you expect them to do. Communication is important in preventing hurt feelings or misunderstandings when emotions are fragile these first few weeks. It is generally best for the new mother to be relieved of all responsibilities except the feeding and care of herself and her baby. This is especially important if she is breastfeeding. Others should assume the chores in the home such as cooking, cleaning, laundry and grocery shopping.

Screening for Syphilis in Pregnancy

Syphilis and other STDs contribute to the transmission of HIV, maternal morbidity and negative pregnancy outcome. In a recent study of

3,591 HIV-negative Malawi women with an active syphilis rate of 3.6 per cent, 21 per cent of perinatal deaths, 26 per cent of stillbirths, 11 per cent of neonatal deaths and 8 per cent of infant deaths were attributable to syphilis.

Testing for syphilis in pregnancy can be undertaken at the antenatal clinic by using the RPR (rapid plasma reagin) test. Staff must be trained, but sophisticated laboratory equipment is not needed for routine RPR testing. Periodically, quality control of RPR testing with laboratory verification using Treponema Pallidum Haemagglutination test (TPHA) should be undertaken to ensure accuracy of RPR testing.

RPR testing for syphilis in pregnancy has been successfully undertaken in refugee camps in Tanzania. Prevalence of syphilis in pregnancy using RPR ranged from 7 to 20 per cent.

Premature births

Most babies are born about 40 weeks after the first day of their mother's last menstrual period. But about 10 percent of babies arrive sooner. A baby born more than three weeks before his or her due date is considered premature. Premature babies have less time to fully develop and mature in the womb. As a result, they're often at increased risk of medical and developmental problems. One of the biggest problems facing premature infants is, under-developed lungs. Your doctor may try to delay your baby's birth if you go into labor earlier than around 34 weeks into your pregnancy (preterm labor). Even a few extra days in the womb can give your baby's lungs a chance to become more mature. But sometimes, inspite of every effort, your baby may be born early. Fortunately, the outlook for premature infants has improved dramatically in recent years. Great advances have been made in the care of premature infants, and even babies born as early as 23 weeks now have a good chance of survival.

Signs and symptoms

It's usually best for a baby to stay in the womb as close as possible to full term. Recognizing the signs of premature labor may help you prevent your baby from being born too soon. The following signs and symptoms can occur as early as four months before your due date:

- Regular contractions of your uterus. At first, contractions seem like a tightening in your abdomen that you can feel with your fingertips.
- Light vaginal spotting or bleeding.
- Menstrual-type or abdominal cramps.
- Low, dull back pain.
- Watery discharge from your vagina. This may be amniotic fluid, the protective liquid that surrounds your baby in the womb. If so, it's a sign that the membranes around your baby have ruptured.

- A feeling of pressure in your pelvis, as if your baby is pressing down.

If you suspect you're in premature labor but haven't had a watery discharge, drink two or three glasses of water and lie down on your left side. This helps improve circulation to your uterus.

Causes

About half of women who go into premature labor do so for unknown reasons. Or, you may have a medical condition that contributes to early labor. These conditions may include:

- A rupture of your bag of waters (amniotic sac). Normally, these membranes that surround your baby rupture during labor or just before labor begins. But sometimes they may rupture weeks or even months before your due date, for no apparent reason. In that case, there's a high risk that your labor will begin within a few days. You and your baby are also at increased risk of infection.
- Certain infections. These include infections of your uterus, cervix or urinary tract.
- Weak cervix. A cervix that opens (dilates) without contractions (incompetent cervix). In a normal pregnancy, your cervix dilates in response to uterine contractions. But if your cervix is weak, it may open just from the pressure on your uterus caused by your progressing pregnancy. The cervix may have been weakened by a previous pregnancy or during a previous surgery involving the cervix, such as a dilation and curettage (D and C) or a biopsy. Other factors that may weaken your cervix include carrying more than one fetus or having too much amniotic fluid (hydramnios).
- Certain chronic diseases. These include high blood pressure, diabetes, kidney disease and hypothyroidism.
- Uterine abnormalities. These include an abnormally shaped uterus or a benign tumor (fibroid) of the uterus.
- A previous premature delivery. Women who have had a premature delivery are at higher risk of going into premature labor again. For many women, though, early labor happens only once.
- Substance abuse. These include smoking, alcohol use, or misuse of other drugs.
- Malnutrition. Women who are undernourished or anemic are more likely to give birth prematurely.
- Other conditions. A fetus with congenital defects or production of an overabundance of amniotic fluid also can contribute to early labor.

- o Urinary tract infection
- o High blood pressure
- o Diabetes
- o Pregnancy and diabetes
- o Hypothyroidism
- o Uterine fibroids
- o Uterine Fibroids Health Decision Guide

Good prenatal care includes regular visits to your doctor throughout your pregnancy to check on both your health and your baby's health. If you're at risk of premature labor, being in weekly contact with your doctor and carefully monitoring your own signs and symptoms can be especially helpful. If you develop any signs or symptoms of early labor, such as bleeding with cramps and pain, a watery discharge from your vagina, or more than five or six contractions an hour, call your doctor or hospital right away. It's a good idea to keep the phone numbers handy, so that you can find them quickly.

Screening and diagnosis

If your doctor suspects premature labor, she will check to see if your cervix has begun to dilate and whether the fetal membranes have ruptured. In some cases, a monitor may be used to measure the duration and spacing of your contractions. Monitoring the length of your cervix with ultrasound imaging may be done. In addition, sampling of the cervical canal for the presence of fetal fibronectin, a glue-like tissue lost with labor, also may help guide your treatment. If it turns out that you're in premature labor, you and your doctor will need to decide whether to try to stop your labor. Considerations include your baby's well-being, as well as your own, along with the risks and benefits of each option.

Complications

Premature labor may create complications for mother, for baby or for both: By itself, premature labor won't put you at any physical risk unless it's the result of another problem, such as a uterine infection. But all treatments used to delay delivery carry some risks. Medications that halt uterine contractions often cause fluid to collect in the mother's lungs. This causes breathing difficulties and can pose a risk for both you and your baby. Other side effects depend on the medication used to stop labor. Some medications can lead to fatigue and muscle weakness. Others may cause a rapid heart beat, blood sugar rise or stomach ulcers. You and your doctor will need to consider your own risk if medications are used to stop labor, as well as the risks to your baby if he or she is born too soon.

If your baby is premature, how well she will thrive depends largely on the baby's gestational age at birth. Risks are greatest for the babies born most prematurely—those born between 23 and 26 weeks gestation. About a third of these smallest survivors, who weigh less than 2 pounds at birth, will have serious medical problems such as cerebral palsy, fluid accumulation in the brain (hydrocephalus), seizures, lasting neurologic problems or developmental delays. Another third will have some less-serious chronic problems, such as mild cerebral palsy, the need to wear glasses and have ongoing eye care, or more mild developmental delays. Other babies born at 23 to 25 weeks do very well at first and may show no signs of problems when they go home from the hospital. But as childhood progresses, many of these children display some difficulties related to their premature birth. In particular, they may not perform as well in school as other children their age.

Premature babies are also at risk of other conditions:

- *Bleeding in the brain (intracranial hemorrhage).* If this occurs, it's usually in the first week to 10 days of life. The more severe the bleeding, the greater the likelihood that the child will develop serious problems, including developmental delays, seizures, learning disabilities and fluid accumulation in the brain.
- *Retinal problems.* Another complication seen in the youngest and most vulnerable premature babies is retinopathy of prematurity (ROP), an abnormal growth of blood vessels in the retina, the light-sensitive inner lining of the eye. ROP probably occurs because the vascular system in the baby's eye hasn't fully developed. Many cases of ROP disappear on their own, but sometimes the condition leads to scarring. The most serious cases may be treated with cryotherapy, a procedure in which an extremely cold instrument is used to help prevent the baby's retina from becoming detached. Sometimes lasers are used in a similar manner to treat ROP.
- *Intestinal problems.* Some premature infants are also at risk of a potentially severe intestinal problem known as necrotizing enterocolitis (NEC). In the most serious cases, this condition can be life-threatening. Infants who have milder cases of NEC need to be fed intravenously and given antibiotics for 1 or 2 weeks.
- *Sudden infant death syndrome (SIDS).* Premature babies are at increased risk of SIDS, a mysterious condition that claims the lives of about 2,500 infants each year.

But not all pre-emies have medical or developmental problems. By 28 to 30 weeks, the risk of these complications is much lower. And for babies born between 32 and 35 weeks, most medical problems are short-term and may even have resolved by the time the baby comes home from the hospital.

- Cerebral palsy
- Hydrocephalus
- Epilepsy
- Sudden infant death syndrome

Treatment

Treatments related to premature birth may focus on women in preterm labor, on babies still in the womb, or on newborns in hospital neonatal (newborn) intensive care units (NICUs). If you're experiencing preterm labor, your treatment depends on how far along you are in your pregnancy and how far your labor has progressed. Sometimes bed rest and extra fluids are enough to stop premature contractions. In other situations, your doctor may recommend certain medications. These may include some medications originally used for treating asthma, such as terbutaline (Brethaire, Brethine, Bricanyl) and ritodrine (Yutopar). These medications relax smooth muscles, including those of the uterus. Magnesium sulfate is a muscle relaxant that is given intravenously. Medications that block the calcium channels in muscle cells can sometimes stop contractions. So can drugs that block the production of substances that stimulate uterine contractions (prostaglandins), such as ibuprofen or indomethacin. Medications often stop labor only for a brief period of time. They are best used to delay labor long enough to accomplish other goals, such as transferring the mother to a facility better equipped to handle premature delivery or allowing other medications to have a beneficial effect on the baby. Although not common, preterm delivery may result from weakness of the connective tissue of the cervix with minimal pressure from uterine contractions. If this occurs, a surgical procedure known as cervical cerclage may be an option. Using strong thread, an obstetrician stitches around the cervix to close it. The thread is removed in the last month of pregnancy.

If your labor can't be stopped, you may receive medications to help prepare your baby for birth. Corticosteroids such as betamethasone can help make your baby's lungs more mature in as short a time as 24 to 48 hours. Hospital NICUs are designed to provide care for premature babies and full-term babies who develop problems after birth. If your premature baby spends time in an NICU, he or she will receive round-the-clock intensive care from doctors, nurses and respiratory therapists specially trained to care for newborns with medical problems. In an NICU, your baby will probably be kept in an incubator, an enclosed plastic bassinet that is kept warm so your baby can maintain normal body temperature. Because pre-emies have immature skin and very little body fat, they often need extra help to stay warm.

At first your baby will receive fluids and nutrients—known as total parenteral nutrition (TPN)—through an intravenous route, and later start milk feedings through a tube that has been passed through her nose. Like many premature infants, your baby may not yet have developed a sucking reflex or may be too weak to suck. When your baby is stronger, you'll likely be able to feed her by breastfeeding or with a bottle. The antibodies in breast milk are especially important for premature infants. Sensors may be taped to your baby's body to monitor blood pressure, heart rate, breathing and temperature. Caregivers may also use ventilators to help your baby breathe. This high-tech equipment may seem overwhelming at first, but it's all designed to help your baby. In a hospital neonatal (newborn) intensive care unit, babies are often first watched unclothed on a warmer bed. Later your baby will probably be kept in an incubator.

As the parent, you play an important role in your baby's life, even though she is in the NICU. Your baby's caregivers will help you learn how to touch and eventually hold your baby in ways that are calming and not overstimulating. Talking or singing softly to your baby, or just providing quiet company, will give great support and comfort. When your baby is ready to eat on his or her own, the nurses will help you learn how to feed your child. Babies are ready to go home when they no longer have medical problems that require continuous hospital care, when their body temperature is stable and when they can nurse well enough to gain weight. Your baby need not reach a specific weight or age before going home.

Pre-emies are more susceptible than other newborns to serious infections, and their illnesses progress more quickly. That's why it's important that they be examined often. A follow-up visit will likely be scheduled soon after you take your baby home so that your doctor can examine the baby and answer any of your new or ongoing questions.

Prevention

Some research suggests that hydroxyprogesterone caproate, a synthetic progestin hormone, may prevent premature labor in women at high risk. Although this treatment has been shown effective in preventing a recurrence of premature labor, more research is needed to confirm this approach before such treatment is widely accepted and used. The risks and complications of this treatment aren't known. Previous experimentation with hormone treatment to prevent premature birth occurred with the use of diethylstilbestrol to prevent miscarriage. This treatment has proven ineffective, and caused reproductive problems in daughters of women who used it. These risks didn't become apparent until more than a decade after treatment was carried out.

Coping skills

Caring for a premature infant can be a great challenge. You'll face many challenges that don't exist for women who have delivered a full-term baby. Like many parents, you may have tremendous anxiety about your baby's health and the long-term effects of early birth. You may also feel angry, guilty or depressed. All of these feelings are normal, and you'll likely find they change from day-to-day. Sometimes you may also experience the anxiety and sadness of postpartum depression—the result of sudden changes in your hormones after pregnancy. You may also find it hard to establish milk production if your baby is too small or too sick to breast-feed at first. In addition, you may need more time to recover physically than you might think. This, combined with your desire to be at the hospital caring for your baby if he or she is in a neonatal intensive care unit, can lead to a great deal of fatigue.

Some of the following suggestions may help during this difficult time:

- Learn everything you can about your baby's condition. In addition to talking to your doctor and your baby's caregivers, read books on premature birth and look for information on the Internet.
- Take care of yourself. Get as much rest as you can and eat a healthy diet. You'll feel stronger and better able to care for your baby.
- Seek good listeners for support. Talk to your partner or spouse, your friends, family or your baby's caregivers. If you're interested, your nursing staff or social worker may be able to suggest a support group in your area. Many parents find it particularly helpful to talk to other parents who are caring for a preemie.
- Accept help from others. Allow friends and family to help you. They can care for your other children, prepare food, clean the house or run errands. This helps you save your energy for your baby.
- Keep a magazine or book. Record the details of your baby's progress as well as your own thoughts and feelings. Include pictures of your baby, so you can see how much he or she is changing. Photos will also help you feel close when your baby is still in the NICU.

Obstetric complications and role of TBAs: Pakistan experience

Obstetrics complication could be any problems arising in a pregnant woman and have effect on her or the fetus. Normal developmental stages of pregnancy can be disrupted when medical complications develop. There could be many causes of obstetric complications but the most common causes both in developed and developing countries are still prolonged obstructed labor, hypertensive disorders of pregnancy, hemorrhage, sepsis and complications of unsafe abortion, according to Rana Jawad Asghar (*Journal of College of Physicians and Surgeons, Pakistan*, Jan. 1999, Volume 9(1): 55-57).

Maternal mortality rates in developing countries average about 450 per 100,000 live births (goes up to 2000 in some areas, compared with an estimated 30 per 100,000 in developed countries. These rates vary widely between different areas of the same region or country. For example there may be two-fold high mortality in the rural than the urban area. But in some urban slums it may be worse than that in rural area because of poor hygiene and sanitation and over crowding. These people are at high risk of malnutrition and under nutrition. But these urban dwellers have the hospitals and clinics available at a shorted distance. This is yet another question if these services are accessible to them or not. Rural population has a very shortage of health personal or health facilities. In India four-fifths of the population but only one-fifth of the physicians, are in rural areas. In African countries healthcare coverage to rural area is even worse.

According to WHO reproductive health problems account for more than one-third of the total burden of disease in women. The World Health Organization estimates that 500,000 women die every year from complications of pregnancy, including abortion and virtually all these deaths occur in developing countries (99 percent). The major causes of maternal mortality in developing countries are anemia, hemorrhage, eclempsia, infections, abortions, complication of obstructed labor. But these deaths represent only a small proportion of the total morbidity and mortality attributable to the above causes. For every maternal death there are many more women in whom, after childbirth, disabilities develop that impair their general health and reproductive functions with possible reduction in their economic activity. For example, it has been estimated that in sub-Saharan Africa for every maternal death, another 15 women are disabled or permanently crippled by incontinence, uterine prolapse and infertility due to pregnancy of birth related causes. Between two and three million African women are left handicapped from obstetric complications each year. Additionally, some women who survive delivery become chronically ill and eventually die from conditions such as diabetes and infectious hepatitis. The frequency of maternal deaths in a country depends not only on the risk of an average pregnancy, but on the fertility rates as well. Not only do women in developing countries have higher risk of death with each pregnancy; they became pregnant more often. An average woman's lifetime risk of dying a maternal death ranges from 1 in 21 in Africa, to one in 9850 in Northern Europe.

A majority of the births in most developing countries, particularly in the rural areas, takes place at home, usually assisted by relatives or traditional birth attendants (TBAs). Frequent vaginal examination with unclean hands and the application of animal dung and herbal medicines to the vulva or the vagina are some of the practices, which may cause genital infection. Pelvic sepsis may follow after these deliveries or abortions and when untreated (as usually it happens in developing countries) may lead to chronic pelvic inflammatory disease, which is the underlying cause of many cases of infertility, menstrual disorders and ectopic pregnancies.

Interventions

The means to prevent deaths from obstetric complications have existed for decades, antibiotics for infection, cesarean section for obstructed labor, blood transfusion and oxytocic drugs for hemorrhage, sedatives and other drugs for eclampsia. Unfortunately, such treatment is not accessible to most women in poor countries. The large number of TBAs are present in developing countries in most of the rural areas where there are no other healthcare facility exists. And it may take a very long time that these developing countries can afford to provide qualified doctors or nurses to all parts of their population. So it is important to use the immense potential, which lies in the communities themselves for providing basic healthcare, thus making it possible for such communities to improve their capacity for serving themselves. TBAs constitute a large segment of that potential. This has been proved by many studies that by training TBAs in timely recognition and referral of pregnancy/delivery/neonatal complications the health situation can be improved. The major areas of training of TBAs are: increased safety in the TBAs practice, such as cleanliness, especially washing of the hands and clean or sterile cord-cutting procedures, non-interference during labor, care of mothers before, during and after delivery, identification and referrals of mother at risk, doing away with traditional harmful practices and leaving alone or supporting those that contribute to psychosocial support. While TBAs concept is becoming more popular day-by-day there are still some problems to be addressed. Lack of an organized system to supervise trained TBAs. Provide continued training for them, and ensure availability of basic supplies, such as cord care kits. Supervision of TBAs constitutes the major link between them and the formal healthcare system. A shortage of supervisory health personal, inadequate transportation systems and insufficient financial resources, problems cited in WHO survey of the 1972 remains the primary obstacles to the development of good supervision.

Giving emphasis on TBAs does not by any way mean that there is less importance of referral hospitals, medicines and or Gyn and Obs centers staffed by well-qualified doctors and nurses. If there is no transport available for the high-risk mothers, mortality cannot be improved very much, even if the TBAs identify high-risk mothers. Same if we don't have enough and safe medicines available for ailments in pregnancy, the condition may also not change much. In an interesting study in Bangladesh it was found that Neonatal deaths due to Tetanus in highly trained TBA's cases was reduced to 6% (Control 24%) and by vaccinating mothers with Tetanus Toxoid it was reduced to mere 1%. So we cant say that by just training TBAs we can solve all the problems, but by providing all the back-up services we certainly can reduce the high maternal mortality in developing countries. It has also been argued that as 63% of all maternal deaths occur within 24 hours of birth and 80% occur in the first week of birth, so it is very important to increase the awareness of signs and symptoms of obstetric complications among women, family and TBAs. Even though TBAs are not trained in emergency obstetric care, it may be a good idea to start training them in selected aspects of emergency obstetric care.

In terms of its social and economic consequences, anemia is the most important cause of morbidity in non-pregnant women of childbearing age in Asian countries. Giving the TBAs training about picking up the Anemic cases by pallor, very easily identifiable and providing them supplies of iron and vitamin supplements (quite cheap to manufacture) we can reduce some complications by little intervention and little investment. In some regions 74 percent of pregnant women are undernourished and TBA's are the main source of nutritional or dietary advice. By training them in basic nutritional principles there is a real chance to correct the problem to some extent. Maternity waiting house (MWH) is another way to reduce the risk in women who are at high risk of delivery complications and where they wait for the last few weeks of their pregnancy and receive medical supervision. This is not a new concept as they are functioning from beginning of this century in Europe. In the developing countries where they are functioning, the TBAs are the most important source to pickup the high-risk pregnancies and refer them to MWHs.

Access to care

It is a major barrier. We need a well-established network of midwifes or TBAs with the established hospitals. Doctors and TBAs must have very good working relationship to work in partnership. The opposition from Medical staff (doctors, nurses, and midwives) is always a big barrier to implement TBA's training and referral network. But if there are a few people who could listen to the cultural and economic needs of the population, things do change. Provision of FREE ambulances is another factor, which may be difficult but not impossible so that high-risk deliveries could be refereed to hospitals or well equipped Gyn and Obs centers without wasting time and also considering that the family may be too poor to afford the ambulance. While discussing obstetrics problems we also should not forget the social, societal and hidden causes of poor health of women in these countries. Unless we address these issues the idea to improve health of women in developing country is quite far fetched. Until the society understand the importance of women health it may be a difficult issue to allocate resources for women health in economies, which are already dying under the burden of heavy debts, corrupt or puppet rulers and waging civil wars. Unless health officials or policy-makers can project these deficiencies or weaknesses in a dramatic way it may be very difficult to have the attention of power full sections of the society to this issue. We have to emphasize that women's status is pivotal towards a sustainable development for the future. Targeted programs are needed to improve nutrition, health, literacy and employment prospects of women.

The cultural status of women plays an important role in depriving her otherwise accessible healthcare. Then there are social and religious beliefs that may complicate the situation more. At some places in South Asia women are discouraged to go outside home (thus deprived of medical supervision) in pregnancy and postpartum. In Africa practices of female circumcision and infibulation must be stopped to decrease high maternal mortality. The easy accessibility to contraceptive methods (may be with the help of TBAs) could easily reduce the high maternal mortality and Obstetric complications by reducing the risk associated with pregnancy and childbirth.

When to go home after delivery?

Look for the following:

1. Mother

1. Afebrile
2. No evidence of chorioamnionitis
3. *Blood loss < 700 cc
4. *Labor < 24 hours
5. Blood pressure stable
6. Fundus firm
7. Absence of tenderness in calves
8. Lochia—saturating < 1 pad/2 hours
9. Voiding without difficulty
10. Ambulating without assistance
11. RH status determined and RhoGam given, if appropriate
12. If necessary, hepatitis status determined and the patient is available for follow-up
13. Rubella status determined and rubella immunization repeated, if appropriate
14. Hemoglobin checked
15. Evidence that pre-eclampsia is resolving, if present
16. Pain control is adequate to allow mother to care for baby

2. Infant

1. *Apgar 7 or greater at 5 minutes
2. *Gestational age 37-42 weeks
3. *Birth weight 6 lbs-9 lbs. 5 oz (2700-4300 grams)
4. Vital signs:
    1. temp. 98.6-100.4 F (rectally or equivalent)
    2. heart rate 90-150
    3. respiratory rate 30-60
5. Must have voided prior to discharge
6. Must have had a bowel movement prior to discharge
7. Sucking and feeding must have observed ability to suck and swallow prior to discharge
8. *Physical examination normal
9. Blood tests:
    1. Metabolic screening per state law, metabolic screening must be done prior to the fifth day after birth. If done prior to 24 hours after birth, the parents or legal guardian must be notified of the need to have it retested before the 14th day after birth.
    2. Baby's blood type determined and noted on the cord blood sample
10. Circumcision (may be performed after discharge, if wanted)
11. Baby discharge weight appropriate
12. Safe environment for the baby

3. Psycho-Social

1. Support system:
    1. transportation must be available
    2. a responsible party is available to assist the mother in an emergency
    3. basic physical supplies for the infant must be present
    4. housing with heat and sanitation facilities
    5. an emergency plan is in place if a phone is not available
2. Relationship between mother and infant:
    1. absence of hostile/negative comments toward the infant
    2. mother holds baby face-to-face
    3. interaction between the mother and baby is present
3. Under these circumstances mothers and babies may require in-patient days in excess of those indicated by medical criteria. While additional in-patient days do not change these circumstances, they may be necessary to make special arrangements:
    1. Prenatal care not initiated by 28 weeks gestation or characterized by frequent missed appointments
    2. Presence of the following:
        1. history of severe postpartum or other depression (consider when the depression was not previously addressed with counseling, etc.)
        2. current medical illness
        3. battering during this pregnancy
        4. drug and/or substance abuse during the pregnancy
        3. Patient is younger than 16 years
4. Depression affect.

3

Abortions and Miscarriages

Through history, women have practised different forms of birth controls and abortions. These practices have generated intense moral, ethical, political and legal debates, since abortion is not merely a techno-medical issue but "the fulcrum of a much broader ideological struggle in which the very meaning of the family, the state, motherhood and women's sexuality are contested" (Petchesky, R.P., 1986). Women have overtly or covertly resorted to abortions, but their access to services has been countered by the imposition of social and legal restrictions, many of which have origin in morality and religion. The norms governing the ethics of abortion have been constantly remoulded to suit the times and the social contexts in which these are set. Despite the dissimilarities in their construct, intent and orientation, these norms have invariably been directed to the fulfilment of social needs that do not recognise women's right to determine their sexuality, fertility and reproduction. Even the latest MTP (Medical Termination of Pregnancy) Act, 1971 does not give any freedom to women themselves to seek the end of a pregnancy, that is not required by her, it leaves the decision in the hands of the doctor, who will decide, 'weather or not to administer' the treatment. Thus, the womens' hands have always been tied in the matter of their sexuality or reproduction. Similaly, the PNDT Act that prohibits women to go for sex-determination of it's unborn baby, with the intention of planning her family as per her need or that of her family is also oppressive. This denies her the right to choose the gender of her next child, and thus in the process she is made the beast of burden for carrying repeated pregnancies and delivering female babies one after the other, in the quest for a son—no doubt the society and family demands a son from her. Else, she may be rejected in the house or expelled from her own house or done to death, as borne out by a news item in *The Tribune*, Chandigarh, dated Oct. 12, 2004.

On the other hand, the term "miscarriage" means, the spontaneous termination of a pregnancy before fetal development has reached 20 weeks.

Doctor is the master

Let us review the abortion scenario with reference to India. A brief historical account of the role of the medical profession in criminalising and decriminalising abortion services is followed by a discussion on the politics of abortion in India. The early abortionists in Europe were lay women healers, who practised "medicine" among the peasantry. When the male dominated profession of medicine emerged as a formidable force in the mid-nineteenth century, its doctors went about the task of weakening competition from all 'non-professional' doctors, a majority of whom were women and providers of abortion services. The first organised attack on abortion was thus spearheaded by doctors. The Hippocratic Oath which provides the foundation of medical ethics, prohibits physicians from conducting abortions (MacKinney, L., 1952). It was to this Oath that the medical profession reverted for its rationale on the question of abortion. In its 1859 convention, the American Medical Association (AMA) declared that the practice of abortion should be outlawed. This was followed a decade later by the Church, when in 1869, the Apostolic sedis Pius IX pronounced that abortion was a transgression of the faith and a ground for ex-communication (Hurst, 1991). Thus, by the 1870s, the medical profession and the Church had joined forces in criminalising abortion and succeeded in prohibiting its practise. Accordingly, the induced abortion was allowed only for therapeutic purpose of saving the life of pregnant woman. This decree remained in force for a century, till 1973, when the Supreme Court of U.S.A. initiated the process of liberalisation through its ruling on the Roe *vs.* Wade case. Earlier in the UK, the Abortion Act of 1967 liberalised abortion services up to 28 weeks of pregnancy. British Medical Association (BMA), issued that "the doctor should recommend or perform termination after 20 weeks only if she is convinced that the health of the woman is seriously threatened or if there is good reason to believe that the child will be seriously handicapped" (BMA, 1988: 80). As the process of liberalisation of the law on abortion spread across various countries, international medical organisations were compelled to make their positions clear. Thus, the Declaration of Oslo issued by the World Medical Association in 1970 conceded to the need to provide abortion services. The document stated: "where the law allows therapeutic abortion to be performed, the procedure should be performed by a physician competent to do so in the premises approved by the appropriate authority."

During the era of criminalisation, "therapeutic" abortions were conducted to save the life of the pregnant woman or to prevent maternal mortality. During the era of liberalisation, however, this definition is widened to include potential or expected medical or psychological morbidity and this is articulated in the form of a number of legal conditions. The concept of the risk to women's life is thus broadened and by treating induced abortion as a "therapeutic" intervention, the medical profession is in a position to accommodate induced abortion in its ethical system with few problems while maintaining its monopoly over the process. Liberalisation of this kind does not empower women with a fundamental right to seek abortion, but merely liberalises their access to services at the hands of medical doctors. This helps the social relations within a patriarchal system to remain unchallenged and intact.

Politics of Abortion in India

In India, abortions were prohibited (unless medically indicated) till the Medical Termination of Pregnancy (MTP) Act was passed. The demand for a liberalised law did not originate from the women's movement, which suffered the absence of a strong feminist current until the early 1970s. The result was that the movement of the time was focussed on the subversion of criminal law without an independent charter of political demands. The challenge of persuading policy-makers was taken on instead by demographers and doctors who were, in turn, directed by their professional interests and ideologies. While proponents of family planning and population control favoured liberalisation with a view to lowering the birth rate, the medical profession was concerned about the adverse effects that abortions (conducted under unhygienic conditions by non-qualified, untrained and ill-equipped providers) could have on the health of women.

With the growing emphasis on family planning in the health agenda in the 1960s, academicians interested in population control were prompted to draw a link between liberalisation and population control. In this context, themes such as liberalisation *vis-a-vis* its birth control potential as well as the possible implications of liberalisation on the social and cultural fabric began to appear. Many scholars also calculated how many abortions were required to save a birth. In the mid-1960s, the Government of India appointed a committee under the chairmanship of a medical professional, Dr. Shantilal Shah. A report was submitted on December 30, 1966 and in 1971, the Medical Termination of Pregnancy (MTP) Act was passed by parliament.

Clearly, the MTP Act does NOT ENCOMPASS A FUNDAMENTAL RIGHT to induced abortion, but is limited to the liberalisation of the conditions under which women may have access to abortion services provided by approved medical doctors. Medical liberalisation, therefore, necessitates medicalisation of the liberalised conditions given in the Act. This is done by expanding the earlier medical indication of saving a pregnant woman to include medical and psychological morbidity or the potential of such morbidity if the woman is forced to carry an unwanted pregnancy to full term. Thus from the medical angle, the termination of a pregnancy becomes a "therapeutic" intervention rather than a right. The liberalised law confers a position of predominance on medical doctors, who mediate women's access to abortion services—pregnancies cannot be terminated in approved centres unless they are authorised by doctors. The two considerations that are brought into play are the length and type of pregnancy. According to the Act, the termination of pregnancies up to 12 weeks can be authorised by one doctor while those between 12 to 20 weeks necessitate the opinions of two doctors. The Act also enjoins upon the doctors to take cognisance of the "actual or reasonable foreseeable environment" that run the risk of injuring the pregnant woman's health. In this connection, a pregnancy following rape (marital rape not included) or failure of contraception (for married women) are mentioned as specific indicators in two separate explanatory notes. The other health conditions visualised are "physical or mental abnormalities" that might "seriously handicap" the unborn child.

The current pre-occupation with population control and the dubious motivations of the medical profession have, ironically, lent a liberal interpretation of the law. However, the Act requires that abortion be induced legally only by a registered Medical Doctor "who has such experience or training in gynaecology and obstetrics" and conducted only at a place that is sanctioned by the appropriate authority (if the facilities available follow the standards prescribed in the Rules of the Act). This stipulation is essential and laudable. However, a liberalised law has little meaning for the many women who wish to terminate their pregnancies in the absence of well developed network of abortion facilities. In many situations, when women approach with their request for MTP, due to their inability to bring up the ensuing child, the govenment doctors put them off, by lame excuses. Thus, the MTP Act fails to regard the right to access as a justiciable right and is, therefore, ineffectual in curbing the incidence of illegal abortions.

The issue of abortion and its liberalisation has failed to become an integral component of the agenda of the women's movement, even as the feminist current has gained in strength in the last decade. Perhaps this has happened because of the non-combative stand of anti-abortion votaries. This is not the case in many countries where the movement is pitted against powerful anti-abortion and anti-contraceptive movements which are systematically backed up by orthodoxy and political forces. In some of these countries, abortions are still criminalised. The case of the pregnant 14 year old in Ireland in the not-so-distant past, who set-off massive people's protest (resulting into an over-rule of the legal order) when she was legally prohibited from undergoing abortion in her country (and abroad as well) and the recent killings of few of the medical persons providing abortions services in the U.S. highlight the context in which priorities of the movement are shaped. As a result, abortion and contraception have become important programmatic components of the struggle of feminists.

Restricted access

The fact that behind the seemingly liberal availability of abortion services lies legislation that could be easily invoked to restrict access, is perhaps also not fully appreciated. For the law does not endorse women's legal right to demand abortion but ends up being a regulatory mechanism of doctors and abortion centres. In developed countries, which have liberal laws as well, the gains of the women's movement have been transient. For instance, the 1973 US Supreme Court decision on abortion in the Roe *vs.* Wade case made abortion legally available to women but the subsequent decision in 1989 with the Webster case signalled a retreat from Roe.

However, abortion is not merely an issue of the political and legal rights of women but of their reproductive rights as well. This includes the right to have as well as not to have children. The issue of abortion thus needs to be embedded in the context of women's reproductive needs, sexuality, emotions, health status and, above all, their immediate familial, social, economic, occupational and cultural environment. Abortion is recognised as a traumatic experience for women both physically and psychologically. In fact, socio-psychological support for women undergoing abortion is now considered to be an integral aspect of abortion services in developed countries. Unfortunately, in India, these factors are not properly recognized and the tendency is to adopt a 'conveyer belt' approach to abortion services and research. Thus, women are 'powerless' in the matter of either choosing the gender of the unborn or decision to have or not to have a child.

The Abortion Scenario

A review of the distribution of healthcare services in India brings to light the dominance of the private sector and its urban concentration. This picture is borne out by the skewed distribution of institutions providing healthcare in general. In 1992, rural areas were provided with healthcare services by a network of 22,441 primary health centres (PHCs), which covered an average population of 28,009. Most of these do not have facilities for indoor medical care while some of them have facilities for sterilisation operations and wards for post-operative sterilisation cases. With only 22,013 doctors employed in all these PHCs, there was less than one doctor per PHC! For the same period, there were 11,174 hospitals and 6,42,103 hospital beds, defining a ratio of one hospital for 75,739 persons and one hospital bed for 1,318 persons. However, only 32% of the hospitals (with a ratio of one hospital for 1,76,163 persons) and 19.7% of the hospital beds (with a ratio of one hospital bed for 4,970 persons) were located in rural areas. The public health services are plagued by inadequate facilities and infrastructure, misplaced priorities, inadequate and irrationally utilised finances. An evaluation of the quality of family welfare services provided by 298 PHCs in 199 districts in 18 states and one union territory revealed that only 12% of the PHCs (mostly in Maharashtra), fulfilled the required population coverage norm of 30,000. The study observed a substantial shortage of Auxiliary Nurse Midwives (ANMs), unavailability of oxygen (in approximately 40% of the PHCs) and supportive drugs in emergencies (in 30% of PHCs), inadequate stocks of antibiotics (in 60% of the PHCs), a total absence of records (in one-third of the PHCs) and an absence of a labour room and an operation theatre (in one-fourth to one-fifth of the PHCs). Wherever they existed, they were poorly equipped and managed. What is interesting is that a majority of the PHCs were lacking in functional equipment and/or trained manpower to carry out pregnancy termination even after two decades of the Act (ICMR, 1991).

Dwindling Public health expenditure is a matter of concern

On the other hand, the flourishing private sector, which is founded on the principle of profit-making, is characterised by irrational (often unnecessary) diagnostic, medical and surgical practices, inadequate equipment and facilities, and unstandardised charging practises (Nandraj, S., 1994). Micro-studies on expenditure on healthcare show that the per capita expenditure on healthcare (which is mostly obtained from the private sector) accounts for a substantial proportion of the total consumption expenditure per family. Therefore, access to private health services is restricted by high costs. The private health sector is an unregulated sector, matched by stories in the local press of medical malpractice and negligence.

MTP services are offered in India through a network of institutions in rural and urban areas, in the public and private sectors. The approved centres include teaching hospitals, district hospitals, rural hospitals, Community Health Centres (CHCs), Primary Health Centres (PHCs), as well as privately-run hospitals and nursing homes in urban and rural areas. Information about its distribution between rural and urban areas, between the public and private sectors is not routinely published by the government. However, studies occasionally include databases on the facilities for abortions in a state or in a selected sample. A study analysing data of 46,858 MTPs in Maharashtra over a three year period (1972 to 1975) showed that 93% of the MTPs were conducted in urban areas. 71% of the approved MTP centres in Maharashtra were in the private sector. Nearly half the registered doctors (i.e. 47.2%) and institutions (i.e. 45%) were based in Bombay alone (Rao, V.N. and Pense, G.A., 1975). Another study covering 88 CHCs/PHCs and 55 private clinics in 11 districts of Gujarat showed that 58.7% of the 816 approved abortion centres in Gujarat were run by an essentially private-for-profit non-governmental sector (Barge, S. *et. al.*, 1994). Unpublished data for the state of Maharashtra showed that in 1992-93, 70.3% of all approved centres were in the private sector. However, not all approved centres in the public health services perform MTPs.

In absolute terms, having over six thousand approved institutions and over half a million MTPs may appear to be high but the distributions are highly skewed between states and in the context of utilisation patterns. Three states, viz. Uttar Pradesh, Maharashtra and Tamil Nadu, constituting 32.3% of India's population accounted for 47.7% of the total number of MTPs and 35.6% of the approved institutions. This is compounded by the overwhelmingly urban location of approved institution in all States. Maharashtra having only 9.3% of country's population alone had 22.8% of all institutions in that year. There was one approved institution for 1,22,260 people in 1990-91. The state-wise distribution of approved MTP institutions was relatively good in Maharashtra (one for 50,568) but the worst in Uttar Pradesh (one for 3,27,323), which also accounted for the second highest number of MTPs (17.8%). Three leading states, Maharashtra, UP and Tamil Nadu with little less than one-third of country's population accounted for 45.1% of all legal abortions done since 1972 and 47.7% of them in 1990-91

Legal v. Illegal

Shantilal Shah Committee report, calculated a figure of 3.9 million induced abortions, all of which were illegal, since they preceded legalisation. Another estimate puts the figure as 4 to 6 million (Goyal, R.S., 1978). A multi-centre study conducted between 1983 and 1985 in five States—UP, Rajasthan, Orissa, Haryana and Tamil Nadu—concluded that there were 2.2 illegal abortions per every legal abortion (ICMR, 1989). The latest estimate contends a rate of 3 illegal abortions to one legal abortion in rural areas and a corresponding ratio of 4-5:1 in urban areas (Karkal, M., 1991). We feel that these rates are underestimations. Rough estimates give us a ratio of 8 illegal abortions for one legal abortion. The main reasons for seeking illegal abortions are found to be due to financial strain, poverty and social factors like an unmarried, widowed or separated marital status (Phillips, F.S. and Ghouse, N., 1976). There are two other important studies on the medical consequences of induced (legal and illegal) abortions by the ICMR. The first was conducted in 1981, "Short-term Sequelae of Induced Abortion", and the second, in 1982, was titled, "Septic Abortion." Phillips and Ghouse (1976) found that twigs of Calatropis gigantice was most commonly used by unauthorised providers of abortion services. In their study "Criminal Abortion in Western India", Bhatt and Soni (1973) had found that the introduction of a vegetable stick was the most common practice. Most of the studies conducted before 1980 have found that, at the village level, induced abortion services are predominantly provided by traditional birth attendants, most of whom are illiterate women. A dismaying finding for members of the study team was that women in PHC villages were almost totally unaware about the availability of MTP services at the PHC. The Task Force discovered that ANMs and Lady Health Visitors, who are not authorised to do MTPs, used government and PHC facilities for conducting illegal abortions in connivance with doctors and thus making illegal abortions more rampant. Interestingly, the study revealed that women were aware of different types of unauthorised induced abortion even beyond a four month gestation period. Even when women went to government and PHC doctors they were made to pay fees for services rendered. Above all, the study found that a majority of abortions are still conducted using indigenous methods. Further, it found that amongst literate and unauthorised providers, the proportion of males was significantly high. The providers of illegal abortions are not only indigenous doctors but also qualified doctors who may not have registered themselves for providing MTP services. Similarly, the place where illegal abortions are carried out are not only the homes and clinics of the indigenous and non-qualified doctors, but also well equipped hospitals and nursing homes, which are not registered under the Act. Therefore, all institutions properly registered under the MTP Act are not necessarily hygienic nor are all unregistered centres unhygienic.

For a liberalised law to be effective in providing free, safe and humane abortions on demand, it needs to be accompanied by other social inputs like greater empowerment of women especially in their control over their bodies and their sexuality. In situations where women have relatively better control in decision-making and access to contraception (for example, countries in Eastern Europe, which provide extensive and reliable data) liberalisation is accompanied first by a rising trend in the incidence of induced abortions, which stabilises after a point and finally declines once women improve their skills in avoiding unwanted pregnancies. This has not happened in India.

Secondly, a civil right to abortion does not amount to a social right, which is accompanied by all the necessary enabling conditions that makes it concretely realisable and universally available. Further, a really safe abortion is possible only by embedding abortion services in a full range of social services—healthcare, pre-natal care, safe child birth, child care, safe and reliable contraception, sex education, protection from sexual and sterilisation abuse, etc. These social services must function under the organised vigilance of women's groups to ensure that women do really get access to such services.

Issues of induced abortion

Legal and safe abortion is still far from the reach of many people. Here is a *sadhu* who preaches religion and spiritualism, propagates morals amongst his followers, and is expected to abstain from sex, however, finds it difficult to control his passion and eventually rapes a 13-year old girl in rural Madhya Pradesh. Furthermore, to terminate the pregnancy, another *sadhu* gave crude medicine to the victim that caused damage to her eyesight. She gave birth to a still baby. Where do we go from here?

Although three decades have passed, since the MTP Act was passed, no change is seen even in the basic approach that is largely directed towards achieving the demographic goals, irrespective of the fact that India is a signatory to the Programme of Action adopted in ICDP, 1994. Unlike other health information, getting accurate information on abortion is a bit challenging, particularly in Asian countries. From the best available data, we find that in many countries including India, about 15 per cent of the maternal deaths are abortion-related, excluding spontaneous. WHO says 25 per cent of the pregnancies end in abortion world-wide. Researchers' view legal and illegal abortions in India differently, which varies from three to eight illegal abortions against one legal abortion. A recent nation-wide study, Abortion Assessment Project-India (AAP-I), by CEHAT and Health Watch finds that only 15 per cent of the abortions are conducted in the defined framework of MTP Act as far as the reason for seeking abortion is concerned. It also reflects that 73 per cent of abortions are conducted for pregnancies with less than 12 weeks gestation. It's noteworthy that for avoiding the opinion of more than one qualified doctor, in case of pregnancies of more than twelve weeks duration, some pregnancies could be reported wrongly as 1st trimester ones. Likewise, there could be some false reporting in other aspects just to match with the law. It's bit sad to learn from the AAP-I findings that the average cost of abortion in private sector is 7.5 times higher than the public sector.

MTP Act is Inadequate

Even though abortion has been liberalised in India, the act gives an upper hand to the providers than the abortion-seekers in taking a decision. Likewise, the act also leaves scope for unnecessary delays in case of 2nd trimester abortions as the opinion or consent of second doctor has to be obtained. The unfortunate thing under the present law is that it creates hurdles for qualified doctors of private sector to conduct legal-abortion, like their government counterparts, as there are different criteria to be fulfilled for getting the private abortion centres registered. Hence, there is an immediate need to simplify the registration requirements for private sector that controls 87 per cent of the abortion market; since only 24 per cent of abortions in private sector are certified and legal. Furthermore, the provision of obtaining the guardian's consent for women under 18 years looks like an undesirable chore. However, if one were to look at this provision in connection with the minimum age of marriage, then a lot of questions can be raised. Very few people know that abortion has been legalised, so, the punishments for clandestine abortions may be revised suitably by taking into account the interests of people living in rural and tribal areas. Besides many factors such as national and state level policies on population too contribute towards the sex preference of new-borns, thereby resulting in sex-selective abortions despite the fact that most pregnant women have no-say over it.

In the present context, safe abortions should get top priority that would not only reduce abortion-related morbidity and mortality but also save a great deal of expenditure at different levels. Good medical procedures during the termination of pregnancy as well as quality post-abortion care must be the thrust areas of abortion for public health considerations. Doctors of private sector should have access to similar training programmes like their counterparts in government service. It's bit astonishing to learn from AAP-I that dilatation and curettage (D&C) seems to be the preferred method for nearly 89 per cent of abortions, even among the user of vacuum aspiration the practice of check curettage is common. Urgent action is needed for a complete shift towards vacuum aspiration that is not only less painful but could also help save abortion-related expenses in health sector. Furthermore, the availability and usage of emergency contraceptives should also be encouraged. Although it's a fact that unwanted pregnancies cannot be prevented absolutely, the problem of unmet needs should be properly addressed with the help of contraceptives such as basket-of-choice. Safe abortion should be accessible, available and affordable to every woman in India, irrespective of the place of living and socio-economic condition.

There is also a strong need to train and legally authorise the staff nurses and ANMs to conduct abortions, which would not only reduce dependency upon the doctors of modern medicine, but could also drastically decrease unsafe abortions by quacks. Adequate efforts should be made to enhance public awareness on abortion laws, social-acceptability as well as to mitigate irrelevant perceptions and judgmental attitudes among the providers. The government should no longer look at abortion as a family planning device and must take radical steps to promote reproductive health in the country in line with ICPD declarations. In a multicultural India of 21st century there is hardly any need for policy-makers to be bothered by the conservative attitudes and waste time in debates like whether abortion can be considered as a murder. So, what's wrong if a woman who wants to abort her own pregnancy can get it on request? Likewise, the provision of obtaining mandatory consent in case of under 18 normal women should be revoked, as seeking abortion is purely a woman's right.

Lopsided Approach

In case of spontaneous-abortion, eligible women get benefits like leave and health insurance, why not similar facilities be available for every kind of abortion. A lot of research needs to be done from abortion-seeker's point of view so as to equip us to handle issues like stigma, trauma, emotional security, true-consent, etc. Measures of confidentiality and privacy, particularly in public institutions, must be further strengthened and every abortion-seeker should feel that her dignity is not being taken for granted.

If 676 fully-occupied Airbus 320s crashed every year, killing all passengers on board, that figure—130,000—equals the number of women in India who die every year from complications related to pregnancy, abortion and childbirth. Almost all these deaths can be prevented.

Contributing factors

The underlying causes for maternal mortality are poor health and nutrition, lack of physical access to healthcare (including transportation and finances), medical causes and socio-cultural factors that obstruct and underplay the importance of healthcare for women.

Unsafe Abortions and Maternal Deaths

Worldwide, unsafe abortions contribute to nearly 15 percent of all maternal deaths. Nearly 7 million abortions take place in India annually. For each legal abortion, there are at least 10 illegal induced abortions. Prevention and management of unsafe abortions are essential interventions for safe motherhood. Lack of support from men and other members of the family leads to poor utilization of prenatal, natal and postnatal services by pregnant women. Several studies and reports indicate that men do not pay much attention to the health problems of women. Only 52% of women are involved in decision-making on their own healthcare. One in every four adult women in Asian countries suffers long or short-term illness due to pregnancy and childbirth. For each woman who dies, at least 30 develop chronic debilitating conditions. Between 58-80 percent of pregnant women in Asian countries develop acute health problems, and 8-29 percent develop chronic health problems because of pregnancy. Women lose more disability-adjusted life years, 28 million, to maternal causes in Asian countries than to any other cause. DALYs refer to the number of productive life-years lost due to premature death and disability. When a woman dies, there are significant social and economic losses; families lose her contribution to household management, and provision of care for children and other family members. The economy loses her contribution; and communities lose a vital member whose unpaid labor is often central to community life. Children who lose their mothers suffer the most. One study estimates that in some Asian countries, the risk of death for children under five years doubles or triples if the mother dies. Other studies estimate that children whose mother

Pregnancy-related deaths are preventable

* Every minute, one woman somewhere in the world dies from a complication related to pregnancy or childbirth. This is almost 600,000 women a year, worldwide. Ninety-nine percent of these deaths occur in Asian countries. In India, one woman dies every five minutes from a pregnancy-related cause.

For every three deaths of women in their reproductive years in some Asian countries, one is the result of complications from pregnancy and childbirth. 15 percent of deaths of women in the reproductive age in India are maternal deaths.

Complications related to pregnancy, childbirth and complications arising out of unsafe abortion are leading causes of death in adolescent girls. In India, 50 percent of maternal deaths of girls in the 15-19 years age group are due to unsafe complications arising out of unsafe abortion.

Maternal mortality is not just a health issue; it is a human rights issue.

Several international conventions including the Commission for the Elimination of All Forms of Discrimination Against Women (CEDAW), the International Conference on Population and Development, and the Beijing conference on women have emphasized women's rights to a healthy and safe pregnancy and childbirth.

Maternal mortality is the one public health indicator showing the maximum variation between developed and Asian countries. In developed countries, the maternal mortality ratio (MMR) is 27 per 100,000 live births as compared to 480 in Asian countries. India has an MMR of 540 deaths per 100,000 live births.

The goal of the Programme of Action of the International Conference on Population and Development (ICPD), 1994, is to reduce MMRs in countries with high maternal mortality ratio to 120 per 100,000 live births by 2005 and under 75 by 2015. That goal will not be met.

Every pregnancy, anywhere in the world, faces risk. An estimated 15 percent of all pregnant women develop life-threatening complications.

Women in Asian countries have a 40 times greater risk of dying from pregnancy-related complications and childbirth than those in developed countries. A woman's lifetime risk of dying from pregnancy-related complications or during childbirth is one in 48 in Asian countries; that figure in one in 1800 in developed countries.

have died are 3 to 10 times more likely to die within two years than those who have both parents alive. Motherless children are likely to get less healthcare and education as they grow up. Girls, in particular, suffer because they are forced to drop-out of school to look after younger siblings.

Interventions

Maternal Death is an Avoidable Tragedy. It can be prevented if the women have access to basic and emergency medical care during pregnancy, childbirth and the postpartum period.

Creating positive social environment

It is important to educate families and communities on care for pregnant women, teach them to recognize danger signs during pregnancy, ensure that they make arrangements for finances and transportation, and identify health facilities with essential obstetric care in case of an emergency. These arrangements must be made well in advance. In most Indian households, husbands and mother's-in-law are essential decision-makers. Without their awareness and active participation in ensuring appropriate care for the pregnant woman, the best of health services will be ineffective. Empower women, enhance their decision-making abilities and increase their choices and use of healthcare services. This is critical to ensuring Safe Motherhood.

** These contribute to the Four Delays:

Delay in identifying a complication; delay in making a decision to seek treatment; delay in getting the woman to the healthcare center; delay in receiving quality treatment.

Inadequate nutrition is a significant factor contributing to maternal deaths. In India, the average weight gain of pregnant women is just 7 kg compared to almost 9 kg in Thailand and Philippines and 12 kg in the developed countries. One rural study in Gujarat and Maharashtra found that 90 percent of pregnant women were anemic by WHO standards.

Over 80 percent of maternal deaths in India, as elsewhere in the world, are due to six medical causes: hemorrhage, eclampsia, obstructed labor, sepsis, complications arising due to unsafe abortion and pre-existing conditions such as anemia and malaria. All of these can be treated in a hospital or First Referral Unit that has emergency facilities for obstetric care and skilled medical personnel.

Only 60 percent of rural women and 86 percent of urban pregnant women in India receive antenatal check-ups. Among women who gave birth in the last three years, 67 percent received two doses of TT vaccines, 48 percent received 100 Iron Folic Acid (IFA) tablets and 44 percent received a minimum of three check-ups during the period of pregnancy.

Lack of access and inadequate utilization of healthcare, especially essential or emergency obstetric care (EOC) services is an essential cause of maternal deaths. In India, only 34 percent of deliveries take place in health facilities. In rural areas, three out of four births take place at home.

Absence of trained personnel at delivery is another factor contributing to maternal deaths and complications. Skilled personnel attend only 42 percent of deliveries in India. In some districts, that figure drops to 5-10 percent.

Sixty percent of all maternal deaths occur after delivery; yet, less than 17 percent of women in India receive any postpartum care.

Causes of abortions

1. *Infection*: Viral infections such as rubella, cytomegalic virus, hepatitis virus causes death and expulsion of the foetus. Parasitic infections like malaria and protozoal infections like Toxoplasmosi may produce abortion in early pregnancy. Abortion may be precipitated by high fever.
2. Respiratory disease, heart failure, severe anemia, severe gastroenteritis are other important factors causing abortion.
3. Chronic illness like high blood pressure, chronic kidney diseases and other long standing wasting diseases can lead to abortion.
4. Endocrine factors—An increase association of abortion is found in thyroid disorders and diabetes mellitus.
5. Trauma—Direct trauma on the abdominal wall by bow or fall or other operative trauma may be related to abortion.
6. Congenital malformation of the uterus, cervical incompetence, uterine tumour or fibroid, retroverted uterus are common causes of recurrent abortion.
7. Blood group incompatibility—ABO and Rh incompatibility show a higher incidence of abortion.
8. Premature rupture of the membranes leads to abortion.
9. Some deficiency disorders like folic acid or Vitamin E deficiency may lead to abortion.
10. Defective sperms, which contribute half of the number of chromosomes to the ovum may result in abortion.
11. In many cases the cause can not be traced.

Threatened Abortion

Here the process of abortion has started but has not progressed to a state from which recovery is impossible. The pregnant woman complaint of bleeding from vagina and pain following haemorrhage. A blood investigations like haemoglobin investigations, ABO grouping and Rh typing is done ultra sonogrophy is an important investigation to identify the presence or absence of a normal conceptus.

Bed rest is advised to the patient. For sedation and relief of pain, drugs are prescribed. The patient should limit her activities and avoid heavy work and excitement. Coitus is contraindicated during this period. The patient should report the doctor if bleeding or pain becomes aggravated.

Inevitable Abortion

Here the abortion has progressed to a state from where continuation of pregnancy is impossible. The patient complains of increased vaginal bleeding and aggravation of the pain in lower abdomen. The general condition of the patient is proportionate to the visible blood loss. The process of expulsion is accelerated. If abortion occur before 12 weeks of pregnancy. Suction, evacuation and curettage is done. After 12 weeks of pregnancy the uterine contractions are accelerated by oxytocin drip which leads to expulsion of the abortus.

Missed Abortion

When the foetus is dead and retained inside the uterus for more than four weeks it is called missed abortion. After 12 weeks the retained foetus becomes macerated or mummified. The liquor gets absorbed and the placenta becomes pale, this and may get adherent. There is vaginal bleeding followed by persistent brownish vaginal discharge. The symptoms of pregnancy subside. There is retrogression of breast changes. Uterine growth stops which in fact becomes smaller in size.

Routine blood and urine investigation are done. Ultrasonography is an important investigation in diagnosing missed abortion. Vaginal evaluation is done under anaesthesia if uterus is less than 12 weeks. If uterus is more than 12 weeks induction is done either by oxytocin or prostaglandins.

Septic Abortion

Abortion that is associated with evidence of infection of the uterus and its contents is called septic abortion. About 10% of abortion requiring admission to hospitals are septic. In majority of these cases, the infection occurs following illegal induced abortion but can also occur after

*** Interventions to prevent maternal deaths do work! Sri Lanka, for example, reduced its maternal mortality from 555 deaths per 100,000 live births in the 1950s to 240 in 1960s to 30 in 1994. This was due to a nationwide extension of the healthcare system and expansion of midwifery skills. There has been a marked increase in the proportion of births attended by trained personnel; in 1996, over 94 percent of live births occurred in local hospitals.

Enhance health and nutrition interventions. These cost as little as $3 per woman in Asian countries. Life-saving essential/emergency obstetric care could cost $ 230. Health and nutrition interventions effectively prevent most maternal deaths; half of all infant deaths and the excruciating disabilities inflicted on millions of women.

Ensure access to healthcare facilities, including licensed blood banks. This is critical, because it is the only way to identify and treat complications that could potentially result in an emergency or death. Over half of rural women live in a village that has no health facility. Four out of 10 women are ten or more kms. from the hospital.

Ensure access to ANC. It is the one opportunity to recognize potential problems that pregnant women may face. Studies in India indicate that 72 percent of maternal deaths can be prevented through ANC; of these, 32 percent with proper referral care.

However, since most obstetric emergencies are not predictable, ANC alone will not prevent maternal deaths. A combination of ANC and emergency obstetric care is essential for reducing maternal mortality.

Delay marriage and first pregnancy, prevent unwanted pregnancies through contraceptive use. Enabling women to choose whether, when and how many children they will have is the most cost-effective intervention for Safe Motherhood.

spontaneous abortion. The following symptoms may be present: Fever of at least 100.40f (380 C) for 24 hours or more. Fever can be associated with chills and rigors. There is lower abdominal pain and tenderness. An offensive, purulent vaginal discharge is present. Blood for haemoglobin estimation, complete blood count and blood grouping is done coagulation profile and serum electrolytes are also done. Cervical swab or high vaginal swab is taken to detect the organism microscopically or by culture. X-ray of abdomen and pehis to detect any foreign body left behind in the uterus or abdomen. Hospitalization of the patient is done. Antibiotics, sedatives and pain killers are given to the patient. Antigasgangrene serum and antitetanus serum are given prophylactically. Blood transfusion is done if required.

Evaluation of the uterus is done following antibiotic therapy, vigorous curettage is avoided. The fluid and electrolyte in balance is corrected. Active surgery is indicated if there is pelvic abcess, injury to the uterus or intestine, presence of foreign body in the abdomen, decreased urinary output not responding to conservative treatment.

Under law abortion means the expulsion of the products of conception at any period of gestation before full term. Abortions are classified as natural and artificial. Natural abortion is one that occurs as a direct result of any interference with the pregnancy. Artificial abortions are either legal or criminal. With the liberal provisions of the medical termination of Pregnancy Act, 1971, legal abortions are now more common and criminal abortions less common.

Recurrent Abortions

What may cause recurrent abortions?

Recurrent trauma

For definition purpose 'Recurrent' word is used when a woman aborts consecutively 3 times, before 20 weeks gestation. It is well known that overall 15% of established pregnancies end in miscarriage. The main cause is a problem with the gene cross-over at the time of conception, nothing can be done to prevent it. If all pregnancies are taken into account it is found that up to 60% of pregnancies end in miscarriage—most would just present as a heavier late period. Luckily most of these ladies who have recurrent miscarriage (RM) will go on to have a successful pregnancy the next time—without any kind of tests or treatment. When a woman is investigated majority of the time, no cause is found.

What can make you prone to miscarriage?

There are several diseases and conditions, which can make you prone to miscarriage (i) Systemic Lupus Erythematosus (SLE), which is disease affecting many systems of the body. People affected often have a butterfly-rash over the cheeks and bridge of the nose, (ii) Antiphospholipid antibody syndrome—an immune disease, (iii) Chromosome problems, an unusual gene mismatch occurs, (iv) Womb abnormality—e.g. double-womb or a septum down the middle, (v) Fibroids, (vi) Cervical weakness—may be the cause if miscarriage occurs in 2nd trimester, (vii) Polycystic ovary syndrome—it causes infertility and when this is present with a raised hormone level (LH) there is an increased risk of miscarriage, (viii) Immune problems, (ix) Hormone 'deficiency', and (x) Sexually transmitted diseases.

What is notorious for miscarriage, may not be actually responsible for abortions, viz. Retroversion, infection (toxoplasmosis, listeria, brucella, Chlamydia, herpes simplex and cytomegalovirus), Endocrine or metabolic diseases (hypothyroidism), diabetes mellitus, Crohn's disease, sickle cell or endometriosis, Occupational exposures-herbicide spraying, electro-magnetic fields, chemical inhalation, anaesthetic gases or VDU usage, not resting enough.

Investigations

An ultrasound scan may indicate the presence of PCOD, or structural womb abnormalities. A hysteroscopy involves a look into the womb cavity with tiny telescope to check for the presence of abnormalities or fibroids not seen on scan. Various other investigations of blood, urine, etc. may be done to establish or rule out several conditions, as mentioned above.

Treatment

Treatment is directed at the cause—e.g. genetic counseling, removal of fibroids, cervical stitch. Progesterone supplements have been tried, but have not been shown to be of any benefit. A few people still use them.

Legal Abortions

Legal abortion, under the medical termination of Pregnancy Act, 1971, is allowed on the following grounds:

Therapeutic

This includes conditions where continuation of pregnancy would involve risk to the life of the pregnant woman, or risk of grave injury to her physical or mental health. Thus the indications for therapeutic abortion are organic heart disease with failure, active tuberculosis, severe diabetes, renal failure severe hypertension, acute hepatitis acute pancreatitis, uterine bleedings, malignancy of breast or genital tract, threatened insanity, toxemia of pregnancy, etc.

Eugenic

This include conditions where there is a substantial risk that the child will be born with physical or mental abnormalities making him seriously handicapped there abortion is permitted only within 20 weeks of pregnancy. The indications are : Serious viral infections contracted in first trimester of pregnancy such as german measles, chicken pox, viral hepatitis, etc. Exposure to X-rays and other radiation, Pregnant woman having taken cytotoxic drugs, thalidomide, LSD, etc. Parents have some inheritable mental condition or chromosomal abnormalities, e.g. thalassemia (after fetal blood sampling and chorionic villus sampling).

Humanitarian

This includes cases of rape, as the anguish caused by such pregnancy is presumed to constitute a grave injury to her mental health.

Social

This includes contraceptive failure, and environmental grounds, which are financial difficulties, heart disease wide no help in domestic work, presence of subnormal child needing considerable attention, etc.

In emergency situations any registered medical doctor can terminate pregnancy at any place, irrespective of the duration of pregnancy, if he is of the opinion in good faith that such termination is immediately necessary to save the pregnant woman's life. When there is no emergency a pregnancy can be terminated on the opinion of one registered medical doctor if duration of pregnancy is less than 12 weeks. In case the duration is between 12 and 20 weeks opinions of two registered medical doctors is necessary. The opinion must be in good faith, the doctor must have training in obstetrics and gynaecology, such doctor must be registered for this purpose and the procedure must be carried out at a place approved by the government. Only the woman's written consent is essential and in case of minor or lunatic, the guardian's written consent is essential.

Emergency Contraception

Unwanted pregnancy, within or without marriage is being seen frequently. There are about 11 million abortions in India every year of which 6.7 million are induced and about four million spontaneous. This indicates a ratio of 10-11 illegal abortions for each legal abortion performed, and all this resulting in 15-20 thousand deaths annually. Contraceptive method failure due to various reasons is a common occurrence and contributes to millions of unintended pregnancies each year. Women who experience unprotected sex for whatever reason including condom rupture or slippage, diaphragm dislodgment, breakage or tearing, failed coitus interruptus, IUD expulsion, miscalculation of the safe period, and even sexual assault are among those who can protect themselves from pregnancy by using emergency contraceptives.

While most contraceptives are intended for use before or during intercourse, emergency contraception is that which a woman can use, within a few hours or days after unprotected intercourse to prevent conception. Otherwise known as post-coital contraceptive or 'morning after pills', these regimens work on the idea that the user can start treatment on the morning after unprotected intercourse. What makes emergency contraception different from other contraceptive methods is its use at post-coital stage rather than before or at the time of coitus. However, as its name suggests, its use is not recommended on a regular basis and it is to be used only during 'emergency' situations, which may lead to unwanted conception. The use of emergency contraception is widely accepted even among those who generally oppose contraceptives. The Vatican, for instance, recently lifted a ban on women's use of emergency contraception in the case of rape, recognising contraception in such circumstances as a legitimate form of self-defence. The magnitude of the youth population in India provides another reason for making emergency contraceptives available. Many young men and women are sexually active and have scant or no access to sexuality education, which can guide them to adopt healthy lifestyles and take responsible decisions; emergency contraceptives can be an option for protection against unpremeditated and therefore unprotected intercourse.

The increasing number of reports of child sexual abuse in India, further justifies the need for greater awareness and delivery of emergency contraceptives to prevent unwanted pregnancy. A study done among school children in Delhi showed that 85 percent of the children had been abused within their families and 25 percent of them were cases of serious sexual violation. Statistics reveal that in India, one woman is raped every 54 minutes. Emergency contraception can continue to be used in the treatment of rape victims.

Why Emergency Oral Contraception?

It mainly stops ovulation (release of egg from ovary) but perhaps also works in other ways. Does NOT disrupt existing pregnancy. It seems to prevent about three-fourths of pregnancies that would otherwise have occurred. (Average chance of pregnancy due to one act of unprotected intercourse in the second or third week of the menstrual cycle is 8%; after emergency oral contraceptive it is 2%). The sooner emergency contraceptions are used, the better they prevent pregnancy. Any woman can use emergency oral contraception if she is not already pregnant. Emergency oral contraception should not be used in place of family planning methods. It should be used only in an emergency—for example:

- A woman has had sex against her will or has been forced to have sex in the wedlock or otherwise (rape).
- A condom has broken.
- An IUD (Cu-T) has come out of place.
- A woman has run out of oral contraceptives.
- Sex took place without contraception, and the women wants to avoid pregnancy.

Up to 72 hours after unprotected sex, the woman should take 4 low-dose pills, e.g., MALA-D, OVRAL-L, or 2 "standard-dose", e.g. OVRAL-G combined oral contraceptives, and then take another equal dose 12 hours later. Side effects like nausea can occur. Eat something soon after taking the pills to reduce any nausea. Anti-nausea medicines can reduce the risk of nausea when taken one half-hour before taking emergency contraceptive pills and every 4 to 6 hours thereafter.

There can be vomiting in some cases. If the woman vomits within 2 hours after taking the pills, she may take another dose. Otherwise, she should NOT take any extra pills. Extra pills will not make the method more effective, and they may increase nausea. The next monthly period may start a few days earlier or later than expected. Reassure her that this is not a bad sign.

However, emergency oral contraception is not as effective as most other contraceptive methods. It should not be used regularly in place of another method.

Reasons to see your doctor immediately: If the next period is quite different from usual, especially if it is: Unusually light (Possible pregnancy), Does not start within 4 weeks (Possible pregnancy), Unusually painful. (Possible ectopic pregnancy. But emergency oral contraception does not cause ectopic pregnancy), Unusual vaginal discharge, pain or burning on urination.

Sex selective abortions : Media hype or serious social problem

Barbara Miller coined the phrase, "The Endangered Sex." Amartya Sen used the phrase, "Missing Women." They were referring to those who are also known simply as "never born Girls." These are examples of some of the sensationalist terminology social scientists and activists have been using to highlight the problem of "female infanticide or female feticide" in India. The neutral term "sex-selective abortion" is simpler to use. Here the objective is to tie together several different opinions, facts, interpretations, and arguments in some sort of a thematic analysis that provides readers with a multi-faceted view of the issue(s).

It all started on October 24, 2002 when *The Hindustan Times* carried an article titled 'Death of an Unborn Girl' written by Arundhati Roy Chaudhury. Citing "the dramatic drop in the sex ratio of the girl child population in the 0-6 age group, from 962 girls per 1,000 boys in 1981 to 945 girls/1,000 boys in 1991, and 927 girls/1,000 boys in 2001" as one of the "disquieting trends" that surfaced in the 2001 census, she asks the question: "Are girls being deliberately eliminated? Is technology (ultrasonography, amniocentesis, chorion villi biopsy, foetoscopy, material serum analysis, etc.) assisting in this systematic elimination?" Her reply: "To a great extent, yes."

The article was enough to spark a passionate discussion on the topic. What exactly is Roy recommending? Clearly, she is not against all abortions, she is opposing only female abortions. More specifically, she is focusing on the relative differences in abortion rates by gender, i.e. abortion is fine as long as it is split 50-50 between males/females. Are all abortions wrong? For anyone to raise a voice against female feticide, does the person have to first take a position against all abortions? Why? Are the reasons for any abortion the same as reasons for selective abortion of a female fetus?

What kind of evidence has been presented to suggest that sex-selective abortion is a problem in India? What does research suggest as possible reasons for the declining sex ratios in India? Should we look at the issue of declining sex ratio in India in a global comparative framework? Should we also study the issue of sex-selective abortions in India within the context of a larger debate on abortions in India and elsewhere? Important issues that emerge from the discussions are:

1. Freedom to make decisions regarding one's reproductive choices: Indian women *vs.* Western women.
2. Familial and social pressures to bear a male child/heir.
3. Personally heard stories or lived experiences: Are these anecdotal evidence enough to consider sex-selective abortion an "Indian problem"?
4. Is girl child considered a liability?: Social and economic reasons.
5. Education and empowerment of women.
6. Role of sex-determination technology: Problem or a solution?

Can one argue that in most research on sex-selective abortion in India, researchers look at gender gap in the census figures, and attribute it to practices such as female infanticide and female feticide? And connections are made without fully examining the evidence. One can understand people like Khanna and few other researchers becoming a victim to the Western academic model where everything derogatory about India sells. But for such a large section of the Indian population who believes that selective abortion does take place—how can one explain their mindset?

Prof. Sunil Khanna, an associate professor of Anthropology at Oregon State University's College of Liberal Arts, has conducted extensive research on female feticide and has worked with an activist group in India that is lobbying the government to address the problem. Even Indian doctors writing in medical journals have admitted that it is a common knowledge that selective abortions of females are taking place. One finds it easier to believe that some people may actually choose not to have girls, if they consider them as more of a liability than boys. And if they are given access to inexpensive technology to help them decide whether or not to have one more girl, they may choose to use the technology to avoid having her.

So while some researchers may have been quick in making a connection between declining female to male ratio in India and son-preference as something specific to Indian culture, at best what we have is a tentative hypothesis: if a gender-gap exists, could it be because of selective abortions? Many researchers, activists, and social critics have concluded: Yes, selective abortion is the cause of gender-gap.

But is it due to the selective killings of the sons in those societies, where number of females is higher than males?

The government hospitals and healthcare centres in Dharmapuri and

Salem districts of Tamil Nadu, sport cradles in their campuses, where women are encouraged to anonymously drop-off unwanted female infants. One researcher observed: "About abortions of female fetuses, I am personally acquainted with two women who aborted their third child after sex determination. They were married to an engineer and chartered accountant respectively. They did their sex determination in Bombay and had the abortions performed in Chennai."

"In Bombay, you can find an abortion clinic in almost every corner. How would these clinics thrive if there were no one sustaining them? My maid-servant in India did abort her girl fetus, because she had 4 other girls and wanted a boy. If most people in our society don't see this as a crime, who is going to report it to the authorities? Most people, educated or uneducated have multiple children (mostly girls) in the hope of a boy. I know of a well-educated family who has 7 girls and then decided to stop because of financial constraints (I hope that their education helped them here!)".

"Our maid, in my hometown, has delivered two daughters. Ever since she delivered the second daughter, her husband and mother-in-law have stopped talking to her. They also ill-treat her at home. He has threatened her that he would marry again. My father had to pressurize an elderly and influential person in her locality to make sure things don't get out of hand. So it's only under pressure, and not willingly, that her husband and family are OK with her, for now." "A well-known regional pattern is observed: the Northern and North-western parts of India, including the states of Punjab, Haryana, Rajasthan and Western UP, are areas most unfavourable to the life chances of female children. Other parts of the country, including the East, Central area and the South, exhibit more balanced rates.

Writing in the journal *Feminist Issues*, Manju Parikh notes: "The most disturbing evidence was presented in a study conducted by a sub-committee of the Federation of Obstetricians' and Gynaecologists' Societies of India. Out of 8,000 cases, the study reported that 7,999 were aborted when the test results showed a female fetus (Ravindra, 1986: 21; *The Statesman*, 17 December 1984). Another survey was done by Professor R.P. Ravindra of the Pharmacy College of the S.N.D.T. University of Bombay. In his research on 1000 cases in Bombay, he could not find a single case of a male fetus being aborted, whereas 97 percent of the fetuses identified as female were aborted (Ravindra, 1986:9)." Finally, "another set of comprehensive results was produced by Sanjeev Kulkarni of the Foundation for Research in Community Health. For his report, titled 'Sex-Determination Tests and Female Foeticide in Greater Bombay', he interviewed fifty gynecologists; 84 percent of them admitted that they were performing sex-determination tests. It was estimated that about 50,000 sex-selective abortions were taking place annually in Bombay by 1987. There were 250 abortion clinics in Bombay alone and 600 in the whole state of Maharashtra (Health Monitor, 1988)."

Is it all India bashing by the West?

Sudha and Rajan provide some more evidence collected through surveys and interviews: "A 1982 study in Ludhiana, an urban area in Punjab state, randomly sampled 126 individuals, of whom approximately half each were male and female and most of whom were educated and middle class. All the respondents had heard of the amniocentesis test; 66 per cent of them thought it was intended for sex determination; few knew that it was actually for detecting foetal abnormalities. While 73 per cent of the women and 59 per cent of the men believed that a girl should be aborted if the couple already had two or more daughters, only 25 per cent of the respondents felt that a boy should be aborted if the couple already had two or more sons. The reasons given indicated the nature of male-dominated society, dowry problems, greater responsibilities in bringing up daughters, and social pressure to bear sons. Over 71 per cent of the respondents felt that amniocentesis as a sex determination test should not be banned (Singh and Jain, 1985).

These results were uncannily echoed over a decade later, in rural Maharashtra state, among six villages of Pune district, three with road and access to a health facility, and three others more remote and without these amenities. Results indicated that 49 out of the 67 women interviewed in-depth were aware of ultrasound and/or amniocentesis techniques and 45 per cent of those who knew approved of aborting female foetuses. Only four women were aware that such tests were actually for the detection of foetal abnormalities (Gupte *et al.*, 1997). The spread of awareness of these techniques to rural areas is thus clearly documented.

Based on an ethnographic research in one Haryana Village, Khanna suggests that the availability of new reproductive technologies provided the Shahar-gaon Jat community with an alternate family building strategy to high fertility and sex-specific child mortality. In his study, he found that couples were maintaining a low fertility rate by using contraceptives and achieving the ideal family composition by exploiting reproductive technologies. He concludes: "These family composition strategies limit family size and the number of daughters in a family in the context of an urbanizing economy dominated by an agricultural ethos and patriarchal ideology."

Sabu M. George, Visiting Senior Fellow, Center for Women's Development Studies, New Delhi, India presents one kind of "litigation" evidence: "In February 2000, I filed a public interest litigation in the Indian SC along with two NGOs, CEHAT in Mumbai and MASUM in Pune, against the Union of India and all the State Governments for the non-implementation of the Prenatal Diagnostic Techniques Act, 1994 (PNDT) and for inclusion of all emerging technologies that can be abused to eliminate girls under the purview of the Act. The case is still under consideration, and it is therefore premature to discuss its overall impact. Nevertheless, there have been significant developments. The interim judgment was delivered on 4 May, 2001, and since August 2001 hearings have taken place almost every month. Following the Court's directives, State Governments have undertaken awareness raising on this issue, and the media have been prominently covering the Court proceedings and the follow-up...

"The putative unequal treatment of women is a constant staple of India bashers whether its "dowry deaths", widow remarriage, sati, bride burning and now the latest "whine and cheese" fad—female foeticide..."Killing female babies" is precisely the type of emotive terminology used by the Moral Majority brigade. "This merely obfuscates the discussion." Thus, any meaningful debate about this issue has to take place beyond the field of usual rhetoric wars. "To discuss sensible and implementable solutions to a social crime, we must first admit to its gravity instead of escaping into the bluster of calling it Eurocentric exaggeration or India bashing."

A quick glance at this should put Indian statistics in a larger context:

Country	*Sex-ratio (males per 100 females)*
United Arab Emirates	195
Bahrain	135
Saudi Arabia	115
Oman	113
Samoa	111
Papua New Guinea	109
Jordan	108
Libyan	108
Afghanistan	107
Bangladesh	106
China	106
India	106
Pakistan	106
Sri Lanka	106
Albania	105
Côte d'Ivoire	105
Nepal	105
Iran	105
New Caledonia	105
Dominican Republic	103
Iraq	103
Malaysia	103
Occupied Palestinian Territory	103
Syrian Arab Republic	103
Algeria	103
Costa Rica	103
Niger	102
Nigeria	102
Panama	102
Paraguay	102
Tunisia	102
Turkey	102
Bhutan	102
Guatemala	102

A fact rarely mentioned in this debate is the biological side—that the secondary sex ratio (defined as sex ratio at birth) in humans is typically around 105 males per 100 females. This means that the Indian and Chinese numbers at 106 males per 100 females are much more normal than those of most other countries. Therefore to simplistically attribute all of the sex ratio gap solely to female feticide is ethically and scientifically wrong. It tells only a very small part of the story.

How much is contributed by the dowry mania?

It has often been pointed out that one of the key motivations for sex-selective abortions in India is the institution of dowry, which makes girls more of an "economic burden" than the boys. "Economically a female child is considered a drain on the family purse" (Ramanamma and Bambawale, 1980, as cited in Grant, 1998). Looking at the UAE sex ratio of 195 males to 100 females, one member questioned that statistic giving the reason that in a society that practices mehr, perhaps girls are more valued. But another member quickly pointed out:

> "We may all be so conditioned to believe that dowry = female abortions that . . . automatically assumed that the mehr system would have the opposite impact, i.e. girls would be more valued. It was therefore a shock for her to see that the very societies where mehr is practiced also have the most atrocious sex ratios against females. . . What do we conclude: Either there is no link with mehr but only with dowry? Or that the link with dowry is incorrect?"

So ultimately these are all personal, emotional decisions. The pain gets enhanced when someone is forced by any reason to make this choice. I also believe that anyone who chooses abortion even as a birth-control measure or as a means to keep her independence or looks will eventually have to come to terms with the emotional pain that is caused by these decisions. But I would still want them to have that choice. After that, it is between them and their conscience. The question I would have regarding sex-selective abortion is this—do these women or their families who choose to abort a fetus because it is female ever feel the same guilt or remorse as they would if they had chosen abortion without knowing the sex of the fetus?

If it is wrong to abort a female fetus because of social and family pressures in India, then it should be just as wrong to abort 'any fetus' for social pressures in the West, i.e. career, maintain looks, retirement funds, lack of family support, pressures of single parenthood, forgot to take pill, pregnancy failed to snare husband, date rape, etc.

What the folk songs tell?

Jo hum janati dhia kokhai janamiha

Peeyati mirchi jahar ho Mirchi ke jhaare jhooredhia mari jayiti
Chhoot jayite garhua santaap ho

(Had I known that the foetus was that of a girl, I would have had a drink of hot chillis and killed not only the foetus but also this lifelong curse.)

Chandra grahanwa beti sanjahi laagela
Suraj grahanwa bhinusaar ho,
Dhia grahanwa beti janam se laagela
Jaane kab ugrin hoyee ho

(The lunar eclipse occurs at night, the solar in the day. Eclipse brought about by the birth of a daughter lasts forever.)

Bahurani ke ho gayee bitiya
Khatiya bahire karo
Sasur sunale ki bitiya bhaili
Sir se utaar de lein pagadiya
Khatiya bahiro karo

(The daughter-in-law has produced a daughter. Throw her cot out of the house. The father-in-law should be informed that a girl has been born in the family so that he can remove his turban.)

Can we honestly say that songs like these have no effect on our individual and collective psyche? Can we honestly say that there is no son preference? As Indians living in the diaspora should we become so sensitive to how we, our culture, society, and homeland are portrayed in the Western media and academy, that we stop questioning some of the worst practices prevailing in India?

SPONTANEOUS ABORTION

A spontaneous abortion is the loss of a fetus during pregnancy due to natural causes. The term "miscarriage" is the spontaneous termination of a pregnancy before fetal development has reached 20 weeks. Pregnancy losses after the 20th week are categorized as preterm deliveries. The term "spontaneous abortion" refers to these naturally occurring events, not elective or therapeutic abortion procedures. More specific terms include: missed abortion (a pregnancy demise where nothing is expelled); incomplete abortion (not all of the products of conception are expelled); complete abortion (all of the products of conception are expelled); threatened abortion (symptoms indicate a miscarriage is possible); inevitable abortion (the symptoms cannot be stopped, and a miscarriage will happen); and infected abortion.

Overview, Causes, and Risk Factors

The cause of most spontaneous abortions is fetal death due to fetal genetic abnormalities, usually unrelated to the mother. Other possible causes for spontaneous abortion include: infection, physical problems the mother may have, hormone (endocrine) factors, immune responses, and serious systemic diseases of the mother (such as diabetes or thyroid problems).

It is estimated that up to 50% of all fertilized eggs die and are lost (aborted) spontaneously, usually before the woman knows she is pregnant. Among known pregnancies, the rate of spontaneous abortion is approximately 10% and usually occurs between the 7th and 12th weeks of pregnancy. The risk for spontaneous abortion is higher in women over age 35, in women with systemic disease (such as diabetes or thyroid dysfunction), and women with a history of three or more prior spontaneous abortions.

Diagnosis and Tests

Pelvic examination may reveal moderate thinning of the cervix (effacement), increased cervical dilation, and evidence of ruptured membranes:

- An HCG (qualitative-urine) or HCG (qualitative-serum) test confirms pregnancy.
- Serial HCG (quantitative) values may be drawn at intervals of days to weeks.
- A CBC may be done to determine the degree of blood loss.
- A WBC and differential may be done to rule out potential infection.

An abortion, especially if incomplete or missed, may also alter the results of the following tests:

- Transvaginal ultrasound
- Pregnancy ultrasound
- Estriol—urine
- Estriol—serum
- Serum progesterone
- Fibrin degradation products

Treatment

Treatment for threatened abortion varies from restrictions on some forms of exercise to complete bed rest. Abstaining from intercourse is usually recommended until signs have disappeared.

In the event of spontaneous abortion, the tissue passed from the vagina should be examined to determine the source of the tissue (fetal *vs.* hydatidiform mole) and if any fetal tissue remains in the uterus (incomplete abortion).

Missed abortions that do not abort naturally and incomplete spontaneous abortions may require surgical removal of retained tissue (D and C procedure). Any further vaginal bleeding should be carefully monitored.

Spontaneous Abortion Prognosis

Maternal outcome is good and complications are rare. Waiting a few months before trying to become pregnant again is usually recommended. However, spontaneous abortion can cause some complications:

- Retained dead fetal tissue in the uterus is referred to as an incomplete abortion. This may cause infection and the retained tissue must be removed surgically (D and C).
- An infection may occur after either a complete or incomplete abortion.
- In a missed abortion, the demise of the pregnancy is discovered before the appearance of any symptoms. A, D and C, or a D and E can be performed to remove all of the dead tissue. Some patients choose to await spontaneous expulsion.
- The death of a second or third trimester pregnancy is addressed differently than a first trimester loss. These are usually called intrauterine fetal demises (IUFD). If the dead fetus remains in the uterus for too long, an abnormal activation of blood clotting systems (coagulation and fibrinolytic systems) can develop in response to the release of anti-clotting chemicals from the retained dead fetus. This can adversely affect maternal health.

Prevention

Many of the spontaneous abortions that are caused by maternal disease can be prevented through early (prior to conception) detection and treatment of the disease. Reduced risk of spontaneous abortions has been attributed to early, comprehensive prenatal care and avoidance of environmental hazards (such as X-rays and infectious diseases). Spontaneous abortion naturally occurs after fetal death. The dead tissue is discarded from the uterus and the woman resumes her normal menstrual cycle within a few weeks (usually). It is possible to become pregnant immediately after a spontaneous abortion. However, it is recommended that a woman wait for one or two normal menstrual cycles before attempting another pregnancy. On occasion, the uterus does not expel all of the fetal tissue, in which case it is considered an incomplete abortion. Incomplete spontaneous abortions may require surgical removal of the retained tissue. Pregnancy loss at any gestational age may not be accompanied by prompt expulsion of the dead tissue. Signs of pregnancy decrease, the uterus begins shrinking to its original size, and a brownish or reddish vaginal discharge is often experienced. If spontaneous abortion does not occur in a reasonable amount of time (about 4 weeks), a D and C, or D and E will have to be performed, or labor induced to remove the dead fetus.

When a mother's body is having difficulty sustaining a pregnancy, signs (such as slight vaginal bleeding) may occur. This is a threatened abortion, which means there is a possibility of abortion, but it is not inevitable. A pregnant woman who develops any signs or symptoms of threatened miscarriage should contact her prenatal provider immediately.

Calling Your Doctor

Call your doctor if vaginal bleeding with or without cramping occurs during pregnancy.

Call your doctor if you are pregnant and notice tissue or clot-like material passed vaginally (any such material should be collected and brought in for examination).

Complete Abortion

A complete abortion is an abortion (induced or spontaneous) in which all of the fetal and placental material has been expelled from the uterus before 20 weeks' gestation. This type of abortion generally does not require medical intervention.

MTP

An abortion is a procedure, either surgical or medical, to end a pregnancy by removing the fetus and placenta from the uterus.

Abortion is the termination of pregnancy by any method (spontaneous or induced) before the foetus is sufficiently developed to survive independently. (foetus less than 20 weeks of pregnancy)

Types of Abortions

Abortions can be classified as either of the following:

- Spontaneous, and
- Induced.

Induced Abortion

Out of almost 35 million abortions, which take place annually in the world, more than half of them are illegal and performed by untrained, unskilled persons and done under highly unhygienic conditions.

The Indian MTP Act

To avoid the misuse of induced abortions, most countries have enacted laws, whereby only qualified Gynecologists under conditions laid down and done in clinics/hospitals that have been approved can do abortions. The Medical Termination of Pregnancy Act was enacted by the Indian Parliament in 1971 and came into force from 1 April, 1972. The MTP Act was again revised in 1975.

The MTP Act lays down the conditions under which a pregnancy can be terminated, the persons and the place to perform it. The reasons for which MTP is done, as interpreted from the Indian MTP Act, are:

(i) Where a pregnant woman has a serious medical disease and continuation of pregnancy could endanger her life like:
   - Heart diseases.
   - Severe rise in blood pressure.
   - Uncontrolled vomiting during pregnancy.
   - Cervical/breast cancer.
   - Diabetes mellitus with eye complication (retinopathy).
   - Epilepsy.
   - Psychiatric illness.

(ii) Where the continuation of pregnancy could lead to substantial risk to the newborn leading to serious physical/mental handicaps examples like:
   - Chromosomal abnormalities.
   - Rubella (German measles) viral infection to mother in first three months.
   - If previous children have congenital abnormalities.
   - Rh iso-immunisation link.
   - Exposure of the foetus to irradiation.

(iii) Pregnancy resulting of rape.

(iv) Conditions where the socio-economic status of the mother (family) hampers the progress of a healthy pregnancy and the birth of a healthy child.

Failure of Contraceptive Device irrespective of the method used (natural methods/barrier methods/hormonal methods).

This condition is a unique feature of the Indian Law. All the pregnancies can be terminated using this criterion.

Consent

If married—her own written consent. Husband's consent not required.

If unmarried and above 18 years—her own written consent.

If below 18 years—written consent of her guardian.

If mentally unstable—written consent of her guardian.

A consent assures the clinician performing the abortion that she:

Has been informed of all her options.

Has been counseled about the procedure, its risks and how to care for herself after she chosen the abortion of her own free will.

Person or persons who can perform MTP

Physicians qualified to do MTP are:

(i) Any qualified registered medical doctor who has assisted in 25 MTPs.

(ii) A house surgeon who has done six months posting in Obstetrics and Gynecology.
(iii) A person who has a diploma/degree in Obstetrics and Gynecology.
(iv) 3 years of practice in Obstetrics and Gynecology for those doctors registered before the 1971 MTP Act was passed.
(v) 1 year of practice in Obstetrics and Gynecology for those doctors registered on or after the date of commencement of the Act.
(vi) Whenever the pregnancy exceeds 12 weeks but is below 20 weeks opinion of two registered medical doctors is necessary.

Place where MTP can be performed

Any institutions licensed by the Government to perform MTP. The certificate issued by the Government should be conspicuously displayed at a place easily visible to persons visiting the place.

Methods of Induced Abortion

Abortion can be induced by different methods depending on the weeks of pregnancy completed.

Tests to be done

- A thorough medical examination including blood pressure and weight.
- An internal examination to confirm the duration of pregnancy.
- Urine test for confirmation of pregnancy.
- Routine urine analysis.
- Routine blood counts including hemoglobin estimation.
- Blood group and Rh factor.
- At times, an ultrasound may be required.

First trimester abortion

Surgical methods

(i) Cervical dilatation followed by evacuation of uterus by: Curettage/Suction evacuation/vacuum aspiration/Dilatation and evacuation.
(ii) Menstrual aspiration (MR).

Surgical methods in first trimester

Anaesthesia:

(i) Cervix is numbed (local anesthesia) with an injection so that the patient is pain free. This is given alone or with a sedative.

(ii) General anaesthesia can be given if the lady is apprehensive or has a low pain threshold or in selected cases like unmarried women or if it is her first pregnancy or if she opts for it.

Procedure

The lady is made to lie on her back with her legs raised and placed in stirrups (lithotomy position).

Dilatation and evacuation

Cervical dilatation followed by evacuation of uterus by—curettage/ vacuum aspiration/suction evacuation/suction curettage/dilation and evacuation.

Surgical abortion done in the early pregnancy, that is before 12 weeks is done by first dilating the cervix, which is done by introducing hollow metal rods of increasing diameters and then evacuating the contents of the uterus mechanically by scraping or by suction or both. The procedure takes about 15 minutes.

Advantages

- A single step procedure.
- Safe.
- Possible to carry out Sterilization or insertion of an intra-uterine device.
- Can go home on the same day.
- Can resume working the next day.

Risks

- Reaction to the drugs used in anesthesia.
- Bleeding.
- Infection of the uterus and fallopian tubes.
- Accidental perforation of the uterus.
- Emotional distress.

Menstrual aspiration/Menstrual regulation (MR)

Menstrual aspiration also called minisuction, miniabortion, vacuum aspiration, lunchtime abortion, which is done between 1 to 3 weeks after her failure to menstruate. This procedure is done as an out-patient. A thin plastic tube is inserted into the uterus and its contents sucked out by negative pressure created in a syringe. The procedure takes about 10 minutes to complete.

Advantages

- No hospitalization required.

- Done without anesthesia.
- Surgical risks are minimal.
- Person can go home and resume her normal activities.

Risks

- Failure of the procedure.
- Bleeding.
- Infection

Medical Methods in the first trimester

The main drugs in use today are a group of drugs known as prostaglandin, which can be used through various routes namely by mouth, by injection intramuscularly/intravenously or vaginally. These drugs are used by themselves or in combination with other drugs.

(i) The methotrexate-misoprostol method

A woman receives an injection of methotrexate. Between five to seven days later she returns and inserts suppositories of misoprostol into her vagina. The pregnancy usually ends at home within a day or two. The embryo and other tissue that develops during pregnancy are passed out through the vagina.

(ii) The mifepristone-misoprostol method

Mifepristone also known as RU-486 is antiprogesterone. A woman swallows a dose of mifepristone. She returns in five to seven days and inserts suppositories of misoprostol into her vagina. The pregnancy usually ends at home within four hours. The embryo and other tissue that develops during pregnancy are passed out through the vagina.

Risks

- Mifepristone, Methotrexate and misoprostol cause nausea and vomiting, diarrhea.
- Incomplete abortion may require surgical evacuation.
- Heavy bleeding, which may continue upto 7 days.

In the first trimester abortions the preference is for termination by the surgical method of dilatation and curettage as the drugs are expensive.

These drugs can be misused and hence FDA approval for these agents has not yet been given.

Second Trimester Abortions

Methods of second trimester abortion (13-20 week)

Medical methods using drugs like:

- Ethacridine lactate
- prostaglandin

Surgical methods

- Aspirotomy
- Hysterotomy
- Hysterectomy

Medical Methods: in second trimester

Ethacradine actate

(i) Drug named as Emcredyl or Rivanol

This is a drug that is introduced through a sterile catheter through the vagina into the uterine cavity and placed behind the pregnancy sac. This procedure is not painful. A maximum of 150 ml is installed. It takes between 48 to 72 hours to abort. The procedure is safe, cheap and easily available. To hasten the abortion, ethacridine can be used along with prostaglandin or oxytocin (a naturally available drug to increase uterine contractions).

(ii) Prostaglandin

PG-E2

A gel of prostaglandin called Cerviprime inserted into the mouth of the uterus (the cervix) in the evening in the clinic and the patient is asked to lie down for about half an hour and then allowed to go home. Early the following morning in the hospital a drip of oxytocin is started intravenously. Abortion is usually achieved in less than 24 hrs. and the abortion is complete.

Misoprostol

It is available in tablet form and given by mouth or can be inserted vaginally. Two tablets of Mifepristone is given followed 24 hrs. later by an oral or vaginal dose of misoprostol. The uterus will contract causing cramping followed by the expulsion of the fetus. The cramps and the bleeding will stop after the products have been expelled.

Others

Drugs like urea, hypertonic saline, glucose, which are introduced into the pregnant sac have all been done away with in favour of the above mentioned methods.

Risks

Needs to be in a hospital upto 3 days.

Infection.
Increased bleeding.
Retained products, which may need surgical evacuation.

Surgical Methods in the second trimester

Anaesthesia

General anesthesia can be given depending on the pain threshold/ apprehension of the lady.

Procedure

- Aspirotomy.
- Hysterotomy.
- Hysterectomy.

Aspirotomy

Aspirotomy is a procedure similar to what is done in first trimester. This method can be employed between 13-20 weeks of pregnancy. To help in dilatation of the cervix prostaglandins may be used.

Hysterotomy

Hysterotomy is a major operating procedure where the abdomen is opened. In a hysterotomy the uterus is opened and the contents of the uterus removed directly under vision. This is like a cesarean.

Hysterectomy

In a hysterectomy, the uterus along with the pregnancy is removed in toto. At times hysterotomy or hysterectomy may be necessary because of a failure of a medical induction during the second trimester.

In the second trimester of pregnancy, the procedure followed is by the medical methods rather than by the surgical methods. This is because the risks and the convenience of the medical methods are far less than surgical termination.

An early diagnosis of pregnancy with early termination is safer than in the second trimester.

Counseling

Counseling is normally done by the attending Obstetrician. The aim of counseling is to help her come to a decision as to the need of continuation or termination of the pregnancy and to resolve it in the direction that she chooses.

The purpose of counseling is:

- To allay the anxiety of the person, who intends to undergo the procedure.

- To provide information about the methods, safety, risks, etc.
- To screen for guilt, or any psychiatric ailment.
- To help the lady understand and to cope with her feelings.
- To help her to prevent future unplanned pregnancy.

Description of surgical abortion

A surgical abortion that is performed between 6 and 12 weeks into a pregnancy may be done while the woman is awake. She is given the option of being sedated by medications, or having her cervix numbed with an injection of anesthesia so that she is basically pain-free. Surgical abortion for a pregnancy over 12 weeks is usually done while the woman is sedated, although it can also be performed while the woman is awake. The cervical canal is enlarged (dilated) and a hollow tube is inserted into the uterus. A vacuum (suction) machine is used to remove the tissues (fetus and placenta) from the uterus. Medicines such as oxytocin are sometimes given to cause the uterine muscles to contract and reduce bleeding.

An abortion with medicine can be performed or a pregnancy less than 7 weeks from the first day of the last menstrual period using a combination of medications. The current regimen approved by the FDA includes administration of one dose of Mifepristone (RU486), an antiprogestin, followed by one dose of Misoprostol, a prostaglandin analogue two days later. These medications may be given in the doctor's office, after a thorough history and physical is performed. The experience of abortions with medicines, without surgical intervention is building up.

The need of the hour is to empower women with the right to their sexuality and reproduction, as their fundamental right to choose to have or not to have a child. Presently she is restrained by several factors, viz. medical, social, family, etc.

4

Infertility can make Life Fruitless

The objective of married life and consequent sexual activity is to procreate one's young ones. The life plan of all adult-couples include children, to be their descendants and inherit their legacy. When a couple fails to achieve this primary objective, they are called an infertile couple. So infertility, means inability to bear a child or it may simply be called a failure of the process of procreation. The agony and distress of infertile couples is to be seen, to be believed. When this natural 'wish' fails to materialize—frustration, despair and helplessness are common and with debilitating consequences. It is a situation where the couple is left to pass 'sleepless nights' pondering over the uselessness of their wealth, worth, earnings, professional capability or social life. Infertility can isolate couples, put them through a great deal of mental trauma and strain their marriages. The area of prevention and management of infertility remains a neglected area.

It goes without saying that procreation entails intimate physical and psychological union of a husband and wife, who are in good health. In most cases, such a couple is rewarded with a child in about one year of continuing conjugal relationship. Where there is some defect in the sexual apparatus or in the organs of reproduction either in the male or female, (or problem is there when the two combine) pregnancy may fail to occur. The infertility can occur, even when everything appears normal. Consequently one out of ten couples in India is sterile.

What can go wrong?

Sexual union has been described in our scriptures, as sacrosanct between husband and wife, for the avowed objective of procreation only. However, the sanctity of this sacred relationship has not only been violated with impunity, but this process has been highly abused for passion. So much so, to quench the lust even unnatural methods, objects, persons, animals and techniques have been used, which had no relation to the basic purpose and intent of bearing a child. While womans' body has been the subject of exploitation under duress in many circumstances, of lately the females themselves have resorted to provocative and inviting sexual behaviour for extraneous gains, unrelated to the function of child-bearing. Consequent to such a deviant behaviour, there has been phenomenal rise of sexuality transmitted diseases (STDs) and induced abortions. Many of such encounters result into partial or complete, temporary or permanent loss of reproductive functions.

The concept of 'free sex' has exposed the present generation, especially the youths to the risks of sexually transmitted diseases, which cause devastation of the reproductive apparatus, resulting in permanent infertility, besides chronic ill-health and premature death. In case of AIDS the risk of losing health and early end of life are grave, indeed. While the incidence of syphilis has become less common, with the advent of frequent antibiotics use, several others like Chlamydia and gonorrhoea are still a big problem.

Let us study a few of them.

Chlamydia

As mentioned above, it is one of the most common bacterial sexually transmitted infections (STIs) and is easily transmitted. It usually infects the genitals of both men and women, but can also infect the throat, rectum and eyes. Over 2/3 of women and half of men who have chlamydia have no symptoms. Symptoms include discharge from the vagina or penis and pain on passing urine. It is common in young people. It can cause serious health problems if left untreated. Fortunately, it is easily treated with a course of antibiotics. It is passed from one person to another through sexual activity, viz. vaginal or anal sex, oral sex, when sharing sex toys, and from a mother to her baby during the birth.

Without treatment, the infection can spread to other parts of the body causing damage and serious long-term health problems, e.g. Ectopic pregnancy, Blocked fallopian tubes, Long-term pelvic pain, Early and repeated miscarriages or premature birth, Eye infection or pneumonia in the baby at birth. Similarly, in man it can cause painful inflammation of the testicles, inflammation of the joints, urethra and eyes, etc. Though it is easy to treat with antibiotics, prevention is the best form of treatment. A condom can provide protection from most STIs, if used correctly, every time you have sex.

Gonorrhoea

Gonorrhoea is also a bacterial infection, which infects the genitals, urethra, anus, rectum and throat. More rarely, it can affect the blood, skin, joints and eyes. While it may be silent, often, the symptoms can include discharge from the vagina or penis and pain when urinating. Gonorrhoea can cause serious health problems. However, it's easy to treat with antibiotics. It can spread through Vaginal, oral or anal sex, Close physical contact, Sharing sex toys, Genitals to the eyes by the fingers. In case of females the symptoms are strong smelling discharge, Pain when passing urine, Irritation or discharge from the vagina or anus, low abdominal or pelvic tenderness.

Symptoms in men are white, yellow or green discharge from the tip of the penis, Inflammation of the testicles and prostate gland, Pain when urinating, Irritation or discharge from the anus.

Without treatment, gonorrhoea can spread to other reproductive organs causing damage and serious long-term health problems, viz. Blocked fallopian tubes, Long-term pelvic pain, Ectopic pregnancy, Eye infection to baby at birth. In case of males swelling of testicles and prostate can occur.

Herpes

Genital herpes is caused by the herpes simplex virus and is a painful and common problem. Many people with genital herpes have no symptoms at all. Symptoms include blisters in the genital and anal region, which burst leaving painful sores. There are no treatments to get rid of the virus, although some tablets and self-help measures are useful. Genital herpes doesn't generally cause serious health problems or sterility. Genital herpes is passed on through direct skin contact, mainly during vaginal, oral or anal sex, or kissing. Condoms may help protect against genital herpes.

Serious problems are uncommon. Genital herpes doesn't affect fertility and women can have a normal pregnancy and child-birth. It's not linked to cancer of the cervix, either.

Deviant behaviour and lifestyle can reduce fertility

Several deviations in the behaviour and lifestyle of males as well as females or both can result in sterility. Besides lifestyle factors, there are other causes, maladies, accidents, developmental defects, etc. which can be responsible for infertility and which may be beyond human control. Late marriages, delayed plans for pregnancy, struggle and stress for employment and career advancement, ego clash of the partners—all can lead to infertility. If one or two years of consummation of marriage have elapsed and infertility is well established advise of your friends, such as have fun trying, have faith in God, put a pillow under your hips during intercourse, relax with yoga, have a routine gynae examination need to be ignored. Consult an expert in a sterility clinic. Although most gynaecologists are equipped to treat infertile couples, some restrict themselves only to Infertility and so devote more time to your problem. Such clinics are more suitable for consultation, in case of infertility.

Why Fertility is lower today?

The age of women who want to bear babies has gone up because of the late marriages and fulfiling careers. Men's sperm count has decreased all over the world, probably due to pollution or stress.

Road Block in the long journey

It is the assumption that human beings are remarkably fertile. Most females are capable of conceiving and bearing children beginning in their mid-teen years. While women in civilized societies usually bear children in their 20s and 30s, some women can give birth to a child well into their 40s and beyond. Men can be fertile even in old age. Humans can mate year round and fertility is not restricted to a particular part of the year or to brief episodes of female heat. However, for conception to take place, hundreds of hormonal, chemical, and physical events take place in a precise order. For example, a sperm must form in the testicle, mature in the epididymis, be released into the female vagina, "swim" through the cervical opening, continue through the uterus and into a fallopian tube. In the tube, it must encounter a viable egg within 12 hours of its release, attach it with the egg, penetrate its outer cover and fertilize the ovum within. After staying in the fallopian tube for about two days, the fertilized egg must descend into the uterus, grow and divide for a few more days, and then implant itself on the uterine wall. A disruption, in any of these events and conditions or underlying processes can cause infertility. The sperm may not be viable, it may contain the wrong number of chromosomes, it may have been stored too long. Or sperm is immotile (cannot "swim" correctly). It may be perfectly healthy but not accompanied by enough sperms (men whose semen contains less that 60 million sperms per milliliter frequently have infertility problems). The sperm ducts may be blocked, because of past infection or injury. The man may not be able to ejaculate, or his ejaculation may propel the sperm backward into his bladder rather than out through the penis. Once inside the cervix, the sperm may meet mechanical or chemical roadblocks. A muscle spasm may eject the sperm, the cervical mucus may be too thick to be penetrated, or chemically hostile to the sperm. The fallopian tube may be blocked by scar tissue. The sperm does manage to reach the egg, it may not be able to penetrate its defense (the outer cover) to fertilize it. A fertilized egg may be stuck in the fallopian tube. Or it may not be able to implant successfully in the uterus.

First attempt may not succeed

Only filmy pregnancies occur on a drop of hat. Even the most fertile human couples do not conceive after the first intercourse. In fact, the chance of conception in any given month among fertile couples attempting to conceive is about 20%. In about 30% of infertility cases, the problem can be found in the woman; in another 30%, male factors alone cause the infertility; and in another 30% of cases, both partners have conditions, which render the couple infertile. In the remaining 10% of cases, no clear cause can be found. Women are given physical and pelvic examinations, laboratory tests, and imaging procedures to locate the problem that may be causing infertility. Laproscopy and ultrasound imaging may reveal structural or functional problems. Additionally, some women do not ovulate regularly or at all. Others may produce ovum regularly that are prevented from being fertilized, descending or implanting.

Men are tested for the presence, quantity and quality of their sperms. The most correctable problem (not the commonest) affecting male sperm levels is varicocele, a tangle of veins surrounding testicle. Surgical correction of large varicoceles restore fertility in about two-thirds of such cases. Other causes of male infertility include insufficient hormone levels, blocked tubes, which carry sperm, untreated diabetes or prostate disease and other conditions.

Can fertility be assisted?

After testing is complete, doctors devise a strategy for each couple to restore fertility. Sometimes, small adjustments in sexual frequency and timing may result in pregnancy. Patients are taught to identify the woman's fertile period, so that intercourse can coincide with the most fertile period. Practices that temporarily result in lowered sperm count, e.g. medications, alcohol, drugs, hot tubs bathing, etc. may be stopped. Gonadotrophin treatment to increase the number of female gametes is well accepted, as a part of IVF as well as ICSI. *In-vitro* fertilization (IVF) involves the mixing of sperms and eggs in the laboratory, outside the human body where fertilization takes place, and then the zygote (fertilized egg) is surgically placed in the woman's fallopian tube or the uterus in an effort to establish a pregnancy. One of the most recent developments in ART (assisted reproductive technology) is intracytoplasmic sperm injection (ICSI). This microsurgical procedure involves injecting a single sperm into an egg, allowing men with extremely low sperm counts to become fathers. Future lies in genetics, imaging, and biotechnology to enhance fertility.

Test tube baby debate

While child bearing process used to lie in the domain of complete privacy, by tradition, now the public debate about test tube baby and gestational carrier has brought us in a more modern era. The rapid development of new medical technologies has raised many ethical and legal issues. New reproductive technologies are changing many cherished ideas about family relationships. Today, a child can be born from a donated egg, with donated sperm, from the uterus of a woman who is a "gestational carrier." In this way, a woman with no hereditary link to the offspring may deliver a child, who is also not related genetically to the eventual parents of the child. When all parties agree to such unconventional arrangements, they can try to produce a truly and completely 'Assisted' child.

When fertility treatment results in multiple pregnancies, couples face an ethical dilemma. While it is possible to selectively abort one or more embryos to improve the chances of the survival of one and to reduce the burden on parents of raising several children, this is a difficult decision for couples. Healthcare policy-makers debate whether infertility treatment is a basic right that should be paid for by medical reimbursement, similar to cosmetic surgery? Because infertility raises all these issues, and because the treatment itself may involve considerable time, expense, and loss of privacy, for many couples the procedure is extremely stressful. The role of stem cells and cloning is yet unproven and is controversial.

Beware of the Money Game

Unfortunately, assisted reproduction in cases of infertility have lost human touch. The couples-in-distress are centres, made to pay through their noses. There is no transparency either in diagnostic interventions, or in therapeutic pursuits. The victims are allured through glamorous advertisements and cheated with impunity. There are no checks and no laws for 3000 infertility clinics, operating in a poor country like India. The success rate is low, the claims are tall and unrealistic. We know a large number of so called infertile couples, who succeeded in having a child, spontaneously, but the credit went to treating infertility specialists or Sants and Mahants on the prowl. We also know many couples in double-despair, who parted with lacs of rupees, but remained sterile. Caution and restraint are the watchwords for expectations for the couples.

Legal and ethical issues are complicated

As you know, third party assisted reproduction is a maze and it involves several complications, medical, social, ethical, legal, etc. Even after several attempts, it leaves behind (most) couples clamouring for success. Those couples who succeed to attain pregnancy and those who assist their now found fertility have to be wary of a host of legal and ethical issues.

HOW TO DEFINE INFERTILITY?

When pregnancy does not occur even after one year of regular, unprotected conjugal life after marriage, it is called infertility. It can be due to a variety of factors including endocrine disorders, defects in the reproductive systems, deficient production of sperms or eggs, drugs and toxic chemicals, childhood diseases such as mumps, etc. There has been a recent increase in the number of infertility cases reported throughout the world. While some of the causes are due to natural defects in the process of procreation, many of these are 'man-made' due to reckless and faulty lifestyle, viz. excessive use of alcohol and other intoxicants, smoking of tobacco and other harmful substances, abuse of sex as a perversion, fun, game, with multiple partners or excessive indulgence. More than one factors can also play a role. Males are at fault in about 40% cases. Unexplained infertility is present in 10%, exclusive male factor 25%, failure of ovulation 20%, tubal damage 15% and endometriosis 5%. When a woman fails to bear even her first child it is primary sterility. When she produces one child, but is unable to have a second pregnancy, it is called secondary infertility.

(a) Male factors

In the male, a low sperm count or defective spermatozoa is the major factor. Another well-known factor that contributes to male infertility is the presence of a varicocele, which is a cluster of enlarged veins around the testicle. Varicocele elevates temperature in this part of the body by increasing blood circulation and the higher temperature reduces sperm production. Defects in the male reproductive tract can also be responsible for infertility. Childhood disorders such as mumps may result in permanent damage of the reproductive organs, leading to infertility. The use of certain drugs and toxic chemicals can contribute to infertility.

(b) Female factors

In females, pelvic Infection is the major cause of infertility. It covers a wide variety of infections that can affect the uterus, ovaries, and fallopian tubes. The sites of infection that usually cause infertility are the fallopian tubes, the inflammation of which produces a condition known as salpingitis. Most infections are caused by sexually transmitted diseases (STD). Chlamydia causes a large proportion of salpingitis cases. Gonorrhea is responsible for much of the rest. Attacks of STD can eventually cause scarring, abscess formation, and tubal damage that result in infertility. Endometriosis is responsible for a good number of cases. It results when fragments of the endometrial lining are implanted in other areas of the pelvis, which then develop into cysts and respond to hormonal changes, increasing in size with each menstrual cycle and eventually causing scarring and inflammation. Endometrial implants in the ovaries or fallopian tubes are especially prone to cause infertility. Ovulatory and hormonal problems are responsible for almost 30% of infertility cases in women. These problems result in the failure of the ovarian follicle to rupture, an empty follicle, or entrapment of the egg so that it is not released. Polycystic Ovarian Syndrome (PCO) occurs in 6% of women and is also a major cause of infertility.

(c) Unexplained infertility

Some cases of unexplained infertility may result from early loss of ovarian function. Immune system failure can also cause infertility. Scar tissue that forms after abdominal surgery can restrict the movement of ovaries, fallopian tubes, or the uterus and may cause infertility. Other causes of infertility include a ruptured appendix, diabetes, kidney disease, thyroid disorders, hypertension, drugs, and toxic chemicals. Late marriage, ageing of female, restricted opportunity of intimacy, poor general health of the lady could be some of the other factors. 50-60 percent of infertility cases are due to ovulation problems, pelvic disease, and to cervical problems in the female. About 10 percent of cases have no known cause. If the couple has already had a child or two, it is not unusual to have difficulty conceiving again. Such infertility is more common than primary infertility. So quite often the problems arise in bearing a subsequent child, while the first one may have been born, without any delay.

(d) Find out what's wrong?

A woman usually ovulates on Day 14, that is if you take the day you start your period as Day 1. Your doctor can show you how to take your temperature and check your cervical mucus to find out when you ovulate. Sonographies can pinpoint the exact time.

The egg stays alive for about 24 hours while the sperm stays alive for 48 hours. So you should have intercourse every other day around the time you ovulate—that is Days 10, 12, 14, 16.

How to proceed to find the fault?

- Both will be asked questions and given physical examinations with special reference to your reproductive systems.
- The man's system is analyzed for sperm count, speed, abnormality, consistency, colour and quality.
- Both sets of blood are tested for hormone levels.
- Both sets of blood and urine are tested for infections.

Should all this be clear, things get more difficult:

- If no sperm or very few sperm turn up, the husband should be advised a testicular biopsy under local anesthesia. This is a microscopic examination of tissue, which gives vital information about sperm production.
- A hystero-salpingogram examines the openness of the fallopian tubes of the reproductive system. This can be done by injecting a radio-opaque dye so that any blockage in the womb or fallopian tubes shows up on an X-ray screen.
- An ultrasonography looks into the womb to check the lining of the endometrium and ovulation.
- The serum progesterone level is measured to check the quality of the ovulation.
- A post-coital test determines whether the sperms remain fighting fit through the wife's genital tract. It is done a few hours after intercourse and consists in sucking out a bit of cervical mucus for microscopic examination. If the mucus is normal, the absence of sperm or presence of a few or inactive sperms show that your body reacts to his sperm; thick or hostile mucus signifies an infection, which destroys his sperm.
- A laprascopy, which places a slender lighted telescope device through a tiny incision in the woman's abdomen under general anaesthesia, allows the specialist to examine the tube, ovaries, womb and the inside of the abdomen for signs of defects. Any minor problems can be treated at the same time.
- An endomaterial biopsy under local anaesthesia will remove a small tissue from the womb for further information. Later on you may need some other more sophisticated tests.

Infertility can cause stress and stress can cause infertility. If you are over-ambitious, over-committed, suffer financial distress, have physical inadequacy, fearful, hopeless, anxious, angry, exhausted, depressed, pregnancy may not occur. Sometimes counseling and communicating honestly with your spouse and a relaxed holiday are all that you need to smash the mental block on your ability to add to your family.

HOW THE NATURAL SYSTEM OF PROCREATION WORKS?

The natural system of procreation entails, marriage of a healthy adult male to a female, who is fit and mature enough to bear healthy children. Further it signifies regular and un-restricted co-habitation of the two, with adequate care of the health and medical attention, nutrition, exercise, privacy, conditional satisfaction, materialistic aspirations and peace of mind. Under ideal conditions conception occurs within twelve months in 80-85% of couples who use no contraceptive measures. If pregnancy fails to occur, there is likely to be a defect in either of the partners or both. Approximately in 30% of cases it is found in the man alone, and in another 20% both the man and woman are abnormal. Therefore, the male factor is at least partly responsible in about 50% of infertile couples. This is contrary to popular belief and practice of blaming the 'barren' woman for the ill-luck. Therefore, it is extremely important in the evaluation of infertility to consider the couple as a unit for evaluation and treatment and to proceed with parallel investigation of both, until a problem is uncovered. Many couples experience significant apprehension and anxiety after only a few months of failure to conceive. Obviously, if only female is to be blamed due to a mind-set, and if only she is investigated and treated, the expectation of success would be low.

(a) Masters of Reproductive Orchestra

It would be interesting to observe that the masters of reproductive processes sit higher up in the body, i.e. skull, in the form of Hypothalamus and Pituitary gland and not in the genitals of the two partners. It is the hypothalamus, which gets messages from both the brain above and the testes and ovaries below to regulate the secretion of gonadotropin releasing hormone (GnRH) from hypothalamus. It guides production and release of both luteinizing hormone (LH) and follicle stimulating hormone (FSH) from pituitary gland.

Prolactin also has a complex inter-relationship with the gonadotropins, LH and FSH. In males with hyperprolactinemia, the prolactin tends to inhibit the production of GnRH. Besides inhibiting LH secretion and testosterone production, elevated prolactin levels may have a direct effect on the brain. In individuals with elevated prolactin levels who are given testosterone, libido and sexual function do not return to normal as long as the prolactin levels are elevated.

The hypothalamus

Hypothalamus is the single most important group of cells of the brain, which works round the clock to maintain equilibrium of the temperature of the body and internal environment of the body in every manner. It is a central switchboard of the body or a sort of co-ordinator between brain and pituitary gland (Pituitary is the master gland, which influences all other endocrine glands, the growth, the metabolism, sex characteristics and what not). It also maintains the water balance inside the body and protects in the event of dehydration or over-hydration. It is the hypothalamus, which senses hunger for food and desire for sex. If these areas are damaged the desire for food or sex may disappear or is totally un-regulated. In the event of anger, it prepares the person to fight or flight. Thus most activities of the body are ably controlled by hypothalamus, including the process of procreation, as mentioned above.

(b) Fertility glands

These are the pairs of glands (testes in the male and ovaries in the female), which are responsible for production of sperms (male eggs) and ovum (female eggs), that ultimately meet in the female reproductive apparatus (generally fallopian tube) and initiate fertilization in consequent conception.

Testes

Testosterone is secreted from the Leydig cells of testes in response to LH. The major functions of testosterone (Androgen) in target tissues include: (1) regulation of gonadotropins secretion by the hypothalamic-pituitary axis; (2) initiation and maintenance of spermatogenesis; (3) differentiation of the genital system during fetal development; and (4) promotion of sexual maturation at puberty. In the testes the seminiferous tubules contain all the germ cells at various stages of maturation. These account for 85-90% of the testicular volume and are responsible for production of sperms. Spermatogenesis is a complex process whereby primitive stem cells either divide to reproduce themselves for stem cell renewal or they divide to produce daughter cells that will later become sperms. The entire spermatogenic cycle in humans is 4.6 cycles, each one taking 16 days, which equals to 74 days. LH effects spermatogenesis indirectly in that it stimulates testosterone production. FSH targets Sertoli cells. Sertoli cells offer androgen-binding protein, that cause a high level of testosterone to be maintained in the micro-environment of the Asian spermatozoa. For spermatogenesis to be maintained testosterone is required. However, if spermatogenesis is to be re-initiated after the germinal epithelium has been allowed to regress completely, the FSH and testosterone both are required. The epididymis is intimately involved with the maturation, storage and transport of spermatozoa. Testicular spermatozoa are non-motile and are felt to be incapable of fertilizing ova. Spermatozoa gain progressive motility and fertilizing ability after passing through epididymis. The estimated transit time of spermatozoa through the epididymis in healthy males is approximately four days. The epididymis also serves as a reservoir or storage area for sperm. During emission, secretions from the seminal vesicles and prostate are deposited in the posterior urethra. During ejaculation, the bladder neck and the external sphincter relaxes with the semen being propelled through the urethra. The major volume of the seminal fluid comes from the seminal vesicles and secondarily the prostate. The seminal vesicles provide the nourishing fructose as well as prostaglandins and coagulating substrates.

Ovaries

As mentioned above, pituitary and hypothalamus are the masters of reproductive orchestra (as well as other vital problems in the body, controlled by hormones). Hypothalamus produces GnRH, which act on the pituitary gland for production and their control of secretion of FSH and LH, which are essential for ovulation as well as menstruation. Hypothalamus, in turn, is influenced by brain/mind, e.g. emotional upset can effect all these processes.

FSH controls the ripening of follicles, process of ovulation, as well as activates secretion of oestrogen, and progesterone along with LH. LH level rises within 24-36 hours of ovulation and thus can predict exact time of ovulation, which is of great importance to retrieve ova and arrange, artificial insemination or *in-vitro* fertilization (IVF).

Now LH testing in the urine of a woman, with the help of ova stick has become easy, though still expensive.

Ovaries secrete several hormones for performing various functions. Two important ones are oestrogen and progesterone. Other two are testosterone and androsterdione. The peak level of oestrogen is reached 2 days before ovulation and approximately one day before peak level of LH. It is the oestrogen, which is responsible for feminine characteristics of a girl, viz. texture of skin and hair, shape of female form, development of vagina and other genetic organs, health and development of uterus and fallopian tubes, breast development, bone development, etc. Pogestrone level rises after several days of ovulation and fall in the later part of menstruation cycle, to allow onset of menstrual bleed (which mark the onset of next menstrual cycle). If pregnancy occurs, high levels of progesterone will be maintained, which are essential for continuation of pregnancy. Though testosterone is the principal male hormone, in small quantity it is secreted by ovaries of female also. The same is about andostenedione. After menopause, the level of these hormones may become relatively more.

(c) The menstruation

The menstrual cycle is controlled by two principal female hormones, viz. oestrogen controls the first half, bringing proliferation of endometrium in the lining of uterus and progesterone dominates the second half (secretary phase). It is at puberty that hypothalamus starts the production of GnRH, which sets-up menstrual cycle. At this stage ovaries come into 'life' and that leads to maturation of one dominant Graffian follicle. The process of ovulation occurs under the influence of FSH and LH and female hormones as mentioned above. After ovulation if the pregnancy has not occurred, the level of hormones, esp. progesterone falls towards the end of menstrual cycle and that allows menstrual bleed to occur, with shedding of endometrium.

An average cycle is of 28 days each, out of which later half, i.e. time between ovulation and occurrence of menstruation is fairly constant. The duration of bleeding is 3-5 days and loss of blood is 100-200 cc. A deviation of 2-3 days from 28 days cycle is not uncommon.

(d) The Fertilization

During each month of the menstrual cycle, there is a cyclic increase and decrease of FSH and LH. During the first few days after the beginning of menstruation, concentrations of FSH and LH increase several fold. These hormones cause accelerated growth of 6-12 primary follicles each month. When under the influence of FSH, the group of follicles continue to grow and secrete estrogen. Only one of the follicles becomes mature, i.e. continues to increase it's estrogen production under the influence of increasing level of LH. Small amounts of progesterone are produced by the mature follicle a day or two before ovulation. As the Estrogens is liberated endometrium thickens. Ovulation generally occurs on the 14th day of menstrual cycle due to rupture of mature follicle. Post-ovulatory period is between ovulation and next menses. The ovum passes through one of the fallopian tubes to its onward journey to uterus and if it is fertilized by a sperm in the fallopian tube, it implants in the uterus where it develops into a fetus.

Fertilization occurs if you have intercourse around the time of ovulation, which takes place 14 days before the onset of next menstrual flow. This is a reasonably predictable event. The essentials of fertilization are ovulation, sexual contact during the fertile phase, husband's sperm count adequate, and the mucus in the cervix favorable. Also there must not be any barrier preventing fertilization from taking place, such as blocked fallopian tubes or adhesions around the ovaries preventing the egg from gaining access to the tube and sperm.

If fertilization does not occur, this ovum gets decimated and menstrual flow occurs on the completion of previous cycle from the uterus. It consist of 50-150 ml blood, tissue fluid, epithelial cells derived from endometrium.

FERTILITY IS A TEAM WORK

The common notion that in case of failed fertility, it is the woman who has failed to deliver a child, and hence she is to 'be wholly blamed', is untrue. Child conception is a team work and fertility will require not only each of the husband and wife to be in good health and state of procreation, but also when they are put together, the evaluation of the couple that neither they are incongruous nor incompatible. As a matter of fact, in the first instance one in six couples who are confronted with infertility, half are attributed to the male partner. Being so common, it may seem surprising that it is so seldomly talked about. Male fertility and infertility need not be a cause for shame or undue anxiety, for males, since it is no stigma on their manhood. It is to be further understood that conception requires a team effort and does not always "just happen." It is often necessary, even when both of you are healthy and "normal" to actively plan for a conception. This requires that you understand the female ovulation cycle and that you time intercourse at least during that 4 day window, each cycle when conception is most likely to occur. In some cases, despite both your best efforts and planning, conception may not occur after a year and it will be the time to plan fertility assessment. Again, be prepared for a team effort in which both of the partners participate equally, if success is to be achieved.

In olden days, if a woman failed to provide a successor to the family to inherit the property, she was labeled as BANJH (sterile) and generally abandoned by the husband and his family. Even today's modern society does not take it kindly, if a woman fails to produce a child at all or the child produced is not a male. No effort was made to ascertain the cause of infertility, nor any worthwhile remedial measures were taken. Often some religious or spiritual rituals were performed or some unknown potion of medication administered. Many a times the so-called 'blessings' of a Godman were elicited. The male was never suspected to be lacking or deficient in anything. Many atrocities were perpetuated on infertile woman—until the hapless creature ran away, from home or dumped with a label of ill-omened. Today there is no place for such things—scientific study of both partners is required.

As mentioned, elsewhere, the team effort will entail complete harmony between the couple, opportunity for physical and psychological intimacy, timing of the conjugal union during the fertile period of menstrual cycle, assessment of ovulation and spermatogenesis, assessment of any barriers in meeting of ovum and sperm, assessment of normally of reproductive apparatus of man and the wife and counseling to inculcate positive thinking and hope.

THE LIFESTYLE FACTORS

It is your own lifestyle, which can make or mar your chances of bearing a child—male or female.

(i) Alcohol consumption has been linked to impaired fertility in both men and women. Limiting alcohol consumption is one of the several things you can do to maximize your fertility. Similarly early sexual activity, sex with multiple partners, sexually transmitted diseases, urinary infections, poor sexual hygiene, all expose to temporary or permanent sterility.

(ii) Recreational drugs of abuse, e.g. marijuana, cocaine, barbiturates and heroin can significantly impact female fertility.

(iii) Smoking (even passive smoking) has a negative impact on both male and female fertility. In men, smoking can reduce sperm count and impair sperm motility. In women, smoking has been linked to impaired fertility and increased risk of abortion.

(iv) Use of excessive tea, coffee, soft drinks can reduce fertility. There are studies that link consumption of large amounts of caffeine to increased time to conception, infertility due to endometriosis and tubal disease, and miscarriage.

(v) Reckless use of plant-based products, containing unknown chemicals are best avoided. Various products are taken either to improve health, energy, fertility or for conception of a male child, e.g. Compound Q (Trichosanthin-GLQ233), Chinwood, Simaruba, Pomeganate, Christmas Rose, Safflower, Cassia, Cotton Root, Cats Claw, Castor Oil Plant, Burning Bush, Barberry, Fennel, Goldenseal, Lavender, Male Fern, Calamus, Mistletoe, Pennyroyal, Poke Root, Sage, Cayenne, Tansy, Wild Cherry, Yarrow, Bloodroot, Cypress, Thyme, Celandine, Ephedra, Flaxseed, Juniper, Licorice Root, Mayapple, Passion Flower, Periwinkle, Rhubarb, Cascara Sagrada, Wormwood, St. John's Wart, Echinacea, and Gingko biloba.

Similarly, medicines like steroids, antihistamins, anti-depressants, anti-hypertensives, anti-diabetics, heart ailments and their treatment, ejaculation problems and their treatment can lower fertility. Diseases like tuberculosis, sexually transmitted diseases, head injury, pituitary tumours granulomas, infections any where in the body (even an abscess in the mouth, influenza, upset tummy, urinary problems—all can lower fertility. Also occurrence of hernia or hydrocele or any surgery for their correction can lead to infertility.

(vi) Exercise is certainly an important part of a healthy lifestyle. Exercise imparts benefits to overall health and emotional well-being. Excessive exercise, however, may interfere with a woman's menstrual cycle and cause difficulty in achieving pregnancy. In males, use of tight undergarments, pressure on testicles can reduce fertility. Obesity is a negative factor for both.

(vii) Timing of sexual union around the time of ovulation can be one of the easiest and most effective strategies that can enhance your chances of conception. The man is constantly making sperm, however the woman's fertile period only comes once a month! The 4 important days are 12th to 15th day of menstrual cycle.

(viii) Certain chemicals and pollutants can increase your risk of infertility. Some examples of chemicals that are associated with infertility include pesticides, solvents, heavy metals, and anesthetic gases. If you are an industrial worker, take precautions to minimize exposure.

Another potential occupational hazard is radiation, e.g. medical imaging machines (X-ray and C.T. scan machines) can contribute to infertility.

(ix) It is well known that stress reduces your fertility, since stress affects both your emotional well-being and your sex life. Clearly, a healthy and enjoyable sex life is an important part of getting pregnant. Whether the stress is caused by work, hyper-active lifestlye, or your conscious effort to conceive.

(x) Medicines—intake can affect your fertility. Several medicines, many of them sold over the counter can reduce fertility, e.g. pain killers (use for headaches, menstrual cramps, arthritis, etc.). Valproate (a medication used for epilepsy), Chemotherapy (cancer treatment), anti-hypertensive medicines and others (metoclopramide, methyldopa, cimetidine, haloperidol) Metoclopramide (Reglan®), methyldopa (Aldomet®), cimetidine (Tagamet®), and haloperidol (Haldol®) may interfere with fertility.

(xi) Occupational exposures to pesticides and radiofrequency energy may lead to reduced sperm or ovum counts as well as reductions in some reproductive hormone levels. Now more and more workers are exposed to radiofrequency energy from sources such as communication equipment, microwave ovens and medical or industrial heating devices. These devices can emit high electromagnetic fields (though no radioactivity) and affect fertility in males as well as females. If you work with lead, nickel, insecticides, petrochemicals, polystyrene, benzene, anesthetic drugs, X-rays, etc. These can be lethal to sperm or ovum (also pesticides and other chemicals).

(xii) In case of females, the mania of looking too slim, through crash dieting or too much exercise can affect fertility. Other female factors can be : use of pill for a long time, thyroid disease, use of antidepressant drugs, ovarian cyst, infection due to IUCD, blockage of tube due to previous abortion or sexually transmitted diseases, presence of fibroid in the uterus, cervical infection, immune reaction to husband's semen, prolonged use of antibiotics or other medicines.

EXCLUSIVE MALE FACTORS

Though child bearing is considered a female issue and it is treated as an exclusive domain of mother, in case of failure of fertility, we have also to consider certain factors, which are related to male alone. In men, hormone disorders, illness, reproductive anatomy trauma and obstruction, and sexual dysfunction can temporarily or permanently affect sperm formation or their maturation and prevent conception. Important issues to understand are :

Spermatogenesis

As said above, sperm production takes place in the seminiferous tubules (ducts) of the testes. Sperm development is controlled by the endocrine (hormonal) system because sperm development takes over 2 months. Illness that was present during the first cycle may affect maturity of sperms, regardless of a man's health at the time of examination.

Sperm availability

Several factors can affect sperm development and its supply for reproduction, viz. failure of testes to descend (can impair spermatogenesis), Cystic fibrosis (may cause absence of sperm, vas deferens, or seminal vesicles), Ductal obstruction (caused by repeated infections, inflammations, or developmental defect), Hemochromatosis (metabolic disorder; causes iron deposition in the testes), Hormone paucity, Drugs, Retrograde ejaculation, Sexually transmitted diseases, Sickle cell anemia, Systemic diseases (fever, infection, kidney disease, metabolic disorder; can impair spermatogenesis), Testicular cancer, Testicular trauma (damage to testes), Varicocele, etc.

Retrograde ejaculation occurs when impairment of the muscles or nerves of the bladder neck allows semen to flow backwards into the bladder, instead of ejaculation into the vagina, during 'contact'.

Testicular trauma, resulting from injury, surgery, or infection can trigger an immune response in the testes that may damage sperm. Similarly, infections of the prostate (prostatitis), epididymis (epididymitis), and testicles (orchitis), can cause irreversible infertility if they occur before puberty (see Appendix IV). It may look surprising that male may be responsible for infertility, either exclusively or along with female, in over 50% cases.

ASSESSMENT OF AN INFERTILE COUPLE

In the assessment of causes and circumstances, role of full story of illnesses since birth is important, e.g. undescended testes at birth, delayed puberty or early puberty, occurrence of mumps, injury to testes, exposure to excess oestrogens during the journey in the womb, exposure to internal toxins or polluants outside, too many X-rays or C.T. scan(s) during conception, occupational exposure to chemicals or use of drugs, e.g. chemotherapy, steroids, hormones, sulpha, nitrofurantoin, drugs of abuse or alcohol, associated medical or surgical diseases and their treatments. Even a generalized fever or illness can alter the quality of sperms or ova production. Sexual habits including frequency of intercourse, frequency of ejaculation, use of coital lubricants and the patient's understanding of the ovulatory cycle should be discussed. A history of recurrent respiratory infections and infertility may be associated with the immotility of spermatozoa due to ultrastructural defects. Loss of libido associated with headaches and visual abnormalities may suggest a pituitary tumor. Other medical problems that have been associated with infertility include thyroid

History items	Relevance in azoospermia
History of present complaint	
• Type of infertility (primary, secondary)	Secondary infertility is not congenital
• Duration of infertility	
Sexual history	
• Libido	Reflects testosterone level
• Impotence	
• Frequency of intercourse	
Medical history	
• Recent febrile illness	Depresses spermatogenesis up to 6 months
• Mumps orchitis	Testicular damage
• Venereal disease/epididymitis	Obstruction
• Renal failure	Testicular failure
• Liver failure	Hormonal abnormality
• Chemotherapy/radiotherapy	Testicular damage
• Multiple sclerosis	Ejaculatory dysfunction
• Diabetes mellitus	Ejaculatory dysfunction
• Spinal cord injury	Ejaculatory dysfunction
Surgical history	
• Orchidopexy	Indicative of previous maldescent/torsion
• Vasectomy	Obstruction
• Inguinal hernia repair	Obstruction
• Pelvic/scrotal/urethral surgery	Ejaculatory dysfunction/obstruction
• Prostatectomy	Ejaculatory dysfunction
• Retroperitoneal surgery/sympathectomy Ejaculatory dysfunction	
Testicular history	
• Maldescent	Testicular damage
• Torsion	Testicular damage
• Trauma	Testicular damage
Drug history	
• Cimetidinc	Anti-androgen
• Spironolactone	Anti-androgen
• Anabolic steroids	Inhibit pituitary gonadotrophin secretion
• Gonadotrophin-releasing Hormone agonists	Inhibit pituitary gonadotrophin secretion
• Chemotherapy	Testicular damage
Occupational and recreational exposure	
• Pesticides/herbicides/X-ray	Testicular damage
• Excess heat	Testicular damage
• Radiation	Testicular damage
• Alcohol/drug abuse	Testicular damage
Systems review	
• Headaches/visual disturbance	Pituitary tumours
• Anosmia	Kallmann's syndrome
• Galactorrhoea	Hyperprolactinaemia
• Recurrent respiratory infections	Associated with Young's syndrome
Previous management	
• Investigations	To avoid unnecessary delay or repetition
• Treatment	

disease, seizure disorders, and Liver disease. Interestingly it is not the seizure disorder itself that causes infertility but it is the typical treatment of it with Dilantin (phenytoin).

Patient's Story

The detailed history should include the duration of infertility and whether there have been pregnancies in the past (present and previous partners), as secondary infertility will effectively exclude congenital causes. Sexual history should include frequency and adequacy of intercourse and problems with erection or libido as these are suggestive of testosterone deficiency. Diminution in beard growth and decreased frequency of shaving are other manifestations of testosterone deficiency.

Complete Medical Examination

As referred earlier, fertility is not an issue, related to genitals in isolation, it concerns with whole persons of husband and wife both and their compatibility to each other.

It is better to have a good look onto the male partner and his sex organs. Examination of male and his tests is not complicated. The first look on the husband would give a feel, whether or not he looks like a 'Man', viz. properly developed sexual organs and rich distribution of hair on the face, maxillae or poor development of body frame and muscles. The overall look will be under-development and 'un-manly'. The organs like penis and scrotum will appear infantile. On the other hand, the breast development may be discernible in such a young-man. There may be varicocle in some cases. The cause of under-development may lie higher up, viz. hypothalamus or pituitary.

Hormonal defects

There can be a deficiency of one or more secretions from pituitary or hypothalamus, e.g. deficiency of LH and FSH (Kallmann's Syndrome). Isolated deficiency of LH (fertile eunuch), isolated FSH deficiency (very low sperm count). There is another syndrome called Laurence—Moon—Bardet—Biedel Syndrome, that entails mental retardation, retinitis pigmentosa, polydactyly and hypogonadism—this is due to deficiency of GnRH. In case of pituitary deficiency before puberty, the person is dwarf and does not develop sexual characteristics. When the deficiency occurs in an adult, there is impotence as well as infertility, associated with headaches and visual abnormalities. If pituitary secrets more prolactin than normal, it can affect sexual function as well as reproductive function, i.e. loss of libido as well as loss of spermatogenesis. There are several other rarer problems, which a man can develop due to defects, higher up in pituitary. Similarly, testicular dysfunction can occur due to local causes as well, e.g. defective development, infections, injuries, varicocele, etc. Any ailment, which is chronic and debilitating can lead to infertility, e.g. Kidney failure, liver cirrhosis, defective testosterone formation, diabetes, heart disease, etc.

What can go wrong with sperms?

If the sperms are formed, but either are not transported due to defect in the path or they fail to mature during passage, infertility will result. Similarly, if the sperms are not fully motile and active, they will fail to enter the female ovum and cause fertilization. Even if the sperms are normal in every manner but the male lacks sexual drive or fails to ejaculate or ejaculates too soon, fertility may be excluded.

Semen examination

Get examined the entire quantity of semen, because seminal fluid can affect sperm function and movement. Generally, three semen samples are taken at one month apart to account for variables such as temperature and error. Most specialists prefer three samples that differ no more than 20% from one another. Six sperm factors are analyzed in semen analysis: Concentration (sperm/milliliter; cc), Morphology (sperm shape; normal structure associated with sperm health), Motility (or mobility; per cent sperm movement), Standard semen fluid test (thickness, color), Total motile count (total number of moving sperm), Volume (total volume of ejaculate). If there are less than 60% normal forms, their number is less than 60 million/cmm or less than 60% actively moving Sperms, fertility is subnormal. Even men with normal reproductive tracts and normal hormone systems can have azoospermia (no sperm) due to a lack of sperm-producing tissue in the testes or an obstruction. Obstructions can be viewed with X-ray. The World Health Organization (WHO) has established criteria for normal sperm concentration, morphology, and motility. Total motile sperm count, which should be above 40 million, is calculated by multiplying volume by concentration by motility. The semen fluid test looks at factors that may impede sperm performance. Abnormally thick semen may cause sperm to swim more slowly through cervical mucus, obstructing fertilization. Abnormal sperm shape (i.e., disfigured or multiple heads or tails) usually indicates poor sperm health. Infertility is likely if 60% or more of sperm in semen is abnormally shaped.

Causes of Azoospermia

Pre-testicular azoospermia (hypogonadotrophic hypogonadism)

- Congenital (Kallmann's syndrome)
- Acquired (trauma, tumours, radiotherapy, infections, drug-induced)
- Idiopathic

Testicular azoospermia (testicular dysfunction/failure)

- Congenital (Klinefelter's syndrome, Y chromosome deletion)
- Acquired (radiotherapy, chemotherapy, torsion, mumps orchitis)

- Developmental (testicular maldescent)
- Idiopathic (most common).

Post-testicular azoospermia (ductal obstruction/dysfunction)

- Ductal obstruction in:
- Intratesticular ducts (rete testes)
- Epididymis (post-infection, trauma, surgical damage, Young's syndrome) damage during inguinal hernia repair)
- Ejaculatory duct (congenital cysts, infection, trauma, urethral surgery)
- Ejaculatory dysfunction:
- Anejaculation/retrograde ejaculation (spinal cord injury, multiple sclerosis, diabetes mellitus, bladder neck surgery, prostatectomy, sympathectomy).

Other tests are concerned specifically with sperm's ability to swim through cervical mucus and bind to and penetrate an egg. The postcoital test (PCT), or sperm-mucus interaction test, examines whether the sperm are able to swim through the specific and particular female reproductive tract. This ability is referred to as forward progression. In the middle of the menstrual cycle, the cervical mucus becomes watery. Intercourse is recommended during this time. It is followed, the next day, with an inspection of the mucus to determine if enough semen was delivered to the cervix; sperms are healthy and do not show large numbers of clumped, motionless, or dead cells; and sperm are swimming energetically through the cervical mucus. The sperm penetration assay (SPA), examines the ability of sperm to penetrate the egg by combining it with a hamster egg. The immunobead test looks at semen for the presence of antibodies that damage sperm. Post-ejaculation urinalysis may identify diseases that affect fertility, such as kidney disease, diabetes, and repeated urinary tract infection (UTI). Blood tests identify disorders that impair testosterone, FSH, LH and sperm production.

Physical examination of male

A thorough physical check up of the sub-fertile male is called for by the physician or urologist, to find the invisible causes in the system. Also examination of his genital apparatus can reveal any obvious abnormalities, e.g. testicular shape, size, regularity, epidydmis, vas-defrens, tumor, underdeveloped sex organs and other characteristics, enlarged breast, lack of testosterone, any general abnormality in development, etc. At this stage, it would also be prudent to assess any stress-related symptoms, the underlying causes of stress and the remedies thereof. Stress is an important cause of failure of fertility, when the couple may otherwise be normal.

Antisperm antibodies

Presence of such antibodies can reduce the likelihood of pregnancy. The concentration of antisperm antibodies in the semen influence the degree of impairment. They appear to interfere with sperm function by simply attaching to the plasma membrane of the spermatozoa. Sperm agglutination may be caused by antisperm antibody attachment. Infectons may lead to agglutination of sperm as well.

Immunological defect may also play a role in the pathogenesis of 10-20% cases of "unexplained infertility." It appears that tests capable of detecting antisperm antibodies on living sperms are the most direct way to determine whether significant autoimmunity to sperm exists.

PCT (Post Coital Test)

For fertilization to take place *in-vivo*, the sperm must be able to get past the cervical mucus. The post coital test assesses the ability of sperm to penetrate and progress through cervical mucus. Cervical mucus is examined 2-8 hours after intercourse at the time of expected ovulation. The presence of greater than 10-20 motile sperm per high power field is generally accepted as a normal post-coital test. Post-coital testing is an assay that provides information concerning sexual function, motility of the sperms, the sperm-mucus interaction. A positive result implies normal semen and mucus.

The test of fertilization potential

It has been found that when sperm from normal fertile men are exposed to a known solution of fructose and sodium citrate, 33-80% of the spermatozoa will exhibit swelling. Sperm that are not viable or sperm with non-functioning membranes do not swell. Attempts have been made to correlate this finding to fertilization potential of semen samples. Samples with greater than 62% swelling are able to fertilize ova, whereas less than 60% swelling is observed in samples of inferior semen. This test is currently a research tool.

Histopathological assessment of testes

In Selected cases of severe low count of sperms (normal FSH), primary spermatogenic defects cannot be differentiated from obstructive defect by hormonal investigations. Testicular biopsy may help in such cases. Before biopsy, at least two semen analysis should reveal azoospermia and retrograde ejaculation should be ruled out by examining a post-ejaculatory urine specimen. In certain case vasography may be required to rule out obstruction of the vas deferens, seminal vesicles or ejaculatory ducts.

Imaging Investigation

Color flow Doppler ultrasonography is a superior way to measure the diameters of the spermatic cord veins by imaging these vessels, as well as to quantify and qualify the flow of blood through these veins. It has been shown to be 85% sensitive in the detection of sub-clinical varicoceles. Although vasography has been used to visualize the seminal vesicles and ejaculatory ducts, transrectal ultrasonography is accurate, inexpensive and relatively non-invasive, which can provide detailed images of the seminal vesicles and ejaculatory ducts. Vasography and testicular biopsy may be necessary to rule out testicular failure or proximal obstruction if the transrectal ultrasound study is normal in the azoospermic patient.

Wife

Fertility peaks for both sexes in their mid-twenties and then appears to decline steadily in women over thirty. Also tubal infections, fibroid tumors and endometriosis are more common in older women, which are common causes for infertility. The so-called liberalization of female youth (sex with multiple partners) has played havoc with her fertility, as well as her role as a wife and mother. In a healthy woman, with regular menstrual cycles of 28-35 days, ovulation takes place once every cycle. Some women have fewer fertile periods. If uterus is retroverted, the woman should lie prone, after receiving the semen. If this does not help, surgery may be required. If there are polycystic ovaries (PCO), the conception chances are low, due to irregular ovulation. The sexual contact should be done during fertile period only. The maximum fertile day is 14 days before the onset of next menstrual bleeding.

Physical examination of wife

The assessment of an infertile female is far more elaborate process and is expensive. A good look at the female will be necessary. Whether or not she gives a feminine look? If she has an adequate breast development? What is her age, is it lower than 18 or above 35? If the distribution of hair is on a female pattern or not? If her external genitals are well developed? If her internal examination reveals the presence of normal reproductive organs? If yes, it is possible she is absolutely normal or is just sub-fertile (infertility of male has already been checked). It is also advisable to exclude any general medical or chronic ailments like diabetes or stress, which may be the underlying cause of infertility. Besides routine medical and gynaecological examination, a detailed history and evaluation of female factors will be required. Some of the factors would be common, as described for male. Age of the 'mother to be' is an important criterion in fertility assessment.

The probability of having a baby decreases about 3 to 5 percent each year after the age of 30, and at a faster rate after age 40. By age 40, a woman's chance of becoming pregnant has decreased from about 90 percent to less than 70 percent. At birth, a woman has maximum eggs. As an egg ages, it is more likely to develop a chromosomal abnormality, which may be the other cause of infertility in older women. Older women are also more likely to have other health problems that could interfere with fertility.

We have already discussed the perils of having multiple sex partners. In women, sexually transmitted infection can lead to pelvic inflammatory disease (PID) a common cause of tubal occlusion. Both smoking and alcohol intake may increase the risk of infertility in women. Body fat levels that are 10 percent to 15 percent above normal or a body mass index (BMI) of 27 or higher can impact the reproductive cycle. Obesity is also associated with the body's sensitivity to insulin, a factor, which may be the underlying cause of polycystic ovary syndrome. Similarly, body fat levels 10 percent to 15 percent below normal or a body mass index of 19 or below can shut down the reproductive process. Women at risk include those with eating disorders, such as anorexia, nervosa or bulimia, and women who exercise very intensely, prolonged exposure to high temperatures, industrial chemicals, radiation, or heavy electromagnetic emissions may reduce fertility in women. Stress situations or depression can also effect normal ovulation. In summary take note of any pelvic pain or pain on sexual contact, start a menstrual calender, get a scan of pelvis and ovaries, hormone tests as per advice, rubella antibody titre, weight reduction advice it indicated and counseling about the schedule of co-habitation in the fertile period, test of husband's semen, etc.

Investigations of the woman

Infertility investigations do not follow a rigid schedule of tests. If your periods have stopped (amenorrhoea) you will be required to undergo tests and assays. If, you have a history suggesting that your tubes may be blocked, then a tubal patency test will be required as a preliminary investigation. In most of the cases, no cause is found or none exists. Often when the gynaecologist starts some investigations or writes simple tonics, with a dose of human touch and reassurance, pregnancy occurs. It would be necessary to state that procreation is not a mechanical process, as it is made out to be. Modern working and professional couples may be engaging in sex at will or at whims, but they are neither close to each other nor share intimacy in real sense. Besides physical, it is emotional intimacy as well. Many a times, despite regular sexual union, pregnancy may fail to occur, though both the partners are in normal reproductive health, why? This can be due to the fact that they are not 'intimate couples'.

What is intimacy?

It is not merely the close union of two bodies. It pertains to liking each other, through words, gestures and encompasses tenderness, thoughtfulness, niceness, gentleness, belongingness and oneness. One small sweet gesture inspires reciprocal acts of goodwill. Offer happiness in marriage, not wealth. Luxuries and wealth alone do not bring feeling of intimacy and belonging. Your good 'Bhavna' (intentions) should match with your words and deeds at every step.

Way to intimacy

It is not through the touch of bodies, during conjugal love alone. Think "I reached over, took his hand and squeezed it, and he squeezed back." That hand on back at a dinner party when you knows he is bored. That hug of encouragement as he gives you when you're heading off to a interview. That skin-to-skin sensation is powerful. Physically and chemically, it binds you and makes you feel closer. Forget grand gestures: Think little, personal and sweet. It's a great feeling to know that you're together. The etiquates hold good for all, including yourself. Don't interrupt; say 'please', "thank you", and "I am sorry" when required. Saying 'thank you' when she gets you a glass of water, or 'sorry' when you lose your temper, is such an effortless way to show kindness to each other. It's also a matter of dropping impolite habits. If you have a reason to admire your spouse do not hesitate to express. Do not keep your nice thoughts about husband to your-self. A reminder that we're wise, good looking or fun loving from the person whose opinion we value most—can be all we need to get over self-doubt.

So instead of getting anxious, focus on cheering him up, surprising him with a dinner or gift or just a hug. This can set an optimistic tone for the couple. When your husband is tense, worried, feeling low, do not add to his foul mood. It is this feeling of closeness and kindness, which can break the silence of infertility, with the sweet cry of your baby, in due course. In addition to assuring intimacy one can start with simple investigations and go on to more sophisticated ones, if required.

Basal Body Temperature (B.B.T.)

Keeping a record of your basal body temperature (B.B.T.) is an inexpensive and easy way to determine when and whether you are ovulating. A woman's basal body temperature drops briefly and then rises half a degree following ovulation, and remains elevated until the start of the next period. Maintain a chart. Each chart represents a cycle. The cycle begins from the first day of a period (day 1 of the chart), and continues until the next period begins. When you have completed the first chart, you then commence a new chart. Your body temperature is recorded on the chart when you wake up every morning. The points representing different temperatures are joined up to make a graph. The best temperature charts take the form of a display sheet making up six cycles. Normal BBT is between 96 and 98 degrees. This temperature rises to 97 and 98 degrees after ovulation. If this rise in temperature persists for at least 3 days, it means that ovulation has taken place. The temperature then remains raised until it falls once more with the onset of next period. If there is no ovulation, it will remain low. Maintain the chart for 3 months. During luteal phase, i.e. 2nd half of cycle the temperature should remain high for 11 days. If there is no ovulation, treatment will be required.

New Test Kits

Now some test kits are available, which you can use yourself and predict when ovulation is going to occur in the next 24 hours. The test measures the level of Luteinizing Hormone (L.H.) in an early morning urine sample by using a specially designed urine dipstick, which changes colour when exposed to increasing amounts of L.H. Ovulation is preceded by a surge in the level of L.H. When the L.H.-surge occurs there is an easily detectable colour change indicating that ovulation is likely to occur within the next 24 hours. Intercourse during this period has a good chance of resulting in conception. As a matter of interest, you could check if the temperature rise indicated in your B.B.T. chart occurs just after you get a positive result in your ovulation predictor. The fact that you can tell in advance that you are going to ovulate, reduces the trial and error element in the process of trying to conceive.

Rubella Antibody Test

Rubella is a mild illness in terms of its symptoms, but can be dangerous for a pregnant woman because the Rubella virus could cause severe abnormalities in the baby. So vaccination against rubella is a must for every woman, before pregnancy is considered. Do not take vaccination, if pregnancy has already occurred. Six to eight weeks after the vaccination, a repeat antibody screening test is carried out to check on your response to the vaccine. If immunity is present, consider pregnancy only after that.

PCT (Post-Coital Test)

It was mentioned earlier in assessing the fertility of male. It assesses the ability of sperm to reach the canal of the cervix and survive in the mucus. One of the signs that a woman is ovulating is that there is a noticeable change in the mucus secretion. At the time of ovulation, the ovaries produce more estrogen as a result of which the mucus secreted by the cervix of the uterus becomes very profuse, clear and watery like saliva. The cervical mucus also becomes more receptive to sperm. A completely normal post-coital test will show very flowing "stretchable" mucus containing a significant number of moving sperms. The sperms must be normal in appearance and moving across the slide and not simply shaking on the spot. A post-coital test is considered negative if no sperm or only dead sperms are found in the mucus. Conception may be impossible. If your post-coital test is found to be negative. It will probably be repeated.

Hormonal assessment

It is often essential to measure the levels of the various hormones in the body, which play essential part in ovulation process. Assays of prolactin. F.S.H., LH estrogen and thyroid hormone levels can be very useful in indicating the cause of your problem. A low progesterone level at day 21 of a 28 day cycle indicates that normal ovulation in this cycle has not occurred. Those with low thyroid functions, raised prolactin level or raised LH level will need the help of an endocrinologist also.

Certain observations may help in fertility evaluation : (i) Lower level of uterine amylase or elevated level of acid phosphatase can lead to lower fertility. This signifies that uterine environment is non-conducive to sperm capacitation, (ii) Use of general anaesthesia in the intervention for GIFT, will have an inhibiting effect on sperm motility, (iii) Over expression of LH (raised level of LH) can lead to infertility as well as increased miscarriage and also is a cause for PCOs, and (iv) Ageing leads to higher fetal loss and the possibility rises from 18 years onwards, as found by serial HCG studies (a placental hormone).

Endometrial Biopsy

The biopsy is generally done 2-3 days before the expected period. A fine suction curette is gently inserted into the uterus to take out small amount of tissue from the inside lining of uterus. It is performed as an OPD test. A biopsy of the endometrium will determine whether its stage of development is in line with the stage of the cycle. If there is a lag of more than 2 days, (e.g. on 26th day of the cycle the endometrium has the maturity of only a 23-day cycle), it may indicate insufficient secretion of progesterone. This could be a possible cause of infertility.

Tubal Patency

We had mentioned earlier that fertilization occurs in the tube, where ovum is present to receive sperm. If it is blocked no conception can occur. Tubal patency tests are undertaken when we suspect that there are blockages in the fallopian tubes. These tests include procedures like Gas Insufflation, Hysterosalpingography (H.S.G.), Laparoscopy, etc. The cause of tubal block and pelvic adhesions is previous infections. Under the cause of Infection can be peritonitis from acute appendicitis, previous abortion, miscarriage or difficult delivery, tubal ligation, STDs, etc. About 15% of women attending any infertility clinic will have a tubal problem.

Gas insufflations involves insertion of a canula into the canal of the cervix and blowing in of carbon dioxide gas into the cavity of the uterus. There will be an increase in pressure of the gas within the uterus, if the tubes are blocked. If the tubes are open, the initial rise in pressure is followed by a sudden reduction as the gas escapes along the tubes and into the abdominal cavity. Since it is not reliable, it is not generally done. Now hysterosalpingography (H.S.G.) is commonly done. Here a special radio-opaque dye is injected into the cavity of the uterus. The dye shows up on an X-ray screen and the doctor is able to see the fluid filling the uterus and then passing along both tubes to enter the cavity of the abdomen. If the dye fails to enter the tubes this may indicate an obstruction. The H.S.G. can pinpoint the site of any tubal obstruction and can also show the presence of any irregularity in the shape of the cavity of the uterus.

Laproscopy is like a telescope, a newer modality, through, which one can see uterus, tubes and ovaries. The presence of adhesions either around the tubes or tethering the ovaries can be easily detected, and their significance assessed. Other pelvic problems such as endometriosis and fibroids will also be revealed. Tubal patency is tested by injecting methylene blue dye into the uterus through the cervix. If the tubes are healthy, the dye can be seen passing along them and escaping through the outer openings of the tubes. The great advantage of laparoscopy over H.S.G. is that it allows the surgeon to have a direct view of the pelvic organs and thereby permits a more accurate assessment of tubal patency and any tubal or ovarian problems.

HOW TO RESTORE FERTILITY?

If a cause could be identified the same will have to be tackled on specific guidelines. If only weak health or poor sex access are the problems, these will have to be corrected. If there is no ovulation or if the ovulation is not regular, drugs can be given to stimulate ovulation. The most common drug is clomiphene; the fertility pill. This safe and effective drug stimulates the ovaries to produce ova. Other treatments include fertility shots, such as human Menopausal Gonadotropin (hMG), and a drug that stimulates the pituitary gland, i.e. Gonadotropin-releasing Hormone (GnRH). Surgery is used to correct any defects of the reproductive tract, both in the male and female.

Modern trends

You have noted a lot of hype about test-tube babies, intra-fallopian transfer, intracytoplasmic sperm injection, etc. but the success rate is disappointing. May be future is promising. *In-vitro* fertilisation and embryo transfer (IVF-ET) and gamete intrafallopian transfer (GIFT) are recently introduced treatments. With IVF-ET, the ovaries are stimulated with drugs to produce several ripe eggs at the same time. The eggs are then removed through laproscope, usually under local anaesthesia, using ultrasound to guide a catheter through the vagina into the abdominal cavity. The eggs are incubated under special conditions and then the sperm is added. Fertilisation occurs in the laboratory, resulting in a test-tube baby. Next, several of the pre-embryos are placed through the cervix into the uterine cavity. This improves the chance of success but also increases the chances of multiple pregnancies. With GIFT, the ovaries are stimulated with drugs, and the eggs are removed using a laparoscope. Then the mixture of eggs and sperm is placed into the fallopian tubes. Open fallopian tubes are necessary for GIFT, but not for IVF-ET. If extra pre-embryos are formed after removing the eggs and processing them, the pre-embryos are sometimes frozen and later transferred into the uterus during future cycles. Another recently developed treatment is intracytoplasmic sperm injection (ICSI), which only requires one sperm to achieve a pregnancy. This treatment can be used for cases in, which the male sperm count is very low, the woman has endometriosis or in cases of unexplained infertility. The success rates for the recently discovered therapeutic modalities are improving. At present, this looks most promising. Counseling and psychotherapy is also essential in the treatment of infertility.

Those with pelvic pain, excessive menstrual bleeding or pain on sexual contact need early referral to a sterility centre.

Interventions in case of male infertility : While details of medical or surgical procedures to correct male sterility would be beyond the scope of this write up, we will mention certain interventions, which will be useful, as a matter of awareness.

(i) Hormone therapy

Since hormones are essential to cause sperm formation and their maturation, any deficiency of hormones can cause infertility and treatment with hormones can undo infertility. There may be deficiency of testosterone secretion from Leydig cells of testes. Give HCG (Pregnyl or profasi-2000 IU). It can be three time a week followed with FSH therapy, as hMG. Pergonal contains 75 IU of FSH and 75 IU of LH per vial, given it three times weekly. It takes months for sperm to appear in the ejaculate after initiation of therapy. An alternative is the use of GnRH is to stimulate LH and FSH secretion. GnRH must be given in a pulsatile manner. The initial dosage is 25-50 ng/kilogram every two hours in a small infusion pump. Both the gonadotropins and GnRH are expensive.

(ii) Treatment for antisperm antibodies

Treatment is difficult. Use of immunosuppressive agents and corticosteroids is risky and generally not effective. Innovative methods of semen manipulation have also been attempted. These have included immediate dilution and washing of the semen following ejaculation, use of sperm surface fragments as immuno-absorbants to remove "unbound" antibody.

This method has also been ineffective. Semen processing and intrauterine insemination have become increasingly popular, but still success is not optimal.

(iii) Varicocelectomy

It is the most common surgical procedure for infertility in males. This operation improves semen quality in about two-thirds of men. It doubles the chance of conception, in those who have been suffering from varicocele and have been now operated.

(iv) Electro-ejaculation

This procedure can be used to produce ejaculation when neurological dysfunction prevents it. An electrical rectal probe generates a current that stimulates nerves and induces ejaculation; semen dribbles out through the urethra and is collected.

(v) Sperm retrieval

This technique is used to obtain sperm from the testes or epididymis when obstruction, congenital absence of the vas deferens, failed vasectomy reversal, or inadequate sperm production causes azoospermia. Using a technique called micro-epididymal sperm aspiration (MESA), a surgeon makes an incision in the scrotum and gathers sperm from the epididymis.

(vi) Sperm washing

This procedure isolates and prepares the healthiest sperm for insemination. Sperm retrieved by various ways may be used in *in-vitro* fertilization (IVF) and intracytoplasmic sperm injection (ICSI).

(vii) Intracytoplasmic sperm injection (ICSI)

Using a tiny glass needle, one sperm is injected directly into a retrieved mature egg, (outside the body) in a laboratory. The egg is incubated and transferred back to the uterus. Fertilization occurs in 50% to 80% of cases and approximately 30% result in a live birth.

(viii) Gamete intrafallopian transfer (GIFT)

This procedure is recommended for couples with unexplained fertility problems and normal reproductive anatomy. Mature eggs and prepared sperm are combined in a syringe and injected into the fallopian tube using laparascopy. Embryos that result from this procedure naturally descend into the uterus for implantation.

(ix) There are several other surgical procedures, which are sometimes required, e.g. reversal of vasectomy, transuretheral resection of ejaculatory duct, microsurgical epididymal sperm aspiration (MESA), ablation of pituitary adenoma, correction of undescended testes and several others. There success rate varies from 5 to 30%. These are difficult and expensive, may be tried in desperate cases.

Interventions for female infertility

Some of the interventions mentioned under male infertility will apply to female also. Basically you can have: (i) Medication to improve fertility, (ii) Surgery to correct a defect, (iii) Insemination of donor or husband's washed sperm, and (iv) Egg donation. These are some of the lines of action that one may follow:

(i) Follicular Tracking (sonography pinpoints the release of the egg), (ii) Hormone therapy (clomiphene citrate and bromocritptine help induce ovulation), (iii) Artificial Insemination by Husband, (iv) Pooled Insemination (to concentrate the semen and pick up best sperms), (v) Split Ejaculate (first and richest part of the ejaculate), and (vi) Intra Uterine Insemination (to collect the fittest specimens from the husband or a donor).

In such cases, the donor is checked for health, family history, fertility, physical characteristics, blood group, AIDS and other STDs. This is called TID, i.e. Therapeutic Insemination by Donor.

Other techniques of ART (Assisted Reproduction Techniques) are:

IVF (In-vitro fertilization)

It can be used in cases of fallopian tube block, endometriosis or where the cause of female infertility is unexplained. It involves fertilization of ovum outside the body, using drugs to produce more eggs, putting husband's or donor's sperm with the eggs, incubation in a dish, insertion back of the fertilized egg, into the tubes or uterus. When the fertilized egg (Gamette) is transferred to fallopian tube, it is called GIFT (Gamete Intra Fallopian Transfer). Presently, several variations of GIFT have been born, e.g. pronuclear stage tubal transfer (PROST), zygote intrafallopian transfer (ZIFT), tubal embryo transfer (TET) and tubal embryo stage transfer (TEST). These involve the *in-vitro* fertilization of human eggs followed by transfer of the embryo back into the fallopian tube.

Gonadotrophin treatment

Chronic anovulation is still a major cause of female infertility (up to 30%) and is also being treated with FSH, when repeated treatment with clomiphene citrate does not result in pregnancy. Most patients suffer from Polycystic Ovary (PCO) syndrome. However, clomiphene has been associated with significant side effects, which might make the use of gonadotrophins as first-line treatment, a realistic alternative. Traditional gonadotrophin preparations are derived from large amounts of postmenopausal (FSH and LH) or pregnancy urine (hCG), which is associated with a considerable number of disadvantages.

Disadvantages of urinary gonadotrophin preparations

- Low purity (< 5%).
- No absolute source control.
- Cumbersome collection of urine.
- FSH always with LH contamination.
- Batch-to-batch inconsistency.
- Low specific activity.

Only the highly purified urinary FSH preparations have a higher purity and specific activity. Certain drug houses have developed FSH, by transfecting Chinese hamster ovary cell lines with plasmids containing the two subunit genes encoding FSH.

Characteristics of Developed FSH

- High purity.
- High specific activity (± 10,000 IU/mg protein).
- Identical amino-acid sequence compared to natural FSH.
- No contamination with urinary proteins of undetermined origin.
- No LH activity.

FSH is indicated for the treatment of female infertility in the following clinical situations : Anovulation (including polycystic ovarian disease, PCOD) in women who have been unresponsive to treatment with clomiphene citrate. Controlled ovarian hyperstimulation to induce the development of multiple follicles in medically assisted reproduction programmes (e.g. *in-vitro* fertilization/embryo transfer [IVF/ET], gamete intrafallopian transfer [GIFT], and intracytoplasmic sperm injection [ICSI].

Contraindications include tumours of ovary, breasts, uterus, pituitary or hypothalamus; pregnancy or lactation; undiagnosed vaginal bleeding; hypersensitivity to any of the substances in the preparation, primary ovarian failure; ovarian cysts or enlarged ovaries, not related to polycystic ovarian disease (PCOD); malformations of the sexual organs incompatible with pregnancy; fibroid tumours of the uterus incompatible with pregnancy.

Follicular development at the beginning of each cycle is believed to only occur if serum FSH concentrations exceed a certain threshold. The number of follicles to ovulate is determined by the length of time that the level of FSH remains above this. The role of LH in follicular development is limited.

Infections

Individuals with genitourinary tract infection should be treated with the appropriate antibiotics. Tetracycline is often the first line drug.

Micromanipulation

Micromanipulation of gametes and assisted fertilization allows the surgical manipulation of sperm and ova. The methods of micromanipulation currently utilized include partial zone dissection (PZD), subzonal sperm injection (SZI) and intracytoplasmic sperm injection (ICSI). Overall, fertilization rates range from a 20-40%, with clinical pregnancy rates reports as high as 30%. In case of ICSI, the best sperm is isolated and injected into an isolated egg. This raises a lot of hope for those couples, where the sperm count of the husband is very low. Lazer Assisted Hatching is used for the eggs of older women and other women, whose eggs have thick outer coating. The coating is removed with laser and the egg is harvested in a dish and allowed fertilization with sperms.

Management of Endometriosis

This condition leads to reduced conception rates at all levels. It interferes with ovarian mobility, release of ovum, tube patency, etc. Treatment with FSH or surgery or laproscopic surgery does help in some cases. Overall the treatment is not satisfactory.

Treatment for PCOs (Polycystic Ovarian Syndrome)

In such cases LH secretion is higher than normal. Obese women should be encouraged to lose weight. After that use of clomiphene or tamoxifen is recommended. It may help in 70-80% cases to induce ovulation and lead to successful pregnancy in 40% cases. Laproscopic ovarian surgery is now, the treatment of choice (70-80% ovulation), where medicine treatment does not help. In some cases diathermy or laser ablation of ovary may be done. The lowest possible dose of medicine or laser should be used (see Appendix II).

Correction of Tubal Blockage

Tubal block of fallopian tubes either due to adhesions, spasm of the opening of uterus to the tube (tubal osteum) or due to surgical ligation is fairly common cause of infertility. It is possible than the investigation called hysterosapingography (HSG), may open the tubes. Recannulization, wherever required, is usually a painless procedure. It can be done as a hysteroscopy procedure or as a laparoscopy. In case of spasm, your tubes were never really blocked. That is one of the problems, which a regular HSG would not detect. If you are scared or in pain, the tubes go into spasm and they appear to be blocked when actually they are not. Sometimes the adhesions and debris can be dislodged with catheter and wire. Sometimes a balloon catheter to dilate the tubes may be required. 85-90% of women will have at least one tube opened. 60% will remain open at 6 months if rechecked. 30-40% will conceive. If one tube is already open, recannulization of the other is not likely to improve the chances of pregnancy, so it may not be attempted to open. Recannulization entails some risks and complications.

Some observations

(i) Tubal transfer of cryo preserved embryo may prove to be optimal ART, in cases of tube block. The success rate has been found to be higher in tubal transfer than uterine transfer.

(ii) Cumulus removal and addition of follicular fluid (FF) (without micromanipulation), leads to better contact of sperm to oocytes and improved sperm motility and thus greater success in fertilization.

(iii) If HSG is normal, study of other structures than tubes and uterus, with the help of a laproscopy and hysteroscopy is called for. HSG can still be done, now as treatment.

(iv) If the underlying cause of infertility is tubal damage, the chances of ectopic pregnancy rise even with ART.

(v) Negative PCT result is common in cases of infertility. *In-vitro* cervical mucus-sperm interaction can check cross-hostiliy. More often it is the cervical mucus hostility, which is responsible for failure of fertility. Stimulation with oestrogen makes the mucus thin.

Hasty use of ART is not called for : There is good news and that is most healthy couples worried about infertility after a year of trying, can conceive during the second year. The couples should be patient and doctors should not intervene too fast with assisted reproductive techniques (ART), unless there are known reasons for a couple not conceiving naturally within a year or two. The cause of decline in fertility with ageing of woman (30-40 years) is primarily due to decline in the per menstrual cycle conception rate and not to an increase in the proportion of couples unable to achieve an unassisted pregnancy. If male partner is over 40 the chances of conception decline further. There is clear increase with age in the number of menstrual cycles needed to achieve pregnancy and in the probability of being classified as clinically infertile (a definition applied after a year of trying to conceive). There is a large amount of normal variability in fertility and many couples having below average, but normal fertility may fail to conceive within a year. This is particularly true for older couples, many of whom fail to conceive within the first year but are successful in the second. Fertility treatment, such as IVF and ICSI, can result in an increased risk of multiple pregnancies, pregnancy complications, low birth weight, major birth defects and long-term disability among surviving infants. In addition, the chance of success with ART decreases with age, while the side effects increase in prevalence. Give nature a chance for a longer period and intervene only if there is a definite cause, which can be dealt with ART or Chinese medicine or any other effort.

SECONDARY INFERTILITY

Secondary infertility is defined as the inability to conceive or maintain a pregnancy after having successfully done so before, and is thought to be more common than primary infertility. Secondary infertility takes most people by complete surprise. For one who have easily conceived, carried, and delivered a baby suddenly finds herself wondering about her fertility to her complete bewilderment.

Emotional Aspects

In most cases, people who have children already and find they are having trouble conceiving or carrying again, report a lack of empathy and misunderstanding from family, friends, and acquaintances who express well-intentioned but hurtful opinions. Secondary infertility also brings with it a new kind of guilt: the guilt for feeling that one child "isn't enough." Folks who have experienced primary infertility and then miscarried are also considered to be in this group. Anyone who conceives relatively easily yet experiences recurrent miscarriage is also categorized as "secondary." Seeking the support of others who have been through it can help shield one from grief and confusion.

Medical Aspects

Many will feel a strong loyalty to their OB/Gynecologist, if it is the same doctor who was associated with prior deliveries. Secondaries should follow the same general rule as primaries, that is, seek specialty care if one year of well-timed intercourse doesn't result in a pregnancy. The transition to a specialist may be difficult emotionally, resulting in a feeling of betraying the gynecologist, but could very well result in correction of any new or previously unknown problems.

Always consider, the ageing reproductive system to be a possible factor. Usual basic work-up of 3 hormones (TSH, FSH, estradiol and sometimes prolactin and LH), semen analysis and hysterosalpingogram is required. Sometimes one finds a couple in which the woman has never really ovulated regularly but who had conceived "easily" in the first instance. They have just been very lucky and probably more sexually active in the beginning of their marriage. Now that they have the 2-3 year old child at home creating a possible interruption or other problems, they just don't have sex often enough to catch the infrequent ovum.

A case of secondary infertility requires as much attention as that of primary infertility and possibly more empathy and more careful investigations, to find the cause. Quite often the society looks at a couple with secondary infertility, with amusement and ridicule.

ADOPTION CAN ERASE THE PLIGHT OF INFERTILITY

Yes, it can, and not a very difficult option, when so many unwed mothers are around! One can never imagine that the plight of infertility and the associated feelings of denial deficiency, defect, want, immense grief, sadness and other low feelings would miraculously turn into a blessing of our lives with adoption. Adoptive parents, who have been waiting awhile to be chosen should be careful not to give way to feelings of inadequacy and inferiority. Adoptive patients should keep in mind that there is a child meant for them; it just may not have been conceived yet.

Families wanting to adopt have "adoption anonymity." Such Parents are looking for a child who resembles the child they wish they could have had by birth—a young, healthy infant of good potential, who looks like them—and their fantasy is that this child will then be "theirs" in the same sense that a biological child would have been. They do not emphasize the fact that their child is adopted, but rather wish to blend into the community and be viewed and treated like any other family.

With adoption the perspective of the adoptive parents change dramatically. It takes some time to get adopted to the new find. There are many emotional upheaves in the minds and many uncertainties at hand. First of all it is the "apprehension" phase, where the question of the adoptive parents is, Can we keep and look-after our child? After quite some time the "integration" phase starts that extends for the rest of the lives of all, who are part of that adoption. During these phases, the adoptive family is coping with the "regular" development tasks of the child, which they have adopted legally, but may take a long time to accept it emotionally.

The emotional right grows out of the parent's increasing comfort with their roles as mother or father to the child. Next is the mutual process by, which the adoptive family and the adopted child come to feel that they belong to each other. The process usually begins when the adopted parents find similarities between the child's appearance or habits. A dairy prepared by the adoptive family is a useful device in family assessment and preparation. Like the genogram or eco-map, such a dairy serves as a way of helping a family focus on aspects of its own history and family dynamics that may be important to consider in terms of adoption. Remember, adoption is not uncommon, and one need not feel nervous about it. For several reasons, adoption is increasing and it need not be considered unnatural. Couples now wait longer to have children, and they often find it more difficult to conceive and carry a healthy baby to term when they reach the age at which they feel ready to be parents. Many researchers believe that long-term use of the IUD and the pill have contributed to this increasing incidence of infertility. Let adoption be taken as a natural alternative for an infertile but willing couple.

One should go ahead for adoption, soon after it dawns on the prospective mother and father that their own biological conception is excluded by the gynecologist. Don't wait until old age for adoption. You can give your best to the child's growth and development only, if you, yourself are in sound physical, mental and financial health.

FREQUENTLY ASKED QUETSIONS (FAQ)

Q: What is Infertility?

Ans. Infertility is a disease of the reproductive system that impairs one of the body's most basic functions: the conception of children. Conception is a complicated process that depends upon many factors: on the production of healthy sperm by the man and healthy eggs by the woman; unblocked fallopian tubes that allow the sperm to reach the egg; the sperm's ability to fertilize the egg when they meet; the ability of the fertilized egg (embryo) to become implanted in the woman's uterus; and sufficient embryo quality.

Finally, for the pregnancy to continue to full term, the embryo must be healthy and the woman's hormonal environment adequate for its development. When just one of these factors is impaired, infertility can result.

Q: What Causes Infertility?

Ans. No one can be blamed for infertility any more than anyone is to blame for diabetes or leukemia. In rough terms, about one-third of infertility cases can be attributed to male factors, and about one-third to factors that affect women. For the remaining one-third of infertile couples, infertility is caused by a combination of problems in both partners or, in about 20 percent of such cases, it is unexplained.

The most common male infertility factors include azoospermia (no sperm cells are produced) and oligospermia (few sperm cells are produced). Sometimes, sperm cells are malformed or they die before they can reach the egg. In rare cases, infertility in men is caused by a genetic disease such as cystic fibrosis or a chromosomal abnormality.

The most common female infertility factor is an ovulation disorder. Other causes of female infertility include blocked fallopian tubes, which can occur when a woman has had pelvic inflammatory disease or endometriosis (a sometimes painful condition causing adhesions and cysts). Congenital anomalies (birth defects) involving the structure of the uterus and uterine fibroids are associated with repeated miscarriages.

Q: How is Infertility Diagnosed?

Ans. Couples are generally advised to seek medical help if they are unable to achieve pregnancy after a year of unprotected intercourse. The doctor will conduct a physical examination of both partners to determine their general state of health and to evaluate physical disorders that may be causing infertility. Usually both partners are interviewed about their sexual habits in order to determine whether intercourse is taking place properly for conception.

If no cause can be determined at this point, more specific tests may be recommended. For women, these include an analysis of body temperature and ovulation, X-ray of the fallopian tubes and uterus, and laparoscopy. For men, initial tests focus on semen analysis.

Q: How is Infertility Treated?

Ans. Most infertility cases—85 to 90 percent—are treated with conventional therapies, such as drug treatment or surgical repair of reproductive organs.

Q: What is *In-Vitro* Fertilization?

Ans. In infertile couples where women have blocked or absent fallopian tubes, or where men have low sperm counts, *in-vitro* fertilization (IVF) offers a chance at parenthood to couples who until recently would have had no hope of having a "biologically related" child.

In IVF, eggs are surgically removed from the ovary and mixed with sperm outside the body in a Petri dish ("in-vitro" is Latin for "in glass"). After about 40 hours, the eggs are examined to see if they have become fertilized by the sperm and are dividing into cells. These fertilized eggs (embryos) are then placed in the women's uterus, thus bypassing the fallopian tubes.

IVF has received a great deal of media attention since it was first introduced in 1978, but it actually accounts for less than five percent of all infertility treated in the United States.

Q: Is *In-Vitro* Fertilization (IVF) Expensive?

Ans. The average cost of an IVF cycle in the United States is $12,400.

Like other extremely delicate medical procedures, IVF involves highly trained professionals with sophisticated laboratories and equipment, and the cycle may need to be repeated to be successful. While IVF and other assisted reproductive technologies are not inexpensive, they account for only three hundredths of one percent (0.03%) of U.S. healthcare costs.

Q: Does *In-Vitro* Fertilization Work?

Ans. Yes. IVF was introduced in the United States in 1981 and from 1985 through 1998 ASRM and its affiliate, the Society for Assisted Reproductive Technology (SART), have counted more than 91,000 births of babies conceived through IVF. Through the end of 2000, more than 212,000 babies have been born in the US as a result of reported ART procedures. IVF currently accounts for about 98% of procedures with GIFT, ZIFT and combination procedures making up the remainder. The average live delivery rate for IVF in 1998 was 29.1 per cent per retrieval—a little better than the 20 per cent chance in any given month that a reproductively healthy couple has of achieving a pregnancy and carrying it to term.

Q: Do Insurance Plans Cover Infertility Treatment?

Ans. The degree of services covered depends on where you live and the type of insurance plan you have. Fourteen states currently have laws that require insurers to either cover or offer to cover some form of infertility diagnosis and treatment. Those states are Arkansas, California, Connecticut, Hawaii, Illinois, Maryland, Massachusetts, Montana, New Jersey, New York, Ohio, Rhode Island, Texas and West Virginia. However, the laws vary greatly in their scope of what is and is not required to be covered. For more information about the specific laws for each of those states.

The desire to have children and be parents is one of the most fundamental aspects of being human. People should not be denied insurance coverage for medically appropriate treatment to fulfil this goal.

Q: Does sexual position matter for fertility?

Ans. In general, when a healthy man and a healthy woman are trying to conceive and if they're both fertile and reproductively "normal", then the position in which they engage sexually, doesn't matter. The healthy sperm must be deposited as close as possible to the woman's cervix when it comes to getting pregnant.

To achieve the deposition of sperms at the opening of cervix, sexual positions that are not conducive to conception are Sitting, Standing, Female on top, Bending over, etc. The natural position for conjugal union is lying down, with male over female. After ejaculation the female should preferably lie down for ½ hour on her back. If her uterus is retroverted then let her lie with face downwards, after intercourse.

Q. How the Infertility occurs?

Ans. Infertility is not a simple inconvenience to the couple, nor it is an application of family planning methods, it is the failure of the reproductive system that impairs the conception of children. Conception is a complicated process that depends upon many factors, viz. production of healthy sperms by the man and healthy eggs by the woman; unblocked fallopian tubes that allow the sperm to reach the egg; the sperm's ability to fertilize the egg when they meet; the ability of the fertilized egg (embryo) to become implanted in the woman's uterus; and good embryo quality. Finally, for the pregnancy to continue to full term, the embryo must be healthy and the woman's hormonal environment adequate for its development. When just any one of these factors is impaired, infertility can result. Infertility affects 10-15% of the population of the reproductive age group.

Q. Woman only is responsible for Infertility?

Ans. About one-third of infertility cases can be attributed to defect in male factors, and about one-third to factors that affect women. For the remaining one-third of infertile couples, infertility is caused by a combination of problems in both partners or, of unexplained origin. Common male infertility factors include azoospermia (no sperm cells are produced) and oligospermia (few sperm cells are produced). Sometimes, sperm cells are malformed or they die before they can reach the egg. In rare cases, infertility in men is caused by a genetic disease such as cystic fibrosis or a chromosomal abnormality. Common female infertility factor is an ovulation disorder. Other causes of female infertility include blocked fallopian tubes, which can occur when a woman has had pelvic inflammatory disease or endometriosis (a sometimes painful condition causing adhesions and cysts). Congenital anomalies (birth defects) involving the structure of the uterus and uterine fibroids are associated with repeated miscarriages.

Q. When is Infertility diagnosed?

Ans. When couples are unable to achieve pregnancy after a year of unprotected intercourse, it is called infertility. The doctor will conduct a physical examination of both partners to determine their general state of health and to evaluate physical disorders that may be causing infertility. Usually both partners are interviewed about their sexual habits in order to determine whether unprotected, unhindered and regular intercourse is taking place.

Q. Does the frequency of sexual act matters?

Ans. Yes, it does. The contact should be regular, but not too much indulgence. It must occur during fertile period, i.e. 12th to 16th of cycle. Woman would not get pregnant if she has sex during or soon after their menstrual periods or in the first 8 or last 8 days of cycle. Too frequent sex or too infrequent sexual encounters will lower the fertility.

If you wait for a week or longer before ejaculating, you may be delivering poor quality sperm. In a man with a fully-functioning reproductive system, new sperms are always being produced and a sexual encounter on an alternative night may be more productive.

Q. How is Infertility treated?

Ans. Most infertility cases respond to conservative methods, i.e. advice about fertile period, sleep, rest, exercise, stress, tonics reassurance, etc. Some require drug treatment or surgical repair of reproductive organs.

Q. What is block of tubes?

Ans. Where woman has blocked fallopian tubes, or where men have low sperm counts, *in vitro* fertilization (IVF) offers a chance at parenthood to couples, who until recently would have had no hope of having a child. In IVF, eggs are surgically removed from the ovary and mixed with sperm outside the body in a test tube. After about 40 hours, the eggs are examined to see if they have become fertilized by the sperm and are dividing into cells. These fertilized eggs (embryos) are then placed in the women's uterus, thus bypassing the fallopian tubes.

Q. Why is *In-Vitro* Fertilization Expensive?

Ans. The average cost of an IVF runs into lakhs of rupees. Like other extremely delicate medical procedures, IVF involves highly trained professionals with sophisticated laboratories and equipment, and the cycle may need to be repeated to be successful.

Q. How long bleeding lasts after an abortion?

Ans. The bleeding will probably continue for about 7-10 days, tailing off toward the end of this time. It shouldn't be heavier than a period, and shouldn't have an offensive odour. Normally your next period will come by 6 weeks or so. If they were irregular before, then it may be longer. Also, your fertility returns before your next period, so if you feel pregnant again a pregnancy test might be required.

Q. I had a D&C—will this cause any problems?

Ans. A D&C (dilatation and curettage) or evacuation is carried out to reduce the chance of infection and ensure that you don't continue bleeding over the following weeks. Very rarely, it can cause infection of the womb lining with persistent discharge or an offensive odour. It is wiser to remain under supervision for 6 weeks, of your doctor if D and C is done. The D&C doesn't weaken your cervix or make you more likely to miscarry in subsequent pregnancies.

Q. How common is miscarriage?

Ans. It is possible that as many as 50% of pregnancies miscarry (even the victim is unaware) before implantation in the womb occurs. Early after implantation, pregnancy loss rate is about 30% (ie this is still before a pregnancy is clinically recognised). After a pregnancy is recognised (between days 35-50), about 25% will end in miscarriage. The risk of miscarriage decreases dramatically after the 8th week as the weeks go by.

Q. Why should I suffer from recurrent miscarriage?

Ans. Many women miscarry more than once in their life. Considering the frequency of miscarriage, about 1 in 36 women will have 2 miscarriages due to nothing more than chance. Any miscarriages after that might prompt your doctors to suggest some tests to ensure that it isn't happening for some other reason.

Miscarriage may be more common after a previous miscarriage, or less common following previously normal pregnancies. The risk of miscarriage is related to the past pregnancy history in the following way:

First pregnancy	5%
Last pregnancy terminated	6%
Last pregnancy a live birth	5%
All pregnancies live births	4%
1. previous miscarriage	20%
2. previous miscarriages	28%
3. previous miscarriages	43%

Q. What may contribute to early pregnancy loss?

Ans. Multiple pregnancy, maternal age (over the age of 40 it is 23.1%), poorly controlled diabetes, scleroderma, fever over 100F, smoking (30-50% increased risk), previous contraceptive pill use (slight reduction in the risk of miscarriage), occupational exposure to solvents increases the risk of miscarriage

Q. When can the couple start trying again after a miscarriage?

Ans. It is normally recommend that you await your first period after going home, and begin trying after that. There is evidence that the risk of miscarriage in the next pregnancy is about 1.5 times higher if one cycle does not intervene the pregnancies.

Q. What can I do to improve my chances of pregnancy?

Ans. Taking in regular exercise, a healthy diet, reducing stress and getting your weight to within normal limits gives you something to concentrate on, and improves chances for long-term fertility. Certainly reducing your alcohol intake and stopping smoking will help, too. Remember to start taking folic acid to help normal development of the baby's nervous system.

Q. Doctors talk of type I defect and type II defect, what does it mean?

Ans. Embryos implant in the endometrium of uterus on 5th day of the ovulation (20-24th day of menstrual cycle. In type I defect (Luteal phase)

defect is in hormones. Ovulation may not occur or menses are defective. In type II, Menstral cycle is normal, but there is abnormal endometrial function, i.e. the ovum does not implant.

Q. I have become pregnant too soon, it will spoil the fun of conjugal life. Should I get it cleaned up?

Ans. No. Don't postpone the child bearing for frivolous reasons. Avoid unnecessary surgery. Cutting into the womb, cervix or lower abdomen can cause scarring, which makes it harder for the sperm to get into your womb subsequently and meet the egg. A man's testicles can also be damaged during urological or hernia surgery. Beat stress, anxiety and overwork. Learn to cope by relaxation techniques such as yoga and meditation. Share your feelings and emotions with your spouse. Prioritise your time to include work, play and holidays. Research shows that stress hormones overpower the enzymes that ensure you produce testosterone, which is necessary to create sperm. Focus on mutual enjoyment, rather than procreation during sex. Don't use abortion or contraception because complications can include blocked tubes following an infection after surgery.

Q. What other care and precautions you will advise for prospective parents?

Ans. Check out any itching or unusual penile or vaginal discharge with your doctor. Use a condom if you have sex outside the marital bed. Take the prescribed amount of antibiotics if you have an infection. Use only plain water without soap for genital hygiene and egg white for lubrication during sex. Don't use the IUCD if you have never conceived because you run the risk of Pelvic Inflammatory Disease. The sperm count is highest if you abstain for a couple of days. Man above woman position, is best for pregnancy. Lie down for five minutes after sex and do not wash for a couple of hours. Take tonics, if prescribed. Safeguard yourself with a lead shield if you are being X-rayed. Avoid overheating or tightness of testes always. Keep your weight near normal and don't be obese. Regular aerobic exercises—swimming, dancing, brisk walking—at least 30 minutes 5 times a week, helps your circulation and balances your hormones while promoting weight loss. Moderate exercise is best. Wear cotton trousers, over cotton boxer shorts and have at least 2 cold showers on hot days. No, this will not dampen your ardour. Get adequate sleep to suit your lifestyle. Stop smoking and curb alcohol. Drink 6 to 8 glasses of water a day to keep your hormones in balance. Eat a balanced diet. Foods that affect your hormones and make it harder for your body to use vitamins and minerals are chemicals, preservatives, fats (that harden at room temperature), too much sugar and salt, over six cups of coffee a day.

Q. Can I choose adoption if pregnancy doesn't occur at all?

Ans. Yes, one can choose adoption. Some parents may agree to give their child in adoption, e.g. a single mother may want her baby to have two stable parents, a couple may feel they're too young or don't have the financial resources to raise a child. Others need to complete their education or are in the midst of career difficulties. Even married Birthparents may feel their relationship is not stable enough for a child or they cannot care for more children. Sometimes under Indian conditions a close relative may agree to part with their own child for the welfare of sterile couple.

Q. Can I be involved in choosing the family of my baby?

Ans. Generally not. Occasionally Yes. You can wait for the opportunity, when you can choose a child of the sex of your choice or from a particular caste, etc.

Q. How much contact can adoptive parents have with the family of biological parents after the birth? Or they should forget about them?

Ans. Many Birth-parents receive letters and photos from the adoptive parents on an ongoing basis, some just periodically. Others have phone conversations and a few actually visit one another. It is better if child is not confused by presenting two sets of parents on a continuing basis. Better to forget about them.

Q. How will I know my baby is in a good family?

Ans. The assessment of adoptive parents, their marital stability, financial situation, lifestyle, and medical history is important for the welfare of the child, similarly, medical history and other biological features of the birth parents are important for information of the adopted child, for the satisfaction of new set of parents.

Q. What rights the adopted baby has?

Ans. The child has all the rights of care, development, health, education, career, inheritance, etc. as that of a biological child.

Q. What are the important terms used in ART (Assisted Reproductive Techniques)?

Ans. (i) Common terms:

IVF: *In-vitro* fertilization (IVF), i.e. the union of egg and sperm is achieved in the laboratory by placing the eggs and sperms, together controlled environmental conditions.

ICSI: Intracytoplasmic Sperm Injection means fertilization of an egg in the laboratory by injecting a single sperm inside it with the help of a sophisticated machine called micromanipulator.

Ovum donation: When the wife has lost the capacity to produce her own eggs, the eggs then have to be borrowed from another healthy young woman.

ET: Embryo Transfer means the process of transferring the embryos, (developed in the lab after IVF/ICSI, etc. into the uterus for implantation).

Q. Who may need IVF and who is eligible for it?

Ans. Woman with tubal block is an absolute primary indication for IVF, Infertility of more than 5 years duration due to any cause, Women with endometriosis (chocolate cysts), Previous ectopic pregnancies, More than 6 cycles of unsuccessful IUI (Intra uterine insemination), Decreased sperm counts than normal but > 5 million/ml, Women with pelvic TB, Women with previous sterilization operation, Failed Tuboplasty, Polcystic ovarian disease, etc.

Q. Who may be benefited from ICSI?

Ans. When husband has an occasional sperm seen in the semen, Presence of antisperm antibodies, Presence of sperms inside the testes when vasa deferentia (male tubes) are blocked, Early cases of testicular atrophy, After sterilization operation, etc.

Q. At what age assisted reproductive techniques (ART) are likely to succeed?

Ans. Chances of success are best with ART techniques if the age of woman is less than 35 years. Above 40 years, the chances of success decrease markedly. Also the chance of abortion and abnormal babies increase with age.

Q. What is essential before undergoing ART procedures?

Ans. Both the husband and the wife need to be investigated thoroughly for the cause of infertility, physical fitness to undertake pregnancy and the IVF procedure and the assessment of the success rate. The egg donor also needs to undergo general physical examination, ultrasound and basic tests to assess the general health. Medical diseases such as hypertension, diabetes, etc. need to be diagnosed and treated or controlled before starting the cycle.

Q. How much abstinence is required before semen collection?

Ans. Semen is required after ovum pick up. Couple may abstain from sex for 3-4 days before the procedure. Prolonged abstinence should be avoided.

Q. What is the success rate of ART?

Ans. In women less than 35 years of age maximum of 50% success can be expected. The overall average all over the world is less than 50% or may be 20-30%. The success cannot be guaranteed. Those centres, which claim guarantee are only misguiding the people.

Q. What are the problems with ART?

Ans. Emotional stress, high costs; time consuming treatment and lower success rate, lack of guaranteed cure and risk of multiple pregnancies are the common problems.

Q. Who can donate the female gamete, i.e. ova?

Ans. Any young healthy woman can donate eggs.

Q. Who can donate sperm?

Ans. Generally it is taken from husband's semen or testes. When this source cannot be made available, a donor or cyo-preserved semen may be used in ART techniques.

5

Diseases and Medical Conditions in Women's Prime of Life

The role of women has changed considerably over the last 100 years—For example, 42% of the workforce are women. Surveys show that 54% of working women aged 18-59 years are responsible to look after the children under the age of 12 years. During last 100 years, women's health improved and life expectancy increased from 51 to 81 years. In India and other Asian countries pregnancy-related causes dominate the scene, besides infections. On the positive side, for comparison, see Appendix X: 'A Norway Study on Women's Health'. In that country the status of women's health and life expectancy are reasonably good.

However, in developed countries, cancer is now the number one cause of death, having recently overtaken heart disease, leaving behind reproductive causes. Women live longer than men and therefore experience more disability due to their longer life expectancy. Health surveys show that the most common ailments for women are headaches and the common colds. Healthcare services devoted to women's health and female reproductive needs were at the lowest a few decades ago. But with the help of the feminist revolution in the 1960s and 1970s, as well as the growing concerns of the people, women's health has finally reached maturity. Researchers are now investigating potential treatments for breast cancer and osteoporosis and researching heart disease in women, and drug manufacturers are working to relieve symptoms of premenstrual syndrome (PMS), pregnancy and child birth. In the realm of natural health, naturopathic doctors and herbalists continue to investigate select herbs (dong quai, black cohosh, evening primrose and Vitex) and nutritional supplements traditionally used to combat common ailments among women. Even Ayurveda is taking lot of interest in the matters of woman's health. However, in case of Asian countries like India, a lot remains to be done in the field of reproductive health. See Appendix XI for Ayurvedic point of view about women's health.

The gender roles and biological differences are vast

Biologically a woman's role is vastly different to a man's. Menarche, the onset of menstruation, occurs at as young age as 10-12 years. The reproductive lifecycle continues until the onset of menopause at 50-55 years. The healthy, balanced functioning of the female reproductive system is largely governed by the action of the female reproductive hormones; oestrogen and progesterone. Oestrogen promotes the development and maintenance of female reproductive structures, especially the lining of the uterus. Oestrogen is also essential for the development of female sexual characteristics; such as the breasts. Progesterone works with oestrogen to prepare the lining of the uterus for the implantation of an egg. It also prepares the breast for milk production. Each month a surge in the production of the hormone oestrogen stimulates the release of an egg from one of the two ovaries. The right and left ovaries usually alternate in the release of an egg every month. This egg passes along the fallopian tube, where it may be fertilised. The egg moves to the uterus where, if fertilised, it attaches to the lining and gestation occurs for the next nine months of pregnancy. If the egg is not fertilised, the lining of the uterus (endometrium), breaks down and is shed in a monthly cycle commonly known as menstruation or the period. The hormone oestrogen is higher during the first two weeks of the menstrual cycle, then, once the level has peaked at around day 14, the levels of oestrogen diminish. The level of progesterone is highest during the second two weeks of the menstrual cycle.

Another hormone that plays a smaller role in reproduction is androgen, which is produced in the ovaries, adrenal glands and other tissues. Androgen gets partial credit for the rapid growth spurts girls experience at puberty. Also, during menopause, a woman might lose at least half of her androgen production, which may cause painful symptoms such as vaginal drying and hot flashes.

Nutritional Needs

Women's nutritional needs differ to men's, primarily due to the requirements of the reproductive responsibility. For example, the recommended dietary intake of iron for women is 12-16 mg per day, which for men it is only 7 mg daily. In addition, pregnant women need more iron (up to about 36 mg daily). Older women need less iron. Prior to conception and especially during the first trimester of pregnancy the B group vitamin folic acid is needed in double the quantity than that required for a man. Calcium is also required in larger amounts during pregnancy and lactation. Lifestyle creates special needs—smoking, stress, prescribed drugs, intense physical exercise—all create the need for additional amounts of nutrition.

The cornerstones of preventative health are: a nutritious diet; a healthy level of exercise (not excessive); adequate sleep and relaxation; and sunshine, this last being important for the immune system and production of vitamin D. A healthy diet should provide adequate amounts of antioxidant vitamins and minerals. Antioxidants help protect the body from damage caused by excessive amounts of free radicals. Free radicals are formed as a normal by-product of consuming essential oxygen. They can be generated by many environmental factors such as pollution, sun radiation, cigarette smoke and alcohol. Drugs can increase oxidative damage, as can some food preservatives such as sulphur dioxide and nitmosamine—forming nitrites (typically found in cured or pickled meats). Chlorine in treated water and excess fats in the diet also generate potentially harmful free radicals. Some free radicals are used by the immune system to kill cancer cells and viruses, however, it is the unchecked free radicals that are dangerous and can cause damage to, or even destroy, healthy cells. This could lead to disease or death of the cell, increasing the risk of cancer, heart disease, and degenerative diseases and reducing the length and quality of life. Lifestyle factors clearly influence free radical formation, and supplementing with antioxidant nutrients can provide the nutrient balance that the body needs.

Hormonal swings affect more than just reproduction

Women Researchers from disparate fields find female menstrual hormones influence much more than reproduction. Ask a woman if her period affects her body beyond the reproductive system and she'll probably answer 'yes'. Hormonal swings during a woman's menstrual cycle effect more than just reproduction. John M. Johnson, a physiology professor at the University of Texas Health Science Center, San Antonio, who studies hormonal effects on body temperature regulation says, past studies relied on men as subjects, and not women, to avoid the confounding aspect of the menstrual cycle. Johnson says that this was why he hadn't considered fluctuating-female hormones as a factor, says Susan Brown, a psychology professor at the University of Hawaii, Hilo, "We're bleeding and nobody wants to even think or talk about that." In 1998, epidemiologist Emily White and colleagues from the Fred Hutchison Cancer Center, Seattle, found that mammograms detect cancer more effectively in premenopausal women during the cycle's first two weeks. In the latter half, breast tissue becomes more fibrous and thus opaque most likely due to hormonal fluctuations so it is harder to detect small, early-stage malignancies and several retrospective studies conducted in the United States and Europe during the early 1990s found that high progesterone levels expressed during the luteal phase might contribute to better survival after breast cancer surgery.

Many potential, non-reproductive connections between women's health and menstrual cycle are being studied: metabolic rate, temperature regulation, pain, gastrointestinal function, reaction to insulin in diabetics, and immune function. Susan Manzi, an associate professor of medicine and epidemiology, University of Pittsburgh, notes that 60 percent of women with the autoimmune disease 'lupus' report adverse symptoms suggestive of disease activity during certain times of their cycle. Many say their symptoms worsen at the start of the luteal phase, at ovulation, when progesterone is at its lowest and estrogen is at its highest. But, the data on lupus activity and sex hormones are conflicting. "Since estradiol tends to have more of an immunostimulatory effect and progesterone may have more immunosuppressive characteristics, variations in the levels of these hormones during the menstrual cycle may be important," she says.

"Our hypothesis was that during the follicular phase, women would experience fewer health problems and then during the luteal phase we expected them to experience more," says Brown. Based on the daily diaries of 59 women, who, for three cycles, kept note of general symptoms like runny noses, pimples, herpes cold sore outbreaks, flu-like ailments, and sore throats. Brown found that the participants displayed significantly fewer onsets and contractions of illness during menses. In contrast, the onset of symptoms and contractions of illness peaked during the luteal phase. For example, subjects reported cold symptoms coming on the week before menstruation started. Another area primarily concerns the relationship between pain and the menstrual cycle. For example, Linda A. LeResche, research professor in the department of oral medicine, University of Washington, Seattle, says that researchers "know nothing about clinical pain and cycle with the exception of migraine headache." It's been known for a while that for some migraine sufferers, the headaches come right before, or at the onset of, menstruation.

Roger B. Fillingim, a clinical psychologist and associate professor in the College of Dentistry, University of Florida, Gainesville, also studies how women's perception of pain varies across the cycle. He's currently recruiting women for a study that will look at how interstitial cystitis, a painful bladder condition characterized by increased urinary urgency and frequency, is possibly exacerbated just prior to menstruation. Fillingim's hypothesis: enhanced pain before menstruation occurs because sex hormones affect the neurons in the brain and spinal cord that transmit pain-related information. Another area involving pain is the relationship between bowel disorders and menstrual cycle. "No one has actually measured ovarian hormones and compared them against gastrointestinal symptoms," says Margaret M. Heitkemper, professor and chairperson, department of biobehavioral nursing and health systems, and director, Center for Women's Health Research, University of Washington. Nonetheless, she adds, the evidence is "fairly compelling" that for many women, there is a heightening of symptoms in irritable bowel syndrome (IBS) and other GI tract ailments that occur around the time of menses."I think for many years women were reluctant to talk about symptoms that varied with their cycle," says Heitkemper. "We are beginning to appreciate the full impact of these distressing symptoms.

Premenstrual Syndrome

Premenstrual syndrome (PMS) is a complex interplay of hormonal, nutritional and psychosocial factors. A variety of causes can contribute to the disruption of hormones during the monthly cycle. Emotions, diet and pollutants can disrupt hormone levels so that some women experience high levels of progesterone or estrogen. Other possible theories include a vitamin B6 deficiency, hypoglycemia, a hormone allergy or a psychosomatic problem. Life factors such as reduction in stress, regular moderate exercise, good sleep habits, regular bowel function and good nutrition have been suggested as solutions by both alternative and conventional doctors. Many health doctors have even suggested that the fewer dairy products, refined sugar (including alcohol) and caffeine a woman ingests during the month, the fewer premenstrual symptoms she is likely to experience. Emily Kane, N.D., a naturopathic doctor who practices in Juneau, Alaska, added that caffeine consumption is correlated, in particular, to increased breast tenderness, and sugar and dairy products can impair the absorption of magnesium, the body's natural muscle relaxant. Basic nutrient supplementation may also be helpful in aiding the symptoms of PMS. Kane suggested vitamin B6 to aid in serotonin synthesis and magnesium for muscle relaxation and good elimination. "The lack of B-vitamins, generally speaking, makes it more difficult for the liver to both eliminate excess estrogen and to balance blood sugar," she said. Magnesium is also regarded as helpful in cases of PMS, since it not only relaxes muscles and acts as a gentle laxative but is also necessary for the formation of the brain chemicals dopamine, GABA and serotonin—which all have been implicated to produce particular symptoms of PMS, particularly depression and mood swings. Furthermore, a magnesium deficiency can cause water retention. A study found that 200 mg a day of magnesium reduced fluid retention, breast tenderness and bloating by 40 percent (*J. Women's Health*; 7(9): 1998). Since the body requires adequate amounts of calcium to reap the benefits of magnesium, a combination of magnesium and calcium is essential. Additionally, research points out that women who consume more calcium from their diets are reported to suffer less from severe PMS than those who do not supplement with calcium. A study of 500 women found that 1,200 mg a day of chewable calcium carbonate reduced the physical and psychological symptoms of PMS by nearly 50 percent (*Am J Obstet Gynecol*; 179(2):444-52, 1998).

Herbal medicines have long been used in traditional healing systems to treat various women's conditions. Several herbs have been particularly useful in easing symptoms of PMS. Dong quai (Angelica sinesis), for example, is known in Traditional Chinese Medicine as the female ginseng and has been used to treat menopausal symptoms (especially hot flashes), painful menstruation, lack of or excessive menstrual bleeding and symptoms of pregnancy. Dong quai also possesses anti-inflammatory properties that act as a digestive aid to increase contractions and relax the uterus. The herb may also promote normal hormone balance, which can benefit women experiencing premenstrual cramping and pain. More studies are currently being conducted to further investigate Dong quai's effectiveness, especially since a double-blind study showed that dong quai capsules did not help women with menopausal symptoms (*Fertility Sterility*; 68:981-86, 1997). Another powerful herb that promotes women's health is Vitex, or chaste tree berry, native to the Mediterranean and western Asia. Vitex has been recognized as an herb that balances female hormones and regulates women's menstrual cycles. It stabilizes estrogen and progesterone during a menstrual cycle and corrects menstrual irregularities. By stimulating the pituitary gland to produce more luteinizing hormone, a greater amount of progesterone is produced. A German study (*Therapiwoche Gyn*; 5:60-68, 1992), found that using Vitex once in the morning over a period of several months helps to normalize hormone balance to alleviate the symptoms of PMS. Similarly, a controlled, double-blind study for treatment of PMS (*Phytomedicine*; 4:183-89, 1997) found that vitex is effective. However, Vitex is not a fast acting herb and should be used continuously for four to six months.

Evening primrose oil (EPO) and omega-3 fatty acids have also been considered valuable for the treatment of PMS. Since EPO is rich in essential polyunsaturated fatty acids (gamma-linolenic acid (GLA) and linoleic acid), it serves as a possible remedy for severe symptoms of PMS and the body's overall health. Essential fatty acids (EFAs) are responsible for providing energy, maintaining body temperature, insulating nerves and protecting body tissue. Linoleic acid is used by the body to convert GLA into other substances such as prostaglandins. Prostaglandins are hormone-like substances found in cells and are critical to the body's overall health maintenance. However, prostaglandins need to be replenished as once they serve their purpose, they are destroyed. Omega-3 fatty acids are also being studied for the ability to alleviate PMS symptoms such as swelling, tenderness and irritability experienced during this time. Since these symptoms follow the theory that PMS is inflammation without infection, omega-3 fatty acids remove prostaglandins, from inflammatory precursors such as arachidonic acid, according to Kane.

The Oral Contraceptives and nutrition

Can birth control pills affect nutritional status in women? According to several studies on this topic, the results have been conflicting due to variables that are associated with menstrual cycles, hormone shifts and the body's increased nutritional needs during this time. Research has found that women taking the pill have increased levels of vitamin A and iron and decreased levels of vitamins B6, B12, C and riboflavin. These changes also affect levels of folic acid and zinc. A lower level of vitamin B6 is the most commonly reported nutritional change in pill users. One National Institute of Child Health and Human Development (NICHD) funded study found that lowered levels of B6 during pregnancy and lactation were more common in women who used the pill for more than 30 months and became pregnant within four months after stopping the pill. Nevertheless, it is uncertain whether pill use is a cause of true vitamin B6 deficiency (which is also linked to depression). Other symptoms of vitamin deficiency include weakness, lethargy, dizziness, skin and gum irritations, and an increased susceptibility to infection.

Next to vitamin B6, folic acid is the nutrient most significantly affected by the pill. Changes in folic acid metabolism have been reported in connection with two conditions in pill users. Some women using oral contraceptives have developed a rare but serious anemia condition that may be treated with folic acid supplements. Other women using the pill have experienced changes in folic acid metabolism in cells around the cervix, which may be related to a kind of abnormal cell growth called cervical dysplasia.

Pregnancy and nutrition

The many hormonal and physical changes that take place during pregnancy can make those nine months a trying time. As proper nutrition is essential for a healthy fetus, most doctors are particular about of the properties, dosages and contraindications of remedies that can alleviate cramping, nausea, night sweats and other symptoms that accompany pregnancy. For those looking to supplement the pregnant body naturally, doctors suggest a well-balanced and varied diet that includes fresh fruits and vegetables, whole grains, legumes and fish.

In addition to a healthy diet, most pregnancy nutrition regimens include a proper intake of vitamins and minerals particularly folic acid and calcium. The need for folic acid doubles during pregnancy, since neural tube defects in infants are caused by deficiencies of folic acid. According to a study published in Lancet (338:131-7, 1991), women who were at risk of giving birth to babies with neural tube defects were able to lower their risk by 72 percent by taking folic acid supplements prior to and during pregnancy. Following a host of studies published in 1997 indicating the importance of folic acid in preventing neural tube defects, the government increased its recommended dosage to 400 to 600 mcg. According to Birth Defects Foundation, the most crucial time for an expectant mother to ingest folic acid begins before conception and lasts throughout the first trimester. Another study (*Lancet*; 349(9065):1591-3, 1997) further marked the importance of ingesting folic acid. The study indicated that a greater number of women are genetically at risk for an enzyme defect that causes a vitamin deficiency, predisposing them to having children with a neural tube defect. By ingesting folic acid daily, women can further prevent these defects from occurring. Another important prenatal nutrient proven to prevent defects is calcium. It not only helps the mother maintain good bone strength and density; it also provides the fetus with the necessary nutrients needed to form healthy bones, teeth and nails. Low dietary intake of this mineral can increase the risk of pre-eclampsia, a potentially dangerous condition characterized by high blood pressure and swelling. Calcium supplementation may reduce the risk of pre-term delivery, which is often associated with pre-eclampsia. Calcium may also reduce the risk of hypertensive disorders of pregnancy. The recommended daily dosage is approximately 1,250 mg. Other beneficial nutrients include zinc for Asian the fetus, selenium for maintaining a healthy heart and liver, and iron for producing and expending energy. In one study, 15 of 23 women who were not given extra iron developed an iron deficiency during pregnancy (*Br J Obstet Gynacol*; 90:101-107, 1983). Interested individuals should still seek the advice of their physicians for proper dosage amounts since supplementation with large amounts of iron has been found to reduce blood levels of zinc.

Due to the limited amount of research, there are only a handful of herbs that doctors feel comfortable recommending for pregnancy: crampbark is suggested to prevent miscarriage and ease the nervousness that often accompanies pregnancy; ginger to alleviate nausea; and red raspberry to calm muscle spasms. Dandelion leaf and root may also be helpful in nourishing the system since they are rich sources of vitamins and minerals such as beta-carotene, calcium, potassium and iron. Dandelion leaf's diuretic effect may also stimulate bile flow, which helps with digestive problems associated with pregnancy. Similarly, nettle leaf can provide the body with calcium and iron.

Women's Healthcare in Karnataka: Envisaging a healthy growth

The state-run healthcare system in Karnataka is striving hard to overcome problems such as regional disparities and regain its former standards according to Ravi Sharma, Bangalore. At the same time, health services in the private sector, especially the multi-speciality hospitals, have earned a reputation for themselves. The princely state of Mysore was a pioneer in basic healthcare. In 1806, it was perhaps the first State in the country to take up a vaccination drive against small pox. The State administration set-up a government hospital in Bangalore in 1846, the first public health unit in Mandya in 1929 and the world's first two birth control clinics in 1930. But after Independence, the State of Karnataka, which churns out around 1,800 doctors every year, has been striving to keep up with those standards, especially in the rural areas.

Karnataka, like any other State, is full of regional, even sub-regional disparities in the matter of development. The health infrastructure in certain regions, most notably the State's capital, Bangalore, and to a lesser extent the coastal towns of Mangalore and Manipal, has developed well but other areas, especially the rural areas where 60 per cent of the population lives and the northern districts, have not received sufficient attention from the government and the private sector. Overall, the State has a crude birth rate of 22 (for every 1,000 of the population), a crude death rate of 7.2, an infant mortality rate of 55 per 1,000 live births, a maternal mortality rate of 195 per one lakh live births and a total fertility rate (the number of children born to a woman during her reproductive years) of 2.2. The State's Health and Family Welfare Services has 8,143 sub-centres (that is, one for 5,000 people), 581 Primary Health Units (PHUs), 1,679 Primary Health Centres

The Vanivilas hospital, one of the oldest hospitals run by the Karnataka government

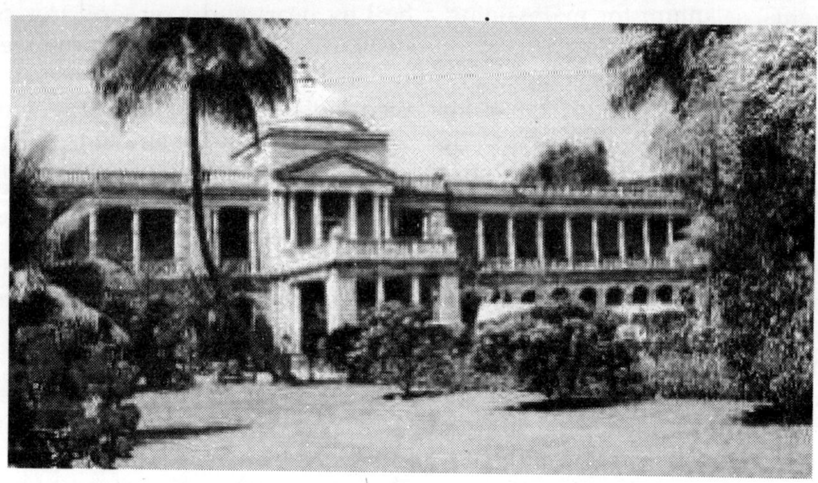

(PHCs), 19 mobile units, 7,304 maternity annexes, 17 urban PHCs and 110 Community Health Centres. While the doctor-population ratio is 1:10,260, the bed to population ratio is 1:1,220. In a novel scheme to improve services, the government has allowed 14 PHCs to be managed by medical colleges and trusts. At these PHCs, 75 per cent of the staff salary is paid by the government and 25 per cent by the private entrepreneur.

Women's services targeted

There are 87 Urban Family Welfare Centres, 124 Urban Health Centres and 24 district-level and 149 taluk-level hospitals. There are 51 other hospitals, including super-speciality hospitals, which treat illnesses like cancer, heart ailments and tuberculosis. As part of the World Bank-funded Karnataka Health Systems Project, the State government has over the past seven years strengthened and upgraded at a cost of Rs. 624 crores the infrastructure in 204 of its taluk and district hospitals. As a consequence, six government hospitals have won ISO-9002 certification. Under the project, user charges are levied in taluk and district hospitals, non-clinical services in some hospitals have been privatised and 44 primary trauma care centres established to provide emergency services to accident victims. Treatment is free for those below the poverty line (BPL) for almost all services in the State government hospitals. For specialised treatments such as cardiac surgeries, BPL families can get up to Rs. 50,000 from the Chief Minister's Relief Fund. The government has also been sanctioning Rs. 50,000 twice a year to each of the district hospitals, which can use the fund to buy from the private sector medical services that are not available with them.

Plenty of doctors, but. . .

There are around 22,000 practising doctors in the State. Of them, 4,197 are working in the State's health institutions and about 15,000 in the private sector. The total bed strength in government health institutions is 43,479 while their outpatient departments serve 60,000 patients every day. There are nearly 2,000 hospitals in the private sector, which interestingly have as many beds as the state sector. According to officials, the shortage of doctors and supervisory staff, financial crunch and an ever-increasing population are some of the major reasons for the state sector's inability to provide a more effective health delivery system. The shortage of doctors, especially specialists, and funds forced the government to hand over in April 2002 part of the management of the Rajiv Gandhi Super Speciality Hospital in Raichur to Apollo Hospitals. Under an agreement, the Karnataka government pays for the maintenance cost of Rs. 3 crores to Rs. 4 crores a year. As a result of the funds crunch only a half of the State's 8,154 sub-centres have permanent buildings. Karnataka has slipped from the sixth place to the seventh in the Human Development Index. And on most human development indices, Karnataka is barely above the all-India average.

In a bid to achieve the "Millennium Development Goals", the new coalition government has decided to make primary healthcare (and primary education) the focus of its development effort. Presenting the new government's first Budget 2004, Deputy Chief Minister Siddaramaiah announced an increase in the Plan outlay for the health sector from Rs. 333 crores to Rs. 377 crores, which would be utilised to improve taluk-level hospitals and the medical infrastructure in impoverished northern Karnataka. The enhanced outlay should partly stabilise the State's falling public health expenditure, which has fallen from 1.02 per cent of the gross state domestic product (GSDP) in 1999 to 0.7 per cent in 2004. Ideally it should reach 2 per cent of GSDP.

Word Bank Project

Under the Rs. 765-crore World Bank-assisted 'Health, Nutrition and Population (HNP) Project' the government hopes to improve and extend the primary healthcare system. The focus of the five-year programme "is to increase access to healthcare for the rural poor and the underprivileged, and to strengthen primary healthcare with community participation."

Says Mohamed Sanaulla, Commissioner, Health and Family Welfare Services: "Our aim is to stabilise and improve facilities. It is a misnomer to say that the services at government hospitals are not good. In fact, our understanding is that, especially in the rural areas, the level of satisfaction among the people is better with the government health service. People are even prepared to pay 'unregistered' (bribe) expenses."

In a bid to ensure effective primary, secondary and tertiary health delivery systems in the State, successive Karnataka governments have implemented a number of measures. The HNP Project seeks to improve the

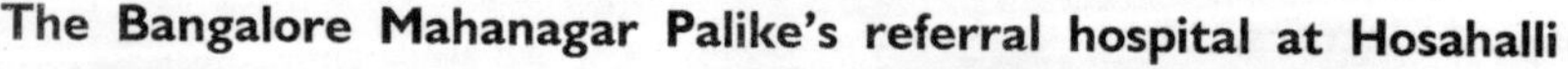

The Bangalore Mahanagar Palike's referral hospital at Hosahalli

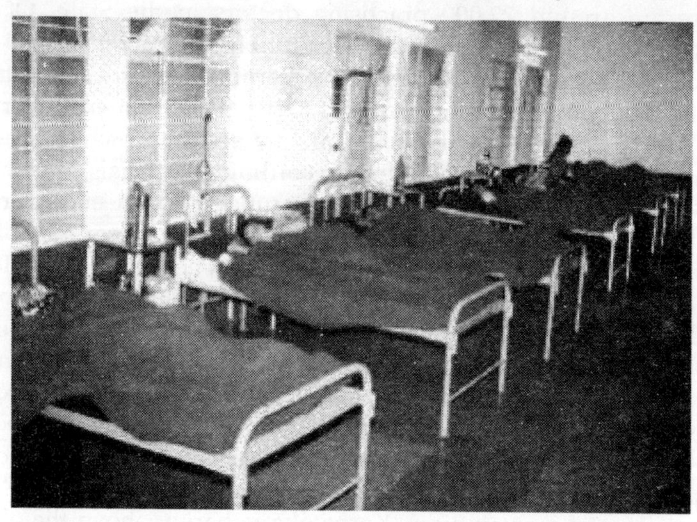

services at the 1,679 PHCs. To be implemented in three districts as a pilot project, this will also aim at increasing public-private participation and introducing an insurance scheme for the common people, with the government subsidising the premiums.

The Rs. 30-crore World Bank-aided Integrated Disease Surveillance Project, spread over five years, is designed to gather initially information regarding communicable diseases such as malaria, cholera, gastroenteritis and typhoid. Information on non-communicable diseases like cancer and hypertension, and trauma care will be compiled later. An information technology network has already been established at the taluk and district levels. The information thus gathered from the district, State and national levels will be analysed and utilised for more effective diagnosis, management and prevention of communicable diseases. The State is also giving shape to the Rs. 15-crore European Union-funded Drug Logistics and Warehousing Project, under, which 14 warehouses will be set-up in the districts. The current system of indenting for packages would be replaced by the indenting for drugs. As part of it telemedicine programme, five private speciality hospitals are being connected via satellite to 25 districts and four taluks hospitals. The system is functioning in two hospitals. The private hospitals have offered free consultations. The Indian Space Research Organisation (ISRO) has set-up the satellite link at a cost of Rs. 35 crores. Karnataka is also hoping to improve the birth rate, infant mortality and maternal mortality parameters in the State when the Government of India's Reproductive and Child Health-Phase II programme is implemented in 2005. The State government has set-up regional diagnostic laboratories in seven districts to conduct sophisticated tests, including CT scans.

India and the World

The profile of diseases contributing most heavily to death, illness, and disability among Indians is changing dramatically. Today, chronic diseases—such as cardiovascular disease (primarily heart disease and stroke), cancer, and diabetes-are among the most prevalent, costly, and preventable of all health problems, however infections have not vanished. Almost 50% of those who die each year, die of a chronic disease. The prolonged course of illness and disability from such chronic diseases as diabetes and arthritis results in extended pain and suffering and decreased quality of life for millions. Chronic, disabling conditions cause major limitations in activity for a large number of people. While Indian figures and that of other Asian countries are not available, the trend in U.S. is evident from the following graphical illustrations.

Most Common, 1999*

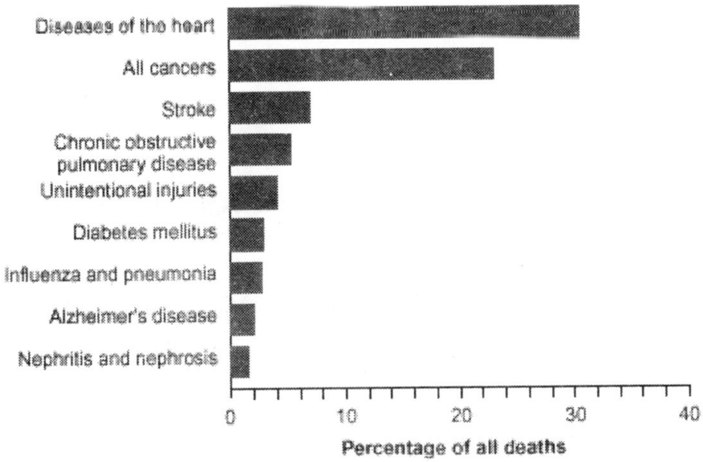

*All data are age adjusted to 2000 total U.S. population.

Causes of Death in the United States

Costs of Chronic Disease

The United States cannot effectively address escalating healthcare costs without addressing the problem of chronic diseases:

- More than 90 million Americans live with chronic illnesses.
- Chronic diseases account for 70% of all deaths in the United States.
- The medical care costs of people with chronic diseases account for more than 75% of the nation's $1.4 trillion medical care costs.
- Chronic diseases account for one-third of the years of potential life lost before age 65.

Actual, 1990†

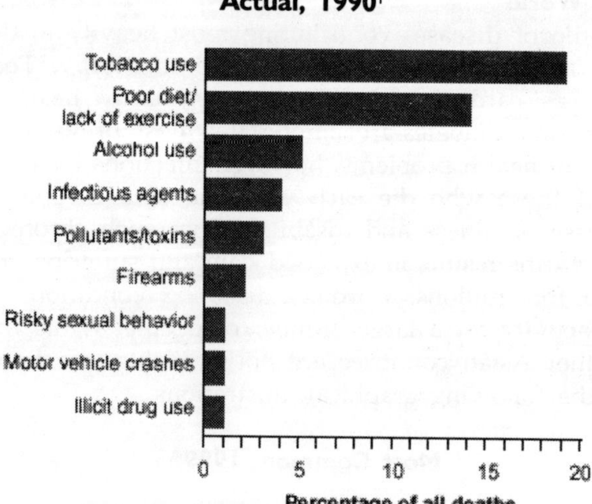

† McGinnis, J.M., Foege, W.H., Actual causes of death in the United States. JAMA 1993; 270:2207-12.

Leading Causes of Disability Among Persons Aged 15 Years or Older, United States, 1991-92

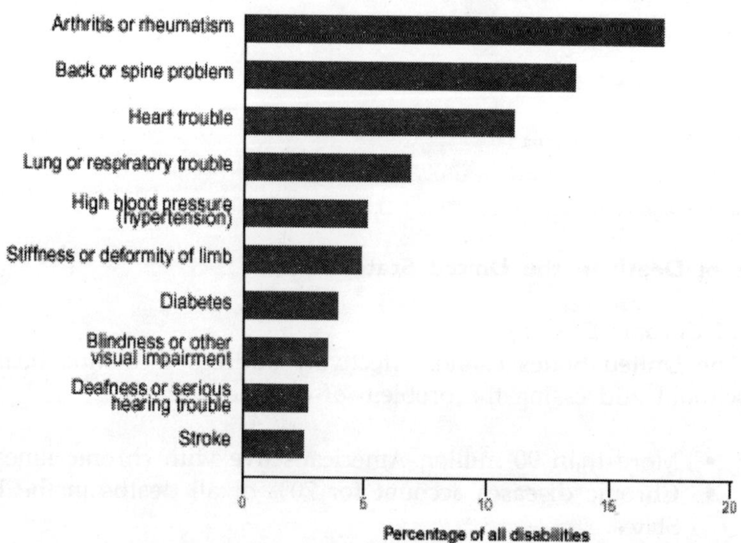

Source: CDC, Prevalence of disability and associated health conditions, United States, 1991-92. MMWR 1994; 43(40): 730-1, 737-9.

- Hospitalizations for pregnancy-related complications occurring before delivery account for more than $1 billion annually.
- The direct and indirect costs of diabetes are nearly $132 billion a year.
- Each year, arthritis results in estimated medical care costs of more than $22 billion, and estimated total costs (medical care and lost productivity) of almost $82 billion.
- The estimated direct and indirect costs associated with smoking exceed $75 billion annually.
- In 2001, approximately $300 billion was spent on all cardiovascular diseases. Over $129 in lost productivity was due to cardiovascular disease.
- The direct medical costs associated with physical inactivity was nearly $76.6 billion in 2000.
- Nearly $68 billion is spent on dental services each year.

Cost-Effectiveness of Prevention

- For every $1 spent on water fluoridation, $38 is saved in dental restorative treatment costs.
- For a cost ranging from $1,108 to $4,542 for smoking cessation programs, 1 quality-adjusted year of life is saved. Smoking cessation interventions have been called the gold standard of cost-effective interventions.
- The direct medical costs associated with physical inactivity was $29 billion in 1987 and nearly $76.6 billion in 2000. Engaging in regular physical activity is associated with taking less

Estimated Per Capita Health Expenditures, by Age and Sex, 1995

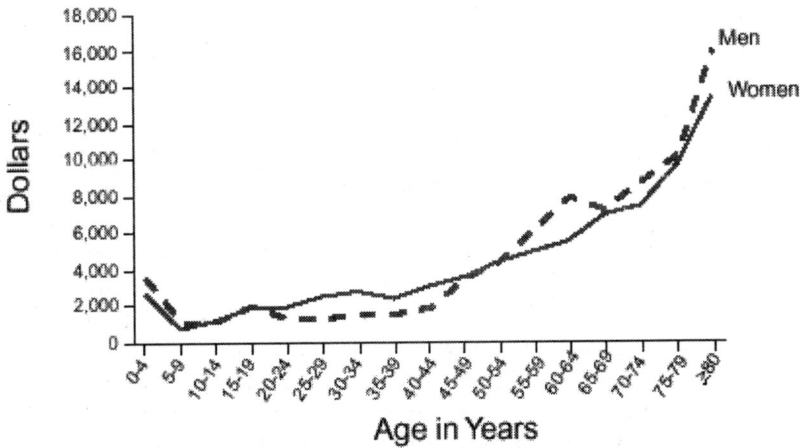

Source: From Baby Boom to Elder Boom: Providing Healthcare for an Ageing Population. Copyright 1996, Watson Wyatt Worldwide.

medication and having fewer hospitalizations and physician visits.

- For each $1 spent on the Safer Choice Program (a school-based HIV, other STD, and pregnancy prevention program), about $2.65 is saved on medical and social costs.
- For every $1 spent on preconception care programs for women with diabetes, $1.86 can be saved by preventing birth defects among their offspring.
- According to one Northern California study, for every $1 spent on the Arthritis Self-Help Program, $3.42 was saved in physician visits and hospital costs.
- A mammogram every 2 years for women aged 50-69 costs only about $9,000 per year of life saved. This cost compares favorably with other widely used clinical preventive services.
- For the cost of 100 Papanicolaou tests for low-income elderly women, about $5,907 and 3.7 years of life are saved.
- After controlling for physical limitation and major socio-economic factors, more than 12% of annual medical costs of the inactive persons with arthritis is associated with physical inactivity. Physical activity interventions may be a cost-effective strategy for reducing the burden of arthritis.

BURDEN OF CHRONIC DISEASES ON MINORITY RACIAL POPULATIONS AND WOMEN

Breast and Cervical Cancer

African American women are more likely to die of breast cancer than are women of any other racial or ethnic group. The incidence of cervical cancer—a 100% preventable cancer—is more than five times greater among Vietnamese women in the United States than among white women.

Anaemia

Anemia is characterized by an insufficient number of haemoglobin and/or red blood cells (RBCs). RBCs carry oxygen from the lungs to tissues throughout the body. All cells require oxygen to function. Red blood cells originate in bone marrow as erythroblasts (a "blast" is a primitive cell that develops into a mature cell). Hemoglobin (Hb), a protein that binds to oxygen, is the main component of red blood cells. Once RBCs become filled with hemoglobin they enter the bloodstream. Healthy hemoglobin holds the oxygen molecules with a precise degree of force. If it binds oxygen molecules in the lungs too loosely, it cannot hold onto them and carry them away. If it binds them too tightly, it cannot release them to tissues. Red blood cell production is stimulated by the hormone erythropoietin (EPO), which is produced in the kidneys. If the kidneys fail to produce adequate EPO, anemia develops. Hospitals use blood supplied by blood banks situated in the same hospital or elsewhere. Blood banks type blood and test the compatibility of donor and recipient blood before transfusion (called cross-matching). Blood types A, B, AB, and O. Whether or not the type is positive or negative depends whether the Rh factor is present on the person's red blood cells. All types can receive O negative blood, but may not be compatible with other types:

- Recipients with A+ blood type can receive A+, A-, O+ and O- blood types.
- Recipients with B+ blood type can receive B+, B-, O+ and O- blood types.
- Recipients with AB+ blood type can receive AB+, AB-, O+ and O- blood types.
- Recipients with O+ blood type can receive O+ and O- blood types.
- Recipients with A- blood type can receive A- and O- blood types.
- Recipients with B- blood type can receive B- and O- blood types.
- Recipients with AB- blood type can receive AB- and O- blood types.
- Recipients with O- blood type can receive O- blood type.

Blood products commonly transfused in Intensive Care Units (ICU) include:

- red blood cells (RBCs)—contain hemoglobin, which carries oxygen to all tissues;
- plasma-straw-colored fluid that carries the blood cells, enzymes, and hormones throughout the body; and
- platelets-cell-like bodies that control bleeding.

Blood banks also test blood for anemia and pathogens (disease-causing bacteria and viruses), including hepatitis viruses B and C, human immunodeficiency virus (HIV), and Treponema pallidum; bacterium that causes syphilis. Despite the many regulations in place to assure the safety of blood supplies, transfusions are not risk free. Possible complications of blood transfusions include—

- allergic reaction (caused by an allergen in the donor blood), and
- hemolytic transfusion reaction (caused by incompatible blood).

Managing patients in ICU requires strategies to minimize blood loss and increase production of blood in bone marrow. Limiting laboratory testing and phlebotomy (drawing blood) are important components of blood management.

Alternative Treatment

Injectable erythropiotin (EPO, e.g. PROCRIT, EPOGEN) is an alternative to blood transfusion to treat critically ill patients with anemia. Exogenous EPO is identical to the natural hormone in its role of stimulating the bone marrow to produce red blood cells. EPO has been used safely in many clinical settings, including chronic renal failure, oncology, and surgery. In the ICU, use of EPO has been shown to reduce the amount of blood transfused by almost 50% at the same time significantly increasing hemoglobin levels.

Backaches

Neck and back pain, especially pain in the lower back, is one of the most common health problems in adults. Fortunately, most back and neck pain is temporary, resulting from short-term stress on the muscles or ligaments that support the spine rather than from a serious injury or medical condition such as nerve damage or kidney disease. The back is an intricate structure of bones, ligaments, muscles, nerves, and tendons. The backbone, or spine, is made up of 33 bony segments called vertebrae:

- 7 cervical (neck) vertebrae.
- 12 thoracic (middle back) vertebrae.
- 5 lumbar (lower back) vertebrae.
- 5 sacral (lowest area of the back) vertebrae.
- 4 coccygeal (coccyx, or tailbone) vertebra (made up of several fused segments).

The vertebrae are arranged in a long vertical column and held together by ligaments, which are attached to muscles by tendons. Between each vertebra lies a gel-like cushion called an intervertebral disc, consisting of semifluid matter (nucleus pulposus) that is surrounded by a capsule of elastic fibers (annulus fibrosus). The spinal cord is an extension of the brain that runs through a long, hollow canal in the column of vertebrae. The meninges, cerebrospinal fluid, fat, and a network of veins and arteries surround, nourish, and protect the spinal cord. Thirty-one pairs of nerve roots emerge from the spinal cord through spaces in each vertebra. The spinal cord and peripheral nerves perform essential sensory and motor activities of the body. The peripheral nervous system conveys sensory information from the body to the brain and conveys motor signals from the brain to the body. Back pain is reported to occur at least once in 85% of adults below the age of 50. Nearly all of them will have at least one recurrence. It is the second most common illness-related reason given for a missed workday and the most common cause of disability. Work-related back injury is the number one occupational hazard.

Risk Factors

Ageing produces wear and tear on the spine that may result in conditions (e.g., disc degeneration, spinal stenosis) that produce neck and back pain. Having a previous back injury puts one at risk for another injury. Physically demanding occupations that require repetitive bending and lifting have a high incidence of back injury (e.g., construction worker, caregiver). Jobs that require long hours of standing without a break (e.g., hairdresser) or sitting in a chair (e.g., keyboard operator) that does not support the back well put a person at risk for neck and lower back injury. Being sedentary (i.e., not exercising regularly or engaging in physical recreation) and being overweight, which increases stress on the lower back, are risk factors. Poor posture, such as slouching in a chair, driving hunched over, standing incorrectly, and using poor body mechanics when lifting and carrying heavy loads are risk factors. Sleeping on a soft or sagging mattress also can lead to back pain. Sports that involve twisting the back, like golf, can result in back injury or worsen existing lower back pain. Joint and/or bone disease (e.g., osteoporosis, arthritis) and infectious disease (e.g., spinal meningitis) can lead to degeneration, inflammation and compression.

Too frequent urination

In people with an overactive bladder (OAB), the layered, smooth muscle that surrounds the bladder (detrusor muscle) contracts spastically, sometimes without a known cause, which results in sustained, high bladder pressure and the urgent need to urinate (called urgency). Normally, the detrusor muscle contracts and relaxes in response to the volume of urine in the bladder and the initiation of urination. People with OAB often experience urgency at inconvenient and unpredictable times and sometimes lose control before reaching a toilet. Thus, overactive bladder interferes with work, daily routine, intimacy and sexual function; causes embarrassment; and can diminish self-esteem and quality of life. Urination (micturition) involves processes within the urinary tract and the brain. The slight need to urinate is sensed when urine volume reaches about one-half of the bladder's capacity. The brain suppresses this need until a person initiates urination. Once urination has been initiated, the nervous system signals the detrusor muscle to contract into a funnel shape and expel urine. Pressure in the bladder increases and the detrusor muscle remains contracted until the bladder empties. Once empty, pressure falls and the bladder relaxes and resumes its normal shape. Overactive bladder affects men and women equally. While the incidence of this common problem is not known in India, the U.S. Department of Health and Human Services has reported that approximately 13 million people in the United States suffer from OAB and other forms of incontinence.

A malfunctioning detrusor muscle causes overactive bladder. Identifiable underlying causes include the following:

- Nerve damage caused by abdominal trauma, pelvic trauma, or surgery.
- Bladder stones.

- Drug side effects.
- Neurological disease (e.g., multiple sclerosis, Parkinson's disease, stroke, spinal cord lesions).

Other conditions can produce symptoms similar to those experienced with overactive bladder, the most common of which is urinary tract infection (UTI) in women.

Three symptoms are associated with an overactive bladder:

- Frequency (frequent urination)
- Urgency (urgent need to urinate)
- Urge incontinence (strong need to urinate followed by leaking or involuntary and complete voiding)

Breast cancer

Breast cancer is malignant abnormal cell growth in the breast. If left untreated the cancer spreads to other areas of the body (called metastasis). Fibrocystic changes (e.g., formation of cysts, scar tissue) may cause benign (i.e., non-cancerous) lumps in the breast. It is important for women to become familiar with their breasts and report changes (e.g., lump, nipple discharge, asymmetry) to their healthcare doctor. Breast cancer is the second most common type of cancer in women and the second leading cause of cancer-related death in women. Approximately 200,000 women in the United States are diagnosed with breast cancer each year, and the disease causes about 40,000 deaths annually. The incidence of breast cancer rises after age 40. The highest incidence (approximately 80% of invasive cases) occurs in women over age 50.

Most breast cancers develop in glandular tissue and is classified as adenocarcinoma. The earliest form of the disease, ductal carcinoma in situ (DCIS), develops solely in the milk ducts. The most common type of breast cancer, invasive ductal carcinoma (IDC), develops from DCIS, spreads through the duct walls, and invades the breast tissue. Invasive lobular carcinoma originates in the milk glands and accounts for 10-15% of invasive breast cancers. Less common types of breast cancer include the following:

- Inflammatory (breast tissue is warm and appears red; tends to spread quickly).
- Medullary carcinoma (originates in central breast tissue).
- Mucinous carcinoma (invasive; usually occurs in postmenopausal women).
- Paget's disease of the nipple (originates in the milk ducts and spreads to the skin of the nipples or areola).
- Phyllodes tumor (tumor with a leaf-like appearance that extends into the ducts; rarely metastasizes).
- Tubular carcinoma (small tumor that is often undetectable by palpation).

- Rarely, sarcomas (cancer of the connective tissue) and lymphomas (cancer of the lymph tissue) develop in the breasts.

Risk Factors

Most women who develop breast cancer have no identifiable risk factors other than their gender. The condition is 100 times more common in women. The growth of breast cancer tumors is often affected by the presence of estrogen and progesterone. The following risk factors result from exposure to these hormones:

- Age (over age 50)
- First pregnancy after age 30
- Long-term (more than 5 years) hormone replacement therapy (HRT)
- Menstruation before age 12
- Menopause after age 50
- Nulliparity (never gave birth to an offspring)

Other risk factors include the following:

- Family history of the disease (mother or sister with premenopausal breast cancer)
- Genetic link
- History of breast biopsy or radiation to the chest
- Moderate alcohol use (2 to 5 drinks daily)
- Obesity
- Personal history of the disease—women with a history of breast cancer are 3 to 4 times more likely to have a recurrence
- Race (slightly more common in Caucasians)
- Sedentary lifestyle.

Approximately 5% of breast cancer cases have a genetic link that results from an inherited mutation in genes identified as BRCA1 and BRCA2. Patients who inherit an altered BRCA1 or BRCA2 gene have an increased risk for Asian premenopausal breast cancer and are more likely to have family members with the condition. Patients concerned about the genetic risk for breast cancer should speak to their healthcare doctor about genetic testing. The cause of breast cancer is unknown.

Toe twisting

A bunion is a bump that develops on the inner side of the foot, near the base of the first toe. It is caused by poor alignment of the metatarsal-phalangeal joint of the big toe (hallux). Physicians call this deformity "hallux abducto valgus" (HAV), a term that refers to the hallux abducting (going away) from the midline of the body. It also refers to twisting of the toe so the inside edge touches the ground and the outside edge turns upward. Essentially, it describes the deviation of the toe toward the outside of the foot. The condition worsens over time leading to discomfort and skin problems, such as corns and lesions, and difficulty walking.

Bunions are one of the most common foot problems. They tend to run in families, suggesting that genetic factors associated with the inherited shape of the foot may predispose people to bunions. Flat feet are unstable and often cause bunions. Body weight is repeatedly transferred to the hallux while walking, and in unstable, flat feet, this transfer of weight allows certain muscles to become stronger than others. This overpowering of muscles causes the toe to bend and deform. Bunions may be caused by excessively tight, pointy-toed, or high-heeled shoes, and shoes that are too small. Women get bunions much more often than men do. Improper shoes exacerbate the underlying cause of flat, unstable feet. Typically, bunions begin as a mild bump or outward bending of the big toe that is only a cosmetic concern at first. However, beneath the surface, strong forces are at work. The forces imparted by the misaligned, outward-bending toe stretch the ligaments that connect the foot bones, pulling against the tendons, gradually drawing the big toe farther out of line. Over time, the big toe continues to twist out of its original position until it no longer lines up properly with its corresponding metatarsal. The end of the metatarsal may become enlarged. Pressure from the first toe can lead to deformity of the metatarsal-phalangeal joint in the second toe, pushing it toward the third toe. In some cases, the second toe may ride up and over, or down and under, the big toe. At this point, the range of motion in the big toe is decreased, a condition called hallux limitus. The condition becomes painful at this stage. The bunion changes the shape of the foot and the biomechanics of walking become altered. Normally, the big toe can bend at least 65 degrees, enabling it to be the last part of the foot to leave the ground during walking. However, with hallux limitus, the big toe cannot function properly and the body weight is transferred to the bunion. A person with uncomfortable bunions gradually begins to compensate by walking in an exaggerated toe-turned-out manner, so the painful hallux does not have to bend as far. This is detrimental because walking with the feet turned out steadily forces the hallux even farther out, causing the bunion to worsen. Without treatment, the deformity eventually becomes disabling.

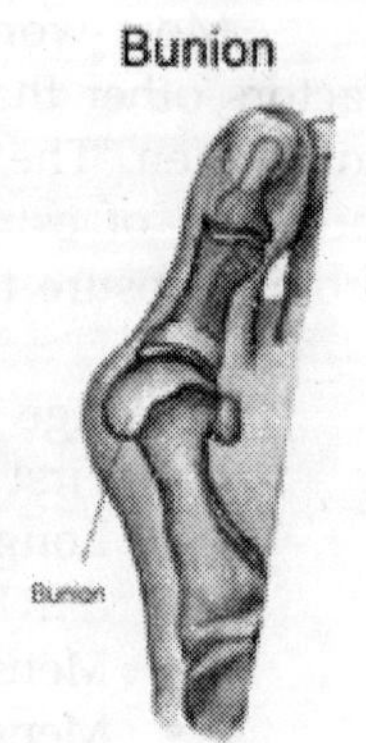

Pre-cancer of uterine cervix

Cervical dysplasia is a term used to describe the appearance of abnormal cells on the surface of the cervix, the lowest part of the uterus. These changes in cervical tissue are classified as mild, moderate, or severe. While dysplasia itself does not cause health problems, it is considered to be a precancerous condition. Left untreated, dysplasia sometimes progresses to an early form of cancer known as cervical carcinoma *in-situ*, and eventually to invasive cervical cancer. It can take 10 years or longer for cervical dysplasia to develop into cancer. Dysplasia can be detected from a Pap smear, the single most important step that a woman can take to prevent cervical cancer. Mild dysplasia is the most common form, and up to 70% of these cases regress on their own (i.e., the cervical tissue returns to normal without treatment). Moderate and severe dysplasia are less likely to self-resolve and have a higher rate of progression to cancer. The greater the abnormality, the higher the risk for Asian cervical cancer. Detecting and treating dysplasia early is essential to prevent cancer. For this reason, most physicians quickly remove suspicious cervical lesions and require frequent Pap smears to monitor for recurrences. Every year, between 250,000 and 1 million women in the United States are diagnosed with cervical dysplasia. While it can occur at any age, the peak incidence is in women between the ages of 25 to 35, i.e. reproductive phase of life and not the menopausal zone. Most dysplasias can be cured with proper treatment and follow-up. Without treatment, 30% to 50% may progress to invasive cancer.

Risk factors increase the frequency of occurrence. Several risk factors have been linked to dysplasia including multiple sexual partners, early onset of sexual activity, cigarette smoking, and sexually transmitted diseases, especially human papillomavirus (HPV) and HIV infection.

HPV Infection

Eighty to ninety percent of women with cervical dysplasia have an HPV infection. Human papillomavirus (HPV) is a group of more than 80 different viral strains. About one-third are sexually transmitted, and some types cause genital warts. HPV infects about 25 million people in the United States, and most of the viral strains are harmless.

However, the NIH Consensus Conference on Cancer of the Cervix and the World Health Organization (WHO) have concluded that several strains of HPV cause cervical cancer. The strains found most frequently in precancerous lesions and in cervical cancer are types 16 and 18. Other strains with high malignant potential include 31, 33, 35, 39, 45, 51, 52, 56, 58, and 68, and together, they account for almost 90% of cancerous lesions and dysplasia in HPV infections. Most HPV infections resolve within 6 months and many women develop immunity. HPV often does not cause symptoms. One study found that nearly one-half of the women infected with HPV had no symptoms and a person may not even know that they are infected. Untreated HPV can result in recurrent and persistent cervical dysplasia and many experts believe that HPV is the main cause for changes in cervical cells that result in dysplasia.

HIV Infection

Women who are infected with HIV are at a greater risk for developing dysplasia. The risk appears to increase as the number of CD4 cells (cells that play a critical role in immune responses) decreases. HIV-positive women also have a higher rate of persistent HPV infections and may be infected with the strains that are associated with severe dysplasia and cervical cancer. Women whose immune systems are suppressed for other reasons, such as by drugs that prevent rejection of organ transplants, are also at greater risk. This suggests that women with weakened immunity are more likely to be infected with HPV and to have a persistent infection that does not resolve on its own.

Smoking

Nicotine and cotinine, chemicals produced from tobacco, have been found in the cervical cells of women who smoke. Men who smoke also excrete these chemicals in their semen, which comes in contact with the cervix during sexual intercourse. Tobacco chemicals may cause alterations in the cells that lead to dysplasia.

High-risk sexual behavior

Having multiple sex partners, having sex with a man who has had multiple sex partners, and engaging in sexual intercourse before the age of 18 are linked to cervical dysplasia. Women in these categories have a greater chance of being infected with HPV or HIV, especially if they do not use a barrier contraceptive such as a condom. These infections put them at higher risk for developing cervical dysplasia.

DES Exposure

Between 1938 and 1971, approximately 5 million pregnant women were prescribed diethylstilbestrol (DES), a synthetic estrogen thought to help prevent miscarriage. Its use was discontinued when researchers found it to be ineffective and dangerous. The daughters of women who took DES have a higher risk for developing cancer of the vagina or cervix, called clear cell adenocarcinoma, and abnormalities of the cervix, vagina, and uterus.

Poor Nutrition

There is growing evidence that certain vitamins, such as folic acid, play a role in cervical health. A poor diet may also cause the immune system to weaken, decreasing the body's ability to fight viruses such as HPV.

Oral Contraceptives

Some research shows that women who use oral contraceptives may be at a higher risk for developing cervical dysplasia. However, it is not clear if the risk is directly attributable to the contraceptives themselves. One reason may be that oral contraceptives interfere with folic acid metabolism in the cells around the cervix, and folic acid may help prevent or improve cervical dysplasia. Another reason may be that women using this method of birth control may have increased exposure to sexually transmitted diseases, compared to those who rely on a barrier method such as a condom.

Cervical cancer

Cervical cancer develops in the lining of the cervix, the lower part of the uterus (womb) that enters the vagina (birth canal). This condition usually develops over time. Normal cervical cells may gradually undergo changes to become precancerous and then cancerous. Cervical intraepithelial neoplasia (CIN) is the term used to describe these abnormal changes. CIN is classified according to the degree of cell abnormality. Low-grade CIN indicates a minimal change in the cells and high-grade CIN indicates a greater degree of abnormality. CIN may progress to squamous intraepithelial lesion (SIL; condition that precedes cervical cancer) or to carcinoma *in-situ* (cancer that does not extend beyond the epithelial membrane). SIL is also classified as low-grade or high-grade. High-grade SIL and carcinoma in situ may progress to invasive carcinoma (cancer that has spread to healthy tissue). Most (80-90%) invasive cervical cancer develops in flat, scaly surface cells that line the cervix (called squamous cell carcinomas). Approximately 10-15% of cases develop in glandular surface cells (called adenocarcinomas). Cancer of the cervix is the most common cancer in women in India and is a leading cause of cancer-related deaths in women in underdeveloped countries. Worldwide, approximately 500,000 cases of cervical cancer are diagnosed each year. Routine screening has decreased the incidence of invasive cervical cancer in the United States, where approximately 13,000 cases of invasive cervical cancer and 50,000 cases of cervical carcinoma in situ (i.e., localized cancer) are diagnosed yearly. Invasive cervical cancer is more common in women middle aged and older and in women of poor socio-economic status, who are less likely to receive regular screening and early treatment. The cause of cervical cancer is unknown. Infection with two types of human papilloma virus (HPV), which is transmitted sexually, is strongly associated with cervical and vulvar cancer and is the primary risk factor. Evidence of HPV is found in nearly 80% of cervical carcinomas. Human immunodeficiency virus (HIV) infection reduces the immune system's ability to fight infection (including HPV infection) and increases the likelihood that precancerous cells will progress to cancer. Sexual activity that increases the risk for infection with HPV and HIV and for cervical cancer includes the following:

- Having multiple sexual partners or having sex with a promiscuous partner.
- History of sexually transmitted disease (STD).
- Sexual intercourse at a young age.

Women who smoke cigarettes are twice as likely to develop cervical cancer. Chemicals in cigarette smoke may increase the risk by damaging cervical cells. Other risk factors include age (the condition is rare in women younger than age 15) and race (invasive cancer rates are higher in Indians). Regular screening with a Pap smear effectively lowers the risk for developing invasive cervical cancer by detecting precancerous changes in cervical cells. Women who do not receive regular Pap smears have a higher risk for the condition.

Early cervical cancer often does not produce symptoms. In women who receive regular screening, the first sign of the disease is usually an abnormal Pap test result. Symptoms that may occur include the following:

- Abnormal vaginal bleeding (e.g., spotting after sexual intercourse, bleeding between menstrual periods, increased menstrual bleeding).
- Abnormal (yellow, odorous) vaginal discharge.
- Low back pain.
- Painful sexual intercourse (dyspareunia).
- Painful urination (dysuria).

Cervical cancer that has spread (metastasized) to other organs may cause constipation, blood in the urine (hematuria), abnormal opening in the cervix (fistula), and ureteral obstruction (blockage in the tube that carries urine from the kidney to the bladder).

Depression

Since its earliest known descriptions dating back to the Old Testament, depression has been observed as a disruption of normal lifestyle. Major depressive disorder is one of two serious mood disorders (the other is bipolar disorder, or manic depressive disorder) that affect every aspect of life. Because there is no mania or elevated mood in major depressive disorder, it is called "unipolar" depression. Depression is the primary cause of suicide. Changes in mood are a natural, normal part of life. People usually recognize, and are comfortable with a change in mood. People with depression, however, often cannot explain the reason for becoming depressed, though they describe it as emotionally painful and saddening.

The predominant symptoms of depression are a general loss of interest and energy, and an inability to experience pleasure. A person with depression typically withdraws from or becomes impaired in social interactions. Apathy toward work, school, relationships, responsibility, and eventually toward important goals, negatively affects the person and the family. The economic cost is significant in terms of lost hours, reduced productivity, and healthcare. The incidence of depression has risen every year since the early 20th century. There are probably many reasons for this, though most studies point to significant socio-economic changes experienced by the present generation. In the United States, one in six people experience a depressive episode during their lifetime. Only 50% of the people who meet the criteria for diagnosis seek treatment for depression, which affects the ability to determine how many people actually suffer from this disorder.

The reported prevalence of depressive disorders varies throughout the world. The lowest rates are reported in Asian and Southeast Asian countries. Percentages represent the lifetime chance that a person will experience a depressive episode that lasts a year or more. For example, Taiwan reports less than 2%, and Korea 3%. Western countries typically report higher rates, such as Canada 7%, New Zealand 11%, and France 16%. The United States has a rate of 6%. Also, countries plagued by protracted civil war, report higher rates of depression. Low rates of depression in Eastern countries such as Taiwan may correspond with low rates of divorce and separation. However, it is possible that, divorce and separation are not publicly acknowledged as often in the East. Culturally-based differences in the perception of symptoms of depression also influence statistics. For example, Eastern people may describe depression as a series of pains, loss of focus, or an imbalance in their energy, rather than as a mental health disorder.

The anomalies of menstruation

Menorrhagia and Metrorrhagia are the two most common irregularities in menstruation. Menorrhagia is meant an excessive or too profuse menstrual flow; by metrorrhagia, a flow of blood between the menstrual periods. Neither one constitutes a disease by itself, but is a symptom of some disease condition. Beyond usual limits, the menstrual flow becomes an actual hemorrhage that, by draining away the life, becomes the source of weakness and disease. This excessive flow, aside from actual local disease, is brought about by excessive muscular exercise during menstruation; by the use of all stimulants, whether alcoholic beverages or quinine; as well as by the thinness of the blood. When the flow is excessive, it needs the physician's attention. Rest in the recumbent position is the first essential; the diet must be plain and unstimulating. The general diseases, which generally cause this condition, are anemia, Bright's disease, malaria, the early stages of tuberculosis, and heart disease. The local causes may be reflex, as powerful emotions; or due to local disease of the uterus and its appendages, as the various inflammations and displacements of the uterus, fibroid tumors, polypi, and cancer. Dysmenorrhea is painful menstruation. The most frequent forms are due to uterine congestion; to mechanical causes, as a narrowing of the cervical canal, particularly at its internal opening, or to a constriction caused by the bending over of the uterus at the junction of the body and the neck; or to ovarian irritation. The pain varies in intensity from slight discomfort to the most intense uterine colic, which is experienced in the lower part of the abdomen. In severe cases the general health becomes undermined, the nervous system gives way, and hysteria and other disorders of the nervous system result. The congestive variety usually occurs in patients who have previously menstruated painlessly. The pain comes on suddenly with the flow and ceases when the flow stops; it is very severe and is generally accompanied by a diminution or a cessation of the flow. There is severe headache, marked diminution in the secretion of the kidneys, and general restlessness. The patient frequently experiences pain in walking, is easily fatigued, has leucorrhoea and an irritable bladder. In ovarian dysmenorrhea the pain precedes the flow for several days and ceases when a free flow is established. The pain is of a dull aching character, and may be felt on one or both sides of the abdomen, as one or both ovaries are involved.

Amenorrhea

In amenorrhea the menstrual flow may not appear for some years after it is normally due; or the flow may cease after some months or years of continuance; or the flow may be abnormally scanty or even absent. The menstrual flow is much later in appearing in some families than in others, so that this may be considered as a family idiosyncrasy; and if the girl's health is good, it need cause no anxiety. If, on the contrary, the girl has severe headaches, or suffers in any way, the physician should be consulted, as the absence of menstruation may be indicative of some serious condition. A scanty flow is often indicative of thinness of the blood; on the other hand, serious anemias often lead to profuse menorrhagias or metrorrhagias. The cause of the profound anemia itself may be insufficient nutrition, overwork, or lack of exercise. Scanty menstruation is often seen to occur in fevers, in the later stages of consumption, in advanced Bright's disease, in malaria, or in any other very serious disease. In these cases it seems to be a conservative process on the part of nature in the run-down state of the system. Great shock sometimes causes a sudden cessation of the flow; and sometimes a sea-voyage, followed by the change of habitat, will cause an obstinate form of amenorrhea. But it cannot be too well understood that, after the menstrual flow has been regularly established, it continues with the greatest regularity throughout the childbearing period, unless the exposure to wet or cold has been sufficiently severe to cause great indisposition on the part of the woman. In this case it is possible that, if the exposure took place just previous to the time of the expected flow, one period may remain out. But except in case of serious illness, for example, typhoid fever, two or more periods do not fail to appear except in the case of pregnancy.

Dysfunctional uterine bleeding (DUB)

Dysfunctional uterine bleeding (DUB) is heavy or irregular menstrual bleeding that is not caused by an underlying anatomical abnormality, such as a fibroid, lesion, or tumor. DUB is the most common type of abnormal uterine bleeding. Most cases of DUB are associated with anovulatory bleeding (menstruation that occurs without ovulation). Anovulatory bleeding is common in women who have just started menstruating and during the several years preceding menopause. When ovulation does not occur, the level of estrogen and progesterone in the uterus is disturbed, leading to DUB. Anovulation, however, does not always lead to DUB and there are other causes as well. Women with ovulatory cycles (cycles that involve ovulation) may also experience DUB. Menstrual cycles vary in duration, frequency, and intensity, making abnormalities difficult to determine. Women who have DUB may experience a variety of patterns of bleeding. A woman who bleeds for longer than a week, bleeds more than every 3 weeks or so, bleeds between periods, or bleeds excessively should see a doctor. DUB is usually painless. Diagnosis involves ruling out other causes of abnormal bleeding. Treatment depends on the intensity and timing of the bleeding, the patient's age, and if she is trying to conceive.

What causes dysfunctional uterine bleeding?

Dysfunctional uterine bleeding (DUB) is caused by the erratic production of hormones. That is why it is more commonly associated with puberty and the menopause. The endometrium (lining of the womb) is stimulated to grow by the hormone oestrogen. If this is not balanced by the presence of progesterone, the endometrium may continue to grow until it outgrows its blood supply. At this point it breaks away and is discharged, causing irregular and sometimes heavy bleeding. If this bleeding is very heavy and very frequent, anaemia can result. Menorrhagia (abnormally long periods) is often a symptom of dysfunctional uterine bleeding. There may also be an irregular bleeding pattern. Other causes of abnormal bleeding patterns, such as endometriosis, fibroids or pelvic inflammatory disease (PID) must be outruled before it can be assumed that the menorrhagia is due to dysfunctional uterine bleeding.

How is dysfunctional uterine bleeding treated?

By definition, dysfunctional uterine bleeding is only said to exist when other causes of abnormal bleeding have been ruled out. Therefore, treatment usually consists of relieving the symptoms of the bleeding so that it does not interfere with a woman's normal life or cause anaemia. This may include taking medications such as the oral contraceptive pill and possibly taking iron supplements to reduce the chances of developing anaemia. In some cases, surgery may be required. In the past, hysterectomy (surgical removal of the womb) was the only surgical option to relieve heavy bleeding in older women. Nowadays, there are a number of options short of hysterectomy, such as endometrial ablation where the lining of the womb (the endometrium) may be removed using a telescopic instrument inserted through the vagina and neck of the womb (cervix). What is endometrium? The endometrium is the mucous surface that lines the inside of the uterus. It is responsive to hormonal changes and contains several layers of cells that vary in appearance and number throughout the menstrual cycle. During the luteal phase (i.e., 2 weeks prior to menstruation), the endometrium is thick, its epithelial cells and glands are enlarged, and the arteries are swollen. At menstruation, the endometrium sheds. Following menstruation, the endometrium regenerates. Menstruation is triggered by a sudden decrease in progesterone and estrogen secretions. The menstrual flow is made up of endometrial cells and tissue, blood, and cervical and vaginal mucus and cells. After menstruation, the increased secretion of estrogen causes cellular growth and the regeneration of the endometrium. This first half of the menstrual cycle is known as the follicular phase. Ovulation (the release of an egg from the ovary) normally occurs 2 weeks after the first day of the last menstrual cycle. After ovulation, the secretion of progesterone stops the growth of the endometrium, balancing out the effects of the estrogen. If conception does not occur, progesterone production declines, and menstrual bleeding begins again.

Normally during the menstrual cycle, the production of progesterone in the latter 2 weeks of the cycle balances out the regenerative effects of estrogen, halting further endometrial growth. In anovulation, the level of estrogen does not decline, and progesterone is not secreted to balance out the effects of estrogen. Endometrial growth does not stop and the endometrial tissue accumulates and thickens, resulting in abnormally heavy bleeding. Also, without progesterone, the endometrium lacks structural support and sloughs-off irregularly, causing heavy and/or irregular periods. Anovulatory periods are common in the 2 or 3 years following menarche (first menstrual period) and during the several years preceding menopause. Up to 80% of menstrual cycles are anovulatory during the first year following menarche. As a woman approaches menopause, she may have 8 to 10 anovulatory periods a year. Women who take oral contraceptives and those on estrogen replacement therapy may also have anovulatory cycles. Stress and illness can also trigger anovulation.

Dysmenorrhea

Dysmenorrhea is the term for painful periods or menstrual cramps. Although menstruation is often painless, many women suffer from discomfort or pain in association with periods at some time during their reproductive years. There are two types of dysmenorrhea:

Primary or spasmodic dysmenorrhea: in this variety no disease or other medical cause can be found for the pain and other symptoms. Primary dysmenorrhea frequently affects women in their teens and early 20s, who have never had a baby.

Features of primary dysmenorrhea: include backache, diarrhoea, dizziness, headache, nausea, vomiting, and a feeling of tenseness. Severe pain occurs only in minority, but their is no doubt that it can be incapacitating. The pain is colicky in nature, usually starts on the first day of the period. It may last for several hours or continue throughout the first and second day. Often the menstrual flow is scanty at first, and then the pain becomes easier when the flow is properly established. The symptoms are caused by prostaglandin, a natural hormone produced by cells in the uterine lining. The level of prostaglandin increases in the second half of the menstrual cycle. When a woman's period begins, the cells in the uterine lining release prostaglandin as they are shed. Women with severe primary dysmenorrhea have significantly higher prostaglandin levels in their menstrual fluid than do other women. The only good thing that can be said about primary dysmenorrhea is that usually the symptoms don't last very long. Some women experience symptoms for up to one or two days, but rarely longer.

Secondary dysmenorrhea is caused by a physical condition. Women who suffer from it tend to be older than those with primary dysmenorrhea. Some conditions that may be responsible for secondary dysmenorrhea are endometriosis (uterine tissue that grows outside the uterus, in the ovaries and other locations). Endometriosis is the most common reason for secondary dysmenorrhea—

1. Adenomyosis (uterine tissue growing into the uterine wall).
2. Endometrial polyps (growths in the uterine lining).
3. Fibroids (growths in the uterus).
4. Narrowing of the cervix (the entrance to the uterus) as it opens into the vagina.
5. Pelvic inflammatory disease (PID).
6. Use of an intrauterine device (IUD).

Features of secondary dysmenorrhea: The type of pain experienced is very variable. It may preced the onset of period for about a week. The pain is often a dull ache felt equally on both sides of the lower abdomen and back, sometimes extending down the thighs.

Tests and treatments

Primary dysmenorrhea, a pelvic examination and/or other tests like an ultrasound examination are done to be sure there's no other cause for the symptoms. If everything is normal, then generally analgesics like aspirin ibuprofen, or naproxen are recommended. The most effective medical treatment is to use the birth-control pill. It acts by stopping the ovulation and decreases prostaglandin levels. Regular exercise can also help minimize pain and cramping.

In case of secondary dysmenorrhea, in these cases the underlying cause must be treated. To find the cause, the doctor may—

- Perform a pelvic examination,
- Ask about the problem and general health,
- Do X-ray and ultrasound examinations.

advise dilation and curettage (D and C), a minor surgical procedure to open the cervix and remove tissue for microscopic testing.

Premenstrual Syndrome (PMS)

PMS consists of various physical and/or emotional symptoms that occur in the second half of the menstrual cycle, after ovulation. It is characterized by premenstrual discomfort in the lower abdomen and back, and in the breasts. All these features precede the period by a week or ten days. Fortunately, a woman obtains relief when her menstrual period begins. Another feature of PMS is a symptom-free time for several days every month, in the first half of the menstrual cycle. Features include physical features like acne, backache, bloating, sore breasts, and headache. Emotional symptoms might include changes in sexual desire, difficulty concentrating, irritability. Women may gain upto a kg. of weight or more in the latter part of the menstrual cycle due to water retention in the body. Emotional stress often contributes to the symptoms. The only saving grace in this problem is that few women experience all these symptoms! Most have a few that recur each month.

The symptoms of certain medical conditions can resemble PMS. These conditions include allergies, depression, diabetes, dysmenorrhea (painful periods), endometriosis, fibrocystic breast disease, and thyroid problems.

There's still some disagreement about what causes PMS, but it definitely seems to be linked to hormones. A relative lack of the hormone progesterone is suspected along with increase in a water retaining substance called anti-diuretic hormone.

The assessment of the emotional and work-related stress is very important. Many women find that a balanced diet and healthy snacks are helpful, as are avoiding caffeine and reducing salt intake. Simple reassurance often does wonders, but often it is necessary to treat the symptoms with various drugs: Diuretics ("water pills") can reduce bloating, Analgesics like ibuprofen, aspirin ease headache or cramps.

Combined oral contraceptives also called the birth control pill may be useful for some women. Evening primrose oil (gamma linolenic acid) is also used widely these days.

Cardiovascular Disease

More than half of persons who die each year of heart disease are women. Heart disease is the leading cause of death for all racial and ethnic groups in the United States. In 1998, rates of death from cardiovascular

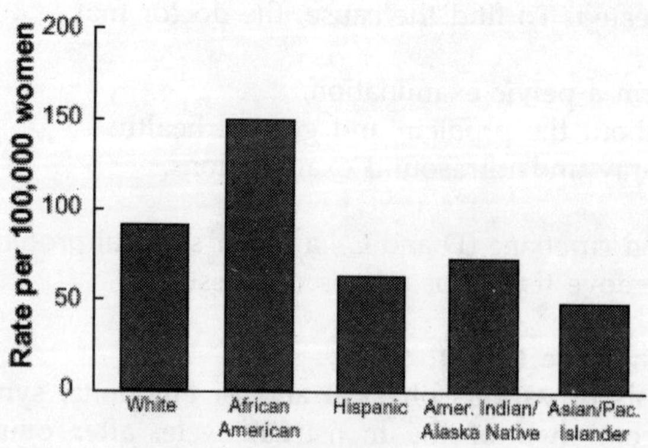

Source: *Journal of Women's Health and Gender-based Medicine*, Vol. 10, No. 8, 2001, pp. 717-24.

disease were about 30% higher among African American adults than among white adults. Age-Adjusted Death Rates for Diseases of the Heart* Among Women, by Race/Ethnicity, 1996-98.

In Asian countries like India, the incidence of cardiovascular diseases is on the rise, due to faulty eating habits and inadequate physical activity

Diabetes

- Diabetes affects more women than men.
- The prevalence of diabetes is 70% higher among African Americans and nearly 100% higher among Hispanics than among whites. The prevalence of diabetes among American Indians and Alaska Natives is more than twice that of the total population, and the Pimas of Arizona have the highest known prevalence of diabetes in the world.

Infant and Maternal Mortality

African American, American Indian, and Puerto Rican infants have higher death rates than white infants. In 1998, the death rate among African American infants was 2.3 times greater than that among white infants.

African American women are four times more likely to die of pregnancy-related complications than are white women, and American Indian and Alaska Native women are nearly twice as likely to die.

U.S. Infant Mortality Rates, by Race/Ethnicity of Mother, 1998

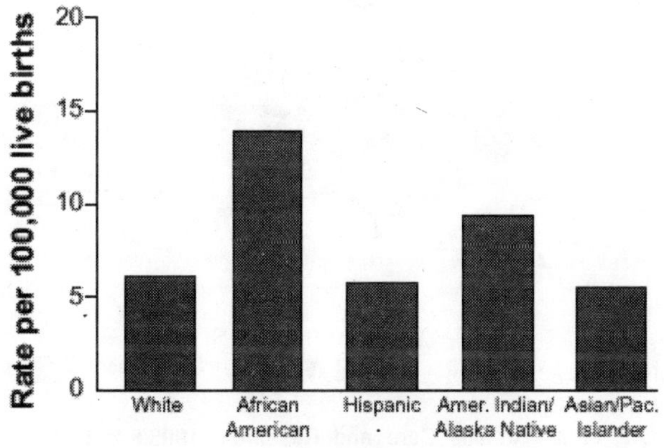

* Average annual deaths per 100,000 women, age adjusted to 1940 U.S. standard population, International Classification of Diseases, 9th Rev., codes 390-398, 402, and 404-29.

Source: CDC, National Center for Health Statistics.

Disability

Life expectancy is higher for women than for men, but women older than 70 years are more likely to be disabled. Arthritis or chronic joint symptoms affect nearly 70 million Americans (about 1 in 3 adults), making it one of the most prevalent diseases in the United States. Arthritis is the leading cause of disability among U.S. adults. It limits everyday activities for more than 7 million Americans. By 2020, an estimated 12 million Americans will be limited in daily activities because of arthritis. Arthritis is not just an old person's disease: nearly two-thirds of people with arthritis are younger than 65 years.

Costs

Each year, arthritis results in 44 million outpatient visits, 750,000 hospitalizations, estimated medical care costs of more than $22 billion, and estimated total costs (medical care and lost productivity) of $82 billion.

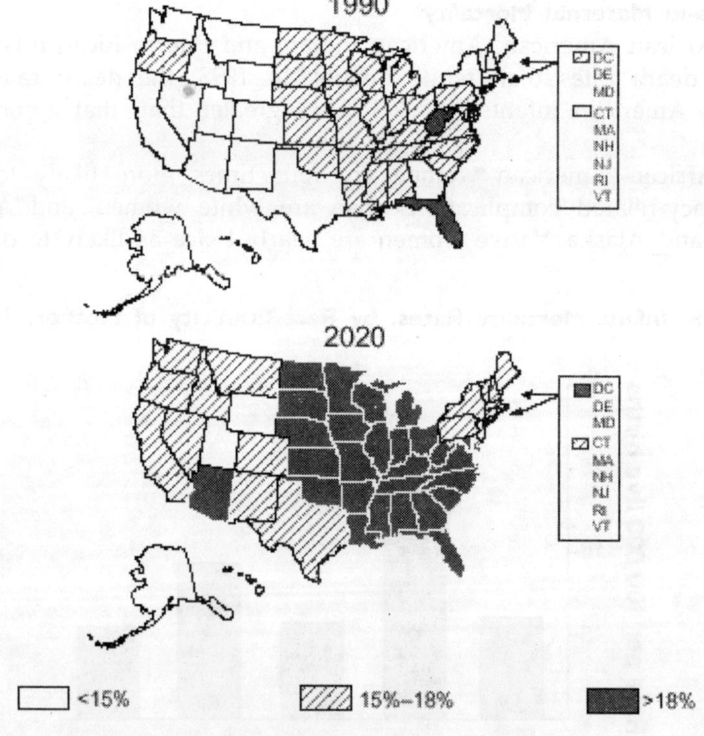

Source: Helmick CG, *et al.* Arthritis Care and Research, 1995:8:203-11.

Examples of CDC Activities

CDC developed the National Arthritis Action Plan in partnership with the Arthritis Foundation and the Association of State and Territorial Health Officials. The plan proposes a national coordinated effort to reduce the occurrence of arthritis and its accompanying disability. In FY 2001, CDC funded arthritis programs in 29 states with the following objectives:

- To develop capacity in state health departments to improve the quality of life of people with arthritis.
- To facilitate prevention and control as called for in the National Arthritis Action Plan.
- CDC and its state partners are working to broaden dissemination of the Arthritis Self-Help Course to build self-management into routine arthritis care and to encourage appropriate physical activity programs for people with arthritis.
- Congress allocated about $11.8 million to CDC in FY 2001 for arthritis control programs. CDC provided grants to state health departments to develop or enhance state-based programs that will decrease the burden of arthritis and improve the quality of life among people with arthritis.
- CDC gives eight state health departments core funding for arthritis control activities and provides limited support to other state health departments for their public health activities related to arthritis.
- CDC conducts arthritis surveillance in all 50 states.

Program Effectiveness

For every $1 spent on the Arthritis Self-Help Program, $3.42 was saved in physician visits and hospital costs.

Cancer Control

The National Comprehensive Cancer Control Program is an integrated, coordinated approach to reducing the impact of cancer that includes monitoring, policy, research, education, programs, services, and evaluation. With 2002 funding of $5.5 million, CDC's National Program provides support and technical assistance to plan and implement comprehensive cancer control activities and programs in 19 states and one tribal organization. Health agencies use this funding to establish broad-based cancer coalitions, provide epidemiological support, and develop and implement a comprehensive cancer control plan. In addition, $3.4 million in supplemental funding has been given to support colorectal, prostate, and skin cancer activities within CCC programs. Comprehensive cancer control is based on the following principles:

1. Scientific data and research are used systematically to identify priorities and inform decision-making.
2. The full scope of cancer care, ranging from primary prevention to early detection and treatment to end-of-life issues, is addressed.

3. Many stakeholders are engaged in cancer prevention and control, including not only the medical and public health communities but also voluntary agencies, insurers, businesses, survivors, government, academia, and advocates.
4. All cancer-related programs and activities are coordinated, thereby creating integrated activities and fostering leadership.
5. The activities of many disciplines are integrated. Appropriate disciplines include administration, basic and applied research, evaluation, health education, program development, public policy, surveillance, clinical services, and health communications.

CCC programs across the country are making significant progress in coordinating and integrating cancer prevention and control. Examples include the following:

Enhancing Infrastructure in Georgia: The Georgia Cancer Coalition, a public-private partnership, was created by Governor Roy Barnes in 2000. With support from tobacco settlement funds, federal grants, and private organizations, the coalition has funded nine rural cancer education and screening projects to develop partnerships to educate citizens and increase cancer screening in rural counties that have breast, cervical, colorectal, or prostate cancer mortality rates above the state average. The Coalition also funded eight projects to improve availability of mammography services for women living in counties that have no mammography facilities.

Assessing the Cancer Burden in Iowa: In 2001, legislation enacted in Iowa mandated the development of the CCC Study Committee. On the basis of the cancer data in Healthy Iowans 2010, the CCC Study Committee used the building blocks model to develop the following priorities:

1. Assess the number of new cases and prevalence of cancer in Iowa.
2. Evaluate the effectiveness of current cancer control efforts in terms of prevention, early detection, treatment, rehabilitation, and quality of life.
3. Identify additional resources for breast and cervical cancer treatment.
4. Evaluate the availability of cancer-related resources and their effectiveness.
5. Focus on prostate, bladder, colorectal, skin, lung, oral cavity and pharynx, breast, and cervical cancers.

The findings of the CCC Study Committee were documented in the CCC Report. The Report identifies priorities for cancer prevention and control in Iowa and serves as the basis for Iowa's comprehensive cancer prevention and control plan. Utilizing Data and Research in the Northwest Tribal Population by linking the records of the Northwest Tribal Registry and the state cancer registries, the Northwest Portland Area Indian Health Board documented an underestimation of cancer incidence among its tribal members (153.5 per 100,000 population prior to linking compared with 267.5 per 100,000 after linking). This work underscores the importance of using high-quality data to assess the cancer burden and eliminate health disparities.

Addressing the Cancer Burden in North Carolina: To address a priority area within the North Carolina CCC plan, the North Carolina Comprehensive Cancer Unit designed a pilot project to conduct colorectal cancer screening in 10 local health departments that service 15 counties throughout the state. The objective of this pilot project was to determine the feasibility of conducting colorectal cancer screening in local health departments. A total of 1,478 participants were counseled and offered fecal occult blood test kits; 706 (48%) completed and returned these kits. Ten precancerous polyps were found and four cancers were diagnosed. An evaluation of this project found local health departments could be useful in raising public awareness about the importance of early detection, as well as encouraging participation in screening programs. North Carolina plans to expand its colorectal cancer screening program as resources become available.

Building Partnerships for Cancer Control in Colorado: Colorado has enlisted the help of a large and varied group of partners both internal and external to the state health department to launch a public education campaign called Sun Smart Tips. The goal of this campaign is to educate national park visitors about the need to protect themselves from the

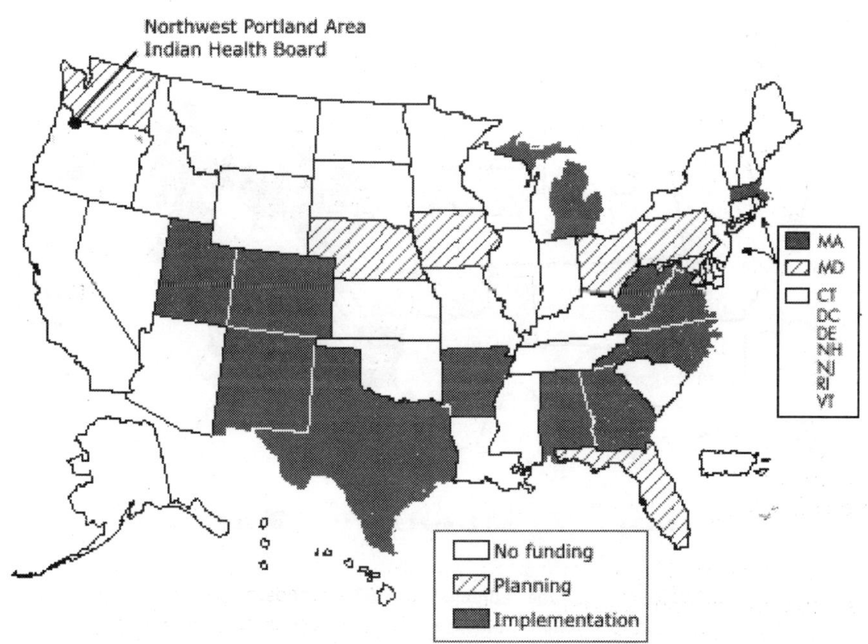

damaging rays of the sun and how best to prevent skin cancer. This campaign resulted from a unique partnership between national park officials and the state health department. Together, Colorado's Comprehensive Cancer Prevention and Control Program, the Mesa Verde National Park, and the park concessioner are educating Colorado residents and visitors from all over the world about the easy steps they can take to protect themselves from the damaging effects of sun exposure.

Preventing Breast and Cervical Cancer

Breast cancer is the second most common cancer among American women (after skin cancer) and the second most common cause of cancer-related death (after lung cancer). According to the American Cancer Society, 203,500 new cases of invasive breast cancer will be diagnosed in 2002, and 40,000 women will die of this disease. The incidence of invasive cervical cancer decreased significantly during the last 40 years, in large part because of early detection. Even so, the American Cancer Society estimates that 13,000 new cases will be diagnosed in 2002, and 4,100 women will die of the disease. Many deaths—which occur disproportionately among low-income women and women from racial and ethnic minority groups—could be avoided by increasing cancer screening rates for all women at risk. Both mammograms and Papanicolaou (Pap) tests are underused by women who are members of some racial and ethnic minority groups, have less than a high school education, are older than 40, or live below the poverty level.

Rates of Death Due to Breast Cancer, 1993-97*

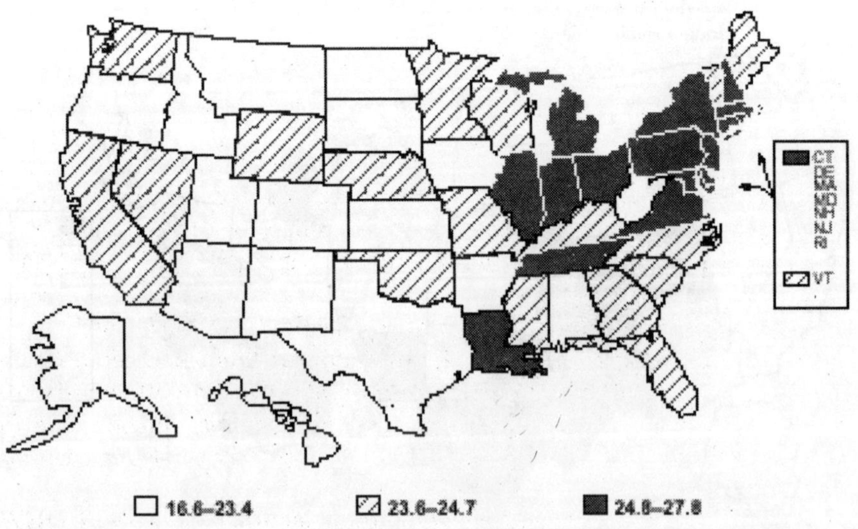

* Rate per 100,000 women, age adjusted to 1970 standard U.S. population.
Source: National Center for Health Statistics, CDC; American Cancer Society.

Costs

According to the National Institutes of Health, in 2002 the overall annual costs for cancer were $170 billion: over $60 billion for direct medical costs, $110 billion in lost productivity. No information is available on the medical or overall costs associated specifically with breast or cervical cancer.

CDC Goals

- To strengthen the capacity to conduct cancer prevention programs in all 50 states, U.S. territories, the District of Columbia, and Native American/Alaska Native Organizations.
- To provide life-saving screening for low-income women through CDC's National Breast and Cervical Cancer Early Detection Program.

Effectiveness of Screening

Mammography is the best way of detecting breast cancer in its earliest, most treatable stage—by about 1 to 3 years before a woman would notice a lump. Timely mammography for women older than age 40 could prevent 15%-30% of all deaths from breast cancer. When breast cancer is diagnosed at a local stage, 97% of women are still alive 5 years later. The 5-year survival rate decreases to 21% when the disease is diagnosed after spreading to other sites. Pap tests detect not only cervical cancer but also precancerous lesions. Detecting and treating such lesions can prevent cervical cancer—and thus prevent virtually all deaths from this disease.

Examples of CDC Activities

- In 2001, CDC funded cancer prevention activities in all 50 states, 6 U.S. territories, the District of Columbia, and 14 American Indian or Alaska Native Organizations.
- CDC's National Breast and Cervical Cancer Early Detection Program (NBCCEDP) screens underserved women for breast and cervical cancer. The NBCCEDP provides clinical breast examinations, mammograms, pelvic examinations, and Pap tests. The NBCCEDP also funds post-screening diagnostic services, such as surgical consultation and biopsy. Now in its 11th year, the NBCCEDP has provided more than 3 million examinations to more than 1.3 million women and diagnosed more than 10,649 breast cancers, 45,154 precancerous cervical lesions, and 700 cases of cervical cancer.
- With $170.5 million in funding in 2001, CDC increased education and outreach programs for women and for doctors, improved quality assurance measures for screening programs, and improved underserved women's access to screening and follow-up services.

Number of Screening Examinations Among NBCCEDP* Participants for Fiscal Years 1991-2000

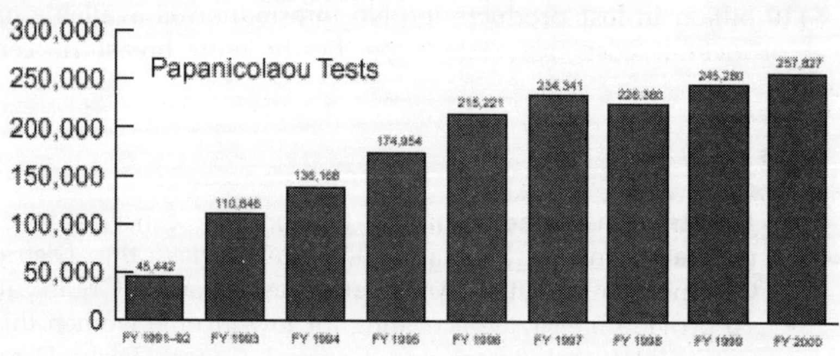

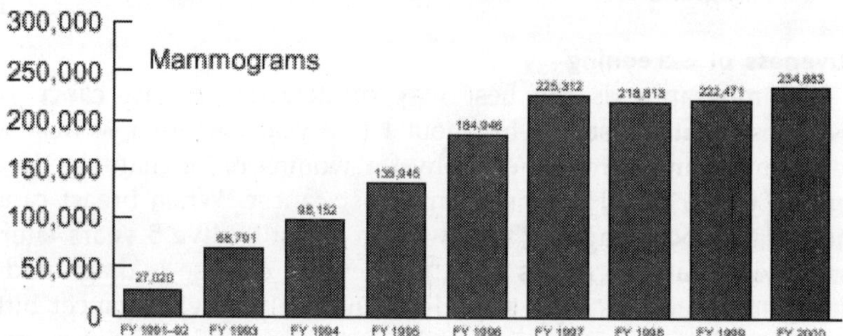

Total Papanicolaou Tests and Mammograms = 3,064,392

* CDC, National Breast and Cervical Cancer Early Detection Program.

Examples of State Activities

Missouri

In collaboration with the Missouri Department of Social Services, the Missouri Breast and Cervical Cancer Control Program hired women who are moving from welfare to work as outreach coordinators to inform women about free breast and cervical cancer screening. To date, these coordinators have referred about 3,400 women for screening, and 12 coordinators have been given full-time employment.

Nevada

Along with Race for the Cure, the Nevada Breast and Cervical Cancer Early Detection Program partnered with Chevron, the Susan G. Komen Foundation, and Mobile-Ray Imaging to offer free mammograms at a local Chevron station. The program provided breast health education, follow-up after an abnormal screening result, and additional mammograms for those who qualified. As a result, hundreds of women were educated about breast and cervical health, and more than 200 underserved women were given a free mammogram.

Preventing Other Forms of Cancer: Colorectal, Ovarian, Prostate, Skin

Colorectal Cancer

Colorectal cancer—cancer of the colon or rectum—is the second leading cause of cancer-related death among men and women in the United States. The American Cancer Society estimates that nearly 56,600 Americans will die of colorectal cancer in 2002.

Ovarian Cancer

Among women, ovarian cancer is the seventh most common cancer and the fifth leading cause of cancer-related death. The American Cancer Society estimates that, in 2002 in the United States, 13,900 women will die of this disease. More whites than blacks get this disease; there is little information about how this disease affects other races.

Prostate Cancer

Among men in the United States, prostate cancer is the second most commonly diagnosed form of cancer and second most common cause of cancer-related death. The American Cancer Society estimates that 30,200 men will die of the disease in 2002. Blacks get prostate cancer more than any other racial or ethnic group. The death rate for blacks is twice as high as that for whites.

Skin Cancer

In the United States, more than 1 million cases of highly curable skin cancer occur annually. The most serious form of skin cancer is melanoma, which occurs 10 times more often among whites than among blacks. Melanoma causes more than 75% of all deaths from skin cancer. If treated early, this disease can usually be cured. Untreated melanoma can spread to other organs, usually the lungs and liver. Although death rates from basal cell and squamous cell carcinomas are low, they can cause considerable disfigurement and damage if left untreated.

CDC Goals

- To increase the number of adults aged 50 or older who are screened for colorectal cancer from 35% to 50%.
- To research the symptoms of ovarian cancer in order to be able to diagnose the disease during its early stages.
- To contribute significantly to the Healthy People 2010 goal of reducing death rate due to prostate cancer from 32.0 to 28.8 per 100,000 men.

To increase to the number of adults and children who regularly use at least one protective measure against skin cancer.

Prostate Cancer (Invasive) Death Rates, by Race and Ethnicity, United States, 1990-98

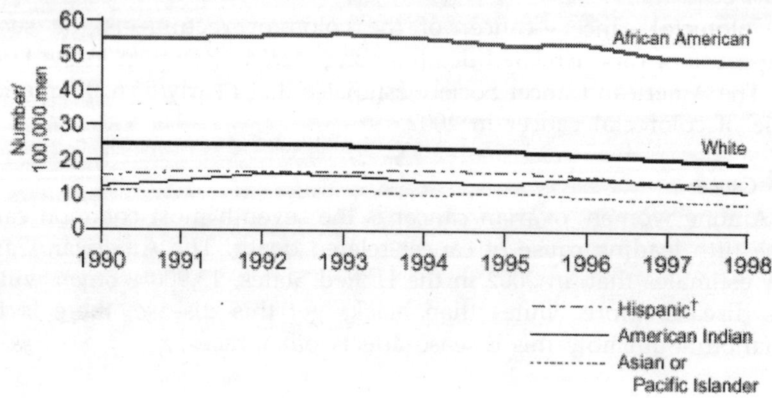

Examples of CDC Activities

Colorectal Cancer

- In partnership with the Centers for Medicare and Medicaid Services, CDC created Screen for Life, a multimedia campaign to promote colorectal cancer screening for men and women aged 50 or older. Screen for Life materials can be ordered or downloaded from the Internet at www.cdc.gov/cancer/screenforlife.
- CDC developed A Call to Action, a Web-based training program to raise primary care providers' awareness and knowledge about prevention and early detection of colorectal cancer.

CDC supports a variety of epidemiological and behavioral research projects to reduce the incidence of colorectal cancer.

Percentage of Adults Aged 50 Years or Older Who Had Colorectal Cancer Screening Tests Within the Recommended Time Interval, 1999

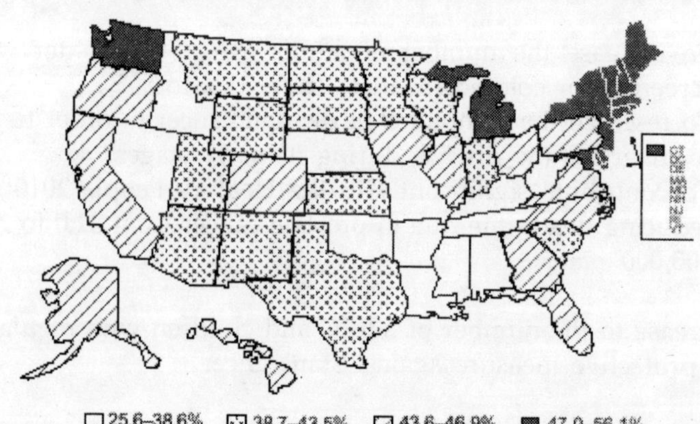

Ovarian Cancer

CDC conducts research or collaborates in research on a variety of issues. For example:

- The factors that distinguish women at stages 1 and 2 from women at stages 3 and 4 of ovarian cancer.
- Ovarian cancer incidence by race.
- The factors that distinguish women with borderline ovarian tumors from women with ovarian cancer.

Prostate Cancer

- Six questions on prostate cancer screening were added to the core questionnaire of the 2001 Behavioral Risk Factor Surveillance System. Answers to these questions are helping determine what proportion of men aged 40 or older were screened for prostate cancer and whether there is an association between race, age, family history of prostate cancer and whether a man gets screened for prostate cancer.
- By collecting prostate cancer data through the National Program of Cancer Registries—especially data on stage of diagnosis, quality of care, and race and ethnicity—CDC and the states can design more effective public health programs to combat the disease. For example:

Skin Cancer

- CDC conducted epidemiologic research to determine national trends in sun protection behavior and attitudes about sun exposure. The findings are being used to target and evaluate skin cancer prevention programs.

CDC's national Choose Your Cover media campaign helps states increase people's awareness about skin cancer and its causes as well as influence social norms regarding sun protection and tanned skin.

CDC and Diabetes spread in USA

Diabetes affects more than 17 million Americans and contributes to over 200,000 deaths a year. Diabetes can cause heart disease, stroke, blindness, kidney failure, leg and foot amputations, pregnancy complications, and deaths related to influenza and pneumonia. About 5.9 million Americans are unaware they have the disease. Among U.S. adults, diagnosed diabetes (including gestational diabetes) increased 61% since 1991 and is projected to more than double by 2050. Type 2 affects 90%-95% of people with diabetes and is linked to obesity and physical inactivity. More than 18% of adults older than age 65 have diabetes. Diabetes affects more women than men.

Costs

The direct and indirect costs of diabetes are nearly $132 billion a year. The average healthcare cost for a person with diabetes in 2002 was $13,243, compared with $2,560 for a person without diabetes.

CDC Goals

- To increase diabetes awareness.
- To promote early detection of diabetes and treatment of its complications.
- To improve the quality of and access to diabetes care.

Diabetes and Gestational Diabetes

Trends Among U.S. Adults Examples of CDC Activities:

- *National Diabetes Prevention Center*. Because diabetes is so common among American Indians, CDC funds a center in New Mexico to develop culturally relevant diabetes prevention strategies for American Indian/Alaska Native communities.
- *U.S./Mexico Border Diabetes Prevention and Control Project*. CDC is working with south-western U.S. border states, Mexican border states, the Pan American Health Organization, and Mexico's Secretariat of Health to assess the burden of diabetes, patterns of care, and barriers to good self-management.
- *Children and Type 2 Diabetes*. CDC and the National Institutes of Health are studying childhood diabetes. SEARCH for Diabetes in Youth is a 5-year, multicenter study to evaluate diabetes cases among children aged 19 years or younger at diagnosis. The target population comprises 4.5 million children, or about 6% of all U.S. children.
- *Diabetes Prevention Program (DPP)*. The DPP is a 27-center randomized clinical trial involving more than 3,200 adults aged 25 years or older. Study participants are African American, Hispanic, American Indian, and Asian American. The DPP evaluated the effectiveness of intensive lifestyle modification, standard care plus metformin, and standard care plus placebo to prevent or delay type 2 diabetes. The results of this first major clinical trial of Americans at high risk for type 2 diabetes are: (1) lifestyle changes reduced participants' risk for type 2 diabetes by 58%, (2) lifestyle changes were effective across all ages and racial/ethnic groups, and (3) those who had standard care plus metformin reduced their risk for type 2 diabetes by 31%.

With FY 2002 funding of $58.3 million, CDC provided limited support to 34 states, 8 territories, and the District of Columbia for core diabetes control programs and more substantive support to 16 states for comprehensive programs.

Epilepsy

Epilepsy is a chronic neurological condition that affects approximately 2.3 million people in the United States—

- Each year, about 181,000 people in the United States are diagnosed with epilepsy; the very young and older adults are the most likely to be affected.
- People of lower socio-economic status, residents of urban areas, and minority populations tend to bear a disproportionate burden.
- Delayed recognition of seizures and inadequate treatment greatly increase the risk for subsequent seizures, brain damage, disability, and death from injuries incurred during a seizure.
- Because of restrictions from certain activities, public prejudice, and public fear of people who have seizures, 20%-30% of people with epilepsy are underemployed.

Costs

The Epilepsy Foundation estimates an annual total cost to the United States of $12.5 billion in direct and indirect costs for epilepsy and seizures.

CDC Goals

- To increase timely diagnosis, effective management, and appropriate treatment for people with epilepsy.

Prevalence of Self-Reported Epilepsy, by Sex and Age Group, United States, 1986-90

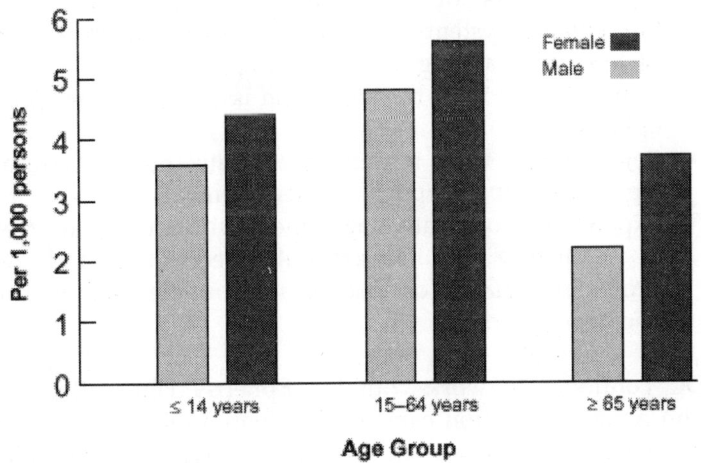

- To develop programs and materials to combat the stigma, discrimination, and misplaced safety concerns related to epilepsy.
- To improve self-management for people with epilepsy.

To promote the ongoing systematic collection, analysis, and interpretation of health data needed to design, implement, and evaluate public health programs related to epilepsy. CDC focuses on improving care, self-management, surveillance, prevention research, communication, information dissemination, and works to strengthen partnerships to promote epilepsy awareness and quality of life for people affected by epilepsy. In 2001, CDC

- Developed sample contract language for health service providers and insurers relating to health service benefits and the provision of those benefits to people with epilepsy.
- Initiated research to analyze population-based data maintained by a managed care organization, and to better assess the incidence, prevalence, and patterns of care of epilepsy in these populations.
- Initiated epidemiologic studies of cysticercosis in selected communities to assess the associated risk of epilepsy and to develop effective primary prevention programs.
- Assessed the needs of parents of children with epilepsy to determine, which products would help them assist their children manage their condition.
- Continued research on the effects of epilepsy and seizures on older people.
- Collaborated on developing a systematic method of evaluating the quality and quantity of research on the care of people with treatment-resistant epilepsy.
- On the basis of data from the Behavioral Risk Factor Surveillance System in Texas, reported on health-related quality of life issues among adults with epilepsy.
- Initiated a study of transportation issues that affect people with epilepsy.
- Began work with a national organization to educate state legislatures about epilepsy and seizures.
- Expanded a cooperative agreement with a national organization to conduct a multifaceted public education and awareness campaign focusing on teenagers and adolescents with epilepsy and their peers.

CDC continues to work with the Epilepsy Foundation and other partners on a communication campaign to help adolescents with epilepsy make decisions about whether, with whom, and when to share information about epilepsy and seizures. CDC will also work with partners to assess the needs of parents in assisting their children with epilepsy in taking appropriate responsibility for managing their condition.

Ageing Population

The life expectancy of Americans increased from 47 years in 1900 to 77 years in 2000. As a result, the number of people in America aged 65 or older increased from 3 million in 1900 to nearly 35 million in 1996—an 11-fold increase. By 2030, the number will have doubled to 70 million when one in five Americans will be older than 65. Although the risk for disease and disability clearly increases with age, poor health is not an inevitable consequence of ageing. People with a healthy lifestyle (i.e., people who get regular exercise, avoid tobacco use, and eat healthily) have half the risk for disability of those who do not have a healthy lifestyle.

Chronic diseases among older adults impose hard demands on the public health system and on medical and social services. Chronic diseases cause disabilities and diminish quality of life. They are also a major contributor to healthcare costs. In 1994, chronic conditions decreased the quality of life for nearly 40% of the elderly not living in institutions—nearly 12 million people. Of those 12 million, 3 million (about 10% of all the elderly) were unable to perform some activities of daily living (e.g., bathing, shopping, dressing, eating). More than 65% of Americans aged 65 years or older have some form of cardiovascular disease; half of all men and two-thirds of all women older than 70 have arthritis.

Costs

Almost one-third of U.S. healthcare costs, or $300 billion each year, are for older adults. Not including the costs of inflation and new

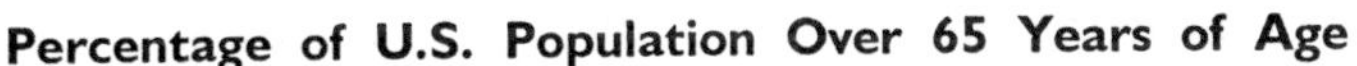

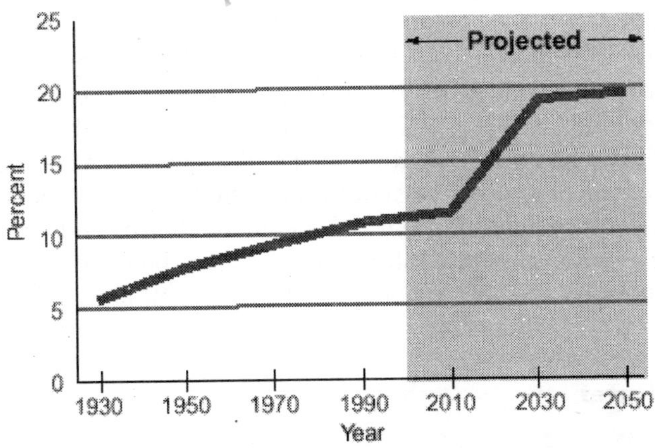

Source: Adapted from Baby Boom to Elder Boom: Providing Healthcare for an Ageing Population.

technology, healthcare spending will increase by 25% between 2000 and 2030 simply because a larger percentage of the population is older than 65.

CDC Goal

To increase the number of Americans 65 or older, who are physically active, eat a healthy diet, and avoid tobacco use.

Program Effectiveness

One example of a worthwhile investment is an arthritis control intervention. According to one Northern California study, for every $1 spent on the Arthritis Self-Help Program, $3.42 was saved in the cost of hospitalizations and visits to physicians.

Examples of CDC Activities

- To combine activities to prevent disease among older adults, CDC is developing new partnerships and strengthening old ones with agencies and organizations that serve older adults. For example.
- CDC brings together the prevention expertise of public health agencies and the ageing services network of the Administration on Ageing.
- Through its Prevention Research Centers network and longstanding partnerships with state health departments, CDC is putting promising prevention strategies into effect in communities across America. For example.

North-west Prevention Effectiveness Center at the University of Washington is working with senior centers to help people older than 65 exercise more, eat well, and preserve their independence.

The health of young people, and the adults they will become, is critically linked to the health-related behaviors they adopt. Certain behaviors that are often established during youth contribute markedly to today's major killers, such as heart disease, cancer, and injuries. These behaviors include tobacco use; unhealthy dietary habits; inadequate physical activity; alcohol and other drug use; sexual behaviors that can result in HIV infection, other sexually transmitted diseases, and unintended pregnancies; and behaviors that result in violence and unintentional injuries (e.g., driving while intoxicated). These behaviors place young people at increased risk for serious health problems, both now and in the future.

Health Challenges

- During the past 20 years, decreases in physical activity coupled with unhealthy eating has resulted in a doubling of the percentage of children and adolescents who are overweight.

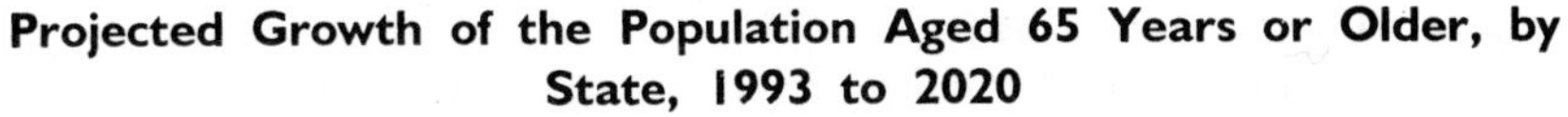

Projected Growth of the Population Aged 65 Years or Older, by State, 1993 to 2020

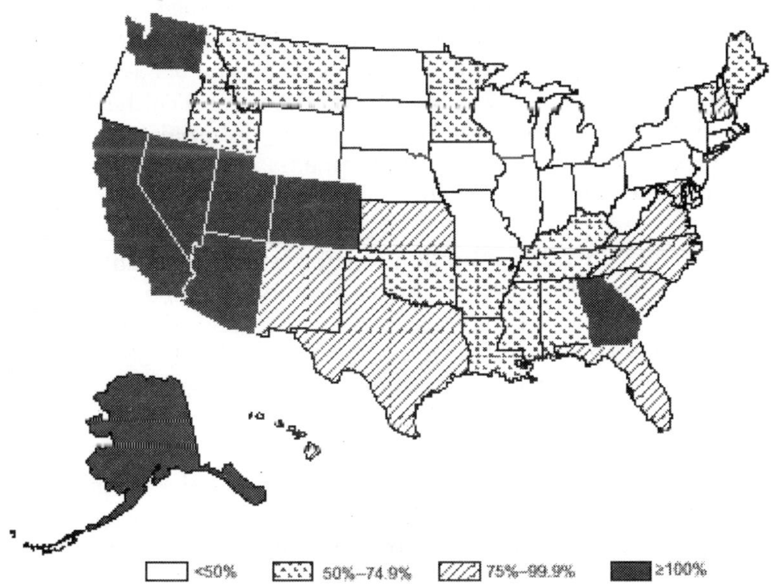

Source: U.S. Bureau of the Census, 1998.

Increases in type 2 diabetes may be one of the first consequences of the epidemic of obesity among young people. CDC Goals

- To provide states with technical and financial assistance for coordinated school health programs.
- To develop model policies, guidelines, and training to assist states in implementing high-quality school health programs.

Effectiveness of Health Education

Rigorous studies show that health education in schools can effectively reduce the prevalence of health-risk behaviors among young people. For example:

- Planned, sequential health education resulted in a 37% reduction in smoking initiation among seventh-grade students.
- The prevalence of obesity decreased among girls in grades 6-8 who participated in a school-based intervention program.
- Students who participated in a school-based life skills training program were less likely to use tobacco, alcohol, or marijuana than were students not enrolled in the program.

Examples of CDC Activities

CDC's Youth Media Campaign is a comprehensive communication approach to promote healthy lifestyles and displace unhealthy, risky behaviors among America's young people. Young people aged 9-13 years will be targeted and encouraged to adopt healthy behaviors, especially physical activity. In FY 2001, CDC granted state and local health education agencies about $7 million for Youth Media Campaign activities. The campaign is supported by national media channels, public/private partnerships, and a national events tour.

- In 1992, while continuing to support HIV prevention education in all states, CDC began to provide funding for coordinated school health programs to reduce chronic disease risk factors: poor eating habits, physical inactivity, and tobacco use. CDC currently supports coordinated school health programs in 20 states.

Heart disease and stroke—the principal components of cardiovascular disease—are the first and third leading causes of death in the United States, accounting for more than 40% of all deaths.

- About 950,000 Americans die of cardiovascular disease each year, which amounts to one death every 33 seconds.
- Although heart disease and stroke are often thought to affect men and older people primarily, it is also a major killer of women and people in the prime of life.

Looking at only deaths due to heart disease or stroke, however, understates the health effects of these two conditions:

- About 61 million Americans (almost one-fourth of the population) have some form of cardiovascular disease.
- Coronary heart disease is a leading cause of premature, permanent disability among working adults.
- Stroke alone accounts for the disability of more than 1 million Americans.
- Almost 6 million hospitalizations each year are due to cardiovascular disease.

Costs

- The economic effects of cardiovascular disease on the U.S. healthcare system grows larger as the population ages. In 2003, the cost of heart disease and stroke is projected to be $351 billion: $209 billion for healthcare expenditures and $142 billion for lost productivity from death and disability.

CDC Goals

- To build a nationwide program to prevent heart disease and stroke.
- To reduce disparities in cardiovascular health among high-risk populations.
- To define geographic variations in the risk factors and the rates of illness and death associated with heart disease and stroke.
- To promote secondary prevention of heart disease and stroke.
- To increase research into heart failure and to develop interventions to prevent it.
- To develop and assess new methods for preventing heart disease and stroke.

Effectiveness of Efforts

Thirty years of research shows that measures such as encouraging healthier lifestyles and increasing early detection and intervention can: (1) prevent heart disease and stroke for those who are healthy, and (2) improve the health of people who have experienced these conditions. For example, people who stop smoking reduce their risk for heart disease rapidly and substantially. Improved nutrition and increased physical activity help to lower high blood pressure. Research done during the 1980s shows that community interventions that change our environment (places where we work, play, learn, or live) are particularly effective in reducing heart disease and stroke throughout the entire community. For example, when a work place adopts a no-smoking policy, all employees benefit whether they smoke or not. From 1987 to 2000, overweight and obesity increased dramatically among U.S. adults, and now obesity has reached epidemic proportions. Nearly 59 million adults are obese, and the percentage of young people who are overweight has more than doubled in the last 20 years. Fifteen percent of Americans aged 6-19 years are overweight.

Effects of Physical Inactivity and Unhealthy Diets

- Poor diet and physical inactivity lead to 300,000 deaths each year—second only to tobacco use.
- People who are overweight or obese increase their risk for cardiovascular disease, diabetes, high blood pressure, arthritis-related disabilities, and some cancers.
- Not getting an adequate amount of exercise is associated with needing more medication, visiting a physician more often, and being hospitalized more often.

Costs

- The direct medical costs associated with physical inactivity was $29 billion in 1987 and nearly $76.6 billion in 2000.

- The annual cost of obesity in the United States is about $117 billion.

CDC Goals

- To increase the amount of physical activity engaged in by adults and children.
- To improve the dietary habits of children and adults.
- To reduce the incidence of obesity and overweight in the United States.
- To devise a comprehensive nutrition and physical activity surveillance system that will evaluate behaviors associated with chronic diseases and obesity.

Effectiveness of Increasing Physical Activity

Modest, regular physical activity substantially reduces the risk of dying of coronary heart disease (the nation's leading cause of death) and decreases the risk for colon cancer, diabetes, and high blood pressure. Physical activity also helps to control weight; contributes to healthy bones, muscles, and joints; helps to relieve the pain of arthritis; and reduces symptoms of anxiety and depression.

Examples of CDC Activities

In FY2001, Congress appropriated $16.2 million to address physical inactivity, poor nutrition, and obesity, which allowed CDC to increase its research program and to provide funding to more states to establish programs.

CDC develops state and community interventions that promote physical activity and good nutrition. For example, CDC—

- Administers WISEWOMAN, a program that screens women for heart disease and other chronic disease risk factors, and refers them to follow-up if needed. WISEWOMAN has 12 programs in 11 states across the country.
- Sponsors Active Community Environments Initiative (ACES), a program to promote walking, biking, and accessible recreation facilities.

In 2001, CDC

- Evaluated insurance reimbursement for obesity interventions and treatments.
- Continued its investigation of the relationships between unhealthy diets, physical inactivity, obesity, and chronic diseases.

Each year in the United States, 500 million dental visits occur. Despite that large number, however, many U.S. children and adults do not have access to dental care and, therefore, receive none. Tooth decay is one of the most common infectious diseases among U.S. children.

Tooth Decay

This preventable health problem begins early: nearly a fifth of 2 to 4-year-olds, more than half of 8-year-olds, and more than three-fourths of 17-year-olds already have tooth decay. Among low-income children, almost half of cavities are untreated, and may cause pain, dysfunction, poor appearance, and underweight-problems that greatly reduce a child's capacity to succeed.

Adults also have serious oral health problems. Almost three of every 10 adults older than 65 years have lost all of their teeth because of cavities or gum disease. Each year, about 30,000 cases of mouth and throat cancers are diagnosed, and more than 8,000 people die of these diseases.

Costs

Nearly $68 billion is spent on dental services each year. More than 108 million Americans do not have dental insurance. For each child without medical insurance, 2.6 are without dental insurance; for each adult without medical insurance, three are without dental insurance.

CDC Goals

- To support state and community programs to prevent oral disease.
- To promote oral health nationwide in communities, schools, and healthcare settings.
- To evaluate the cost-effectiveness of selected preventive strategies.

Effectiveness of Measures to Reduce Oral Disease

Proven preventive measures (e.g., water fluoridation, dental sealants, smoking prevention programs) can reduce oral and dental diseases. However, these measures are often unavailable to those who need them most.

Community water fluoridation prevents cavities and saves money, both for families and the healthcare system. In fact, for large communities of more than 20,000 people where it costs about 50¢ per person to fluoridate the water, every $1 invested in this preventive measure yields $38 savings in dental treatment costs.

Examples of CDC Activities

- In FY 2001, CDC provided $2.3 million to oral health programs

Percentage of Children Who Have Experienced Dental Decay

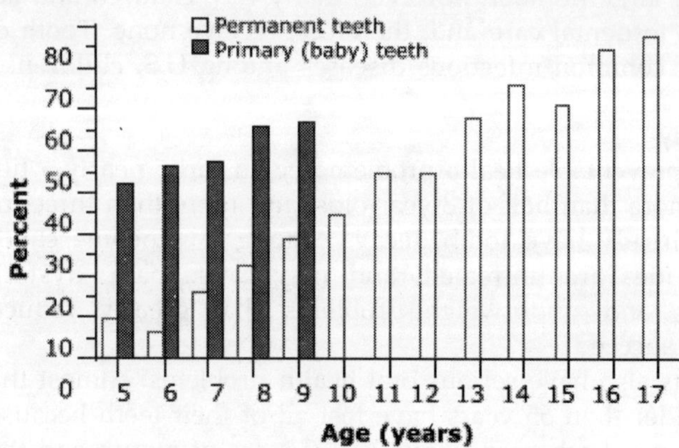

Source: CDC, National Center for Health Statistics, Third National Health and Nutrition Examination Survey, 1988-94.

in 19 states and Palau.

- Provides grants to 10 states and 1 American Indian tribe to assist with community water fluoridation systems.
- Builds and supports the infrastructure of state oral health programs. Five states and one territory now have funding to build core capacity to improve oral health.
- Promotes and supports the integration of oral health components into coordinated school health programs.
- Supports intervention and dissemination research to strengthen the scientific evidence of the benefits of oral disease prevention programs in communities.
- Influences oral health practice and policy by developing and distributing guidelines based on scientific research.

Examples of State Activities

Maine, Rhode Island, South Carolina, and Wisconsin: One proven strategy for reaching children at high risk for dental disease is through school programs that are linked with dental care professionals in the community. In FY 2001, CDC funded programs through the state education agencies in these four states to develop and implement models for improving access to oral health education, prevention, and treatment services for school-aged children who are at high risk for oral disease. CDC will evaluate the applicability of these models to other states.

Wisconsin: "Healthy Smiles for Wisconsin" is a statewide program, supported by CDC, to improve the oral health of Wisconsin children through school and community partnerships. By the 2001 school year, this program enabled 40 new dental sealant programs to be set-up in communities. More than 5,500 school children in 40 counties across Wisconsin received dental sealants through this program in 2001.

Percentage of Americans Aged 65 Years or Older Who Have Lost All Natural Teeth,* 1999

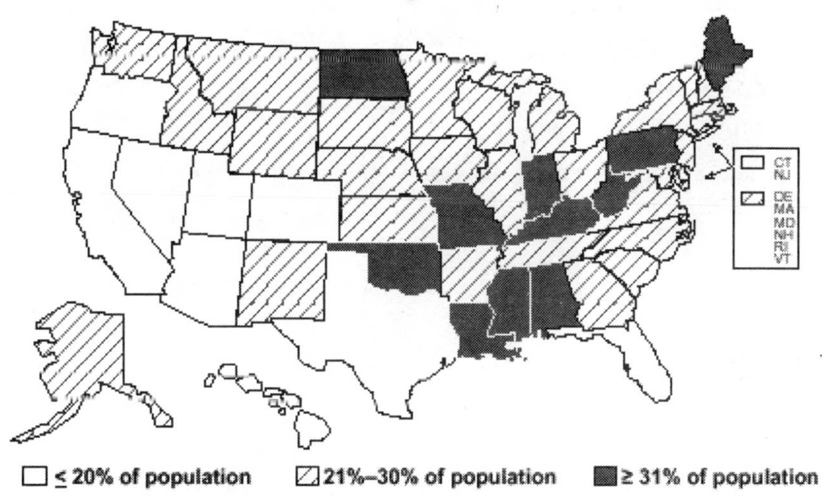

* Healthy People 2010 Goal less than or equal to 20%.
Source: CDC, Behavioral Risk Factor Surveillance System.

Pregnancy-related deaths

Approximately 6 million American women become pregnant each year, and more than 10,000 give birth each day. Each day in the United States, between 2 and 3 women die of pregnancy-related causes. A pregnancy-related death is one that occurs during pregnancy or within 1 year after pregnancy and is caused by pregnancy-related complications. The risk of pregnancy-related complications has not decreased since 1982. The risk of death due to pregnancy varies greatly in different racial and ethnic groups. African American women are 4 times more likely and Hispanic women are 1.7 times more likely than white women to die of pregnancy-related complications. Among women who become pregnant in the United States each year, at least 30% have a pregnancy-related complication. Childbirth is the most common reason for hospitalization in the United States, and pregnancies with complications lead to more costly hospitalizations.

Costs

In the United States, hospitalizations for pregnancy-related complications occurring before delivery account for more than 2 million hospital days each year at a cost of more than $1 billion annually. These figures exclude costs for complications during or after delivery.

Maternal Deaths,* United States, 1987-96

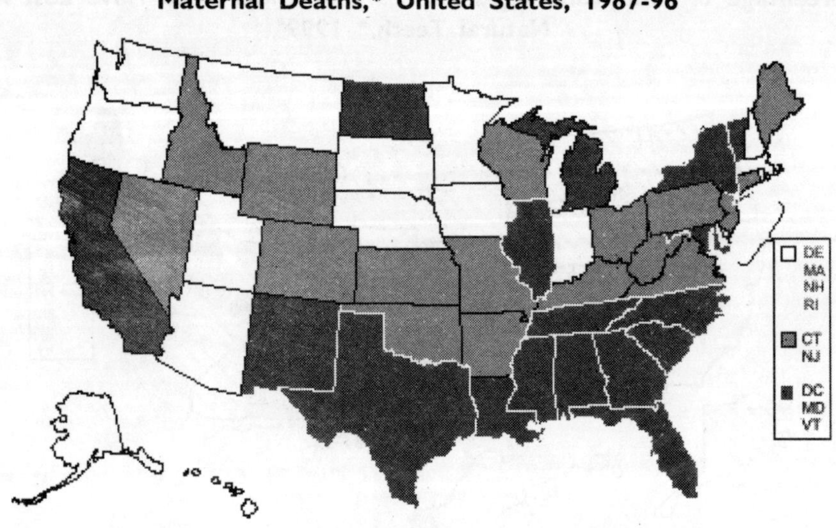

* Deaths during pregnancy or within 42 days after pregnancy, per 100,000 live births.
Source: CDC, National Center for Health Statistics.

CDC Goals

- To promote optimal reproductive and infant health and quality of life.
- To reduce the incidence of pregnancy-related illness and death.
- To identify risk factors for maternal illness and death.
- To examine racial disparities in pregnancy-related death rates.

To explore ways to assist pregnant women at risk for domestic violence.

Examples of CDC Activities

With FY 2001 funding of about $6 million, CDC helped states determine, which women might be at increased risk for pregnancy-related complications and what types of interventions could decrease these risks. Examples of CDC assistance include the following:

The Pregnancy Risk Assessment Monitoring System (PRAMS). CDC and state health departments use PRAMS to collect state-specific, population-based data on maternal attitudes and experiences before, during, and immediately after pregnancy. These data can be used to identify groups of women at high risk for health problems, to monitor changes in health status, and to measure progress toward goals in improving the health of mothers and infants. In 2001, CDC expanded PRAMS to include 32 states and New York City.

Appendix I

Corporate Medical Policy, Maternity Reimbursement

File Name: maternity_reimbursement
Policy Number: ADM9065
Origination: 10/2003
Last Review: 10/2003
Next Review: 10/2005

Description of Procedure or Service

Maternity care includes prenatal care, labor and delivery and post-delivery care. Prenatal care is all care related to the pregnancy before the baby's birth. Post-delivery care is all care for the mother.

Global maternity care includes routine antepartum care, delivery and postpartum care. Other antepartum services such as amniocentesis, cordocentesis, chorionic villus sampling, fetal stress test, and fetal non-stress test are not considered part of global maternity services. They are reimbursed separately.

Benefits Application

Please refer to certificate for availability of benefits. This policy relates only to the services or supplies described herein. Benefits may vary according to benefit design, therefore certificate language should be reviewed before applying the terms of the policy. Elective cesarean delivery (primary or repeat) is not eligible for coverage in the absence of maternity beneifts.

Complications of pregnancy are medical conditions whose diagnoses are distinct from pregnancy, but are adversely affected or caused by pregnancy, resulting in the mother's life being in jeopardy or making the birth of a viable infant impossible and which require the mother to be treated prior to the full term of pregnancy (except as otherwise stated below), including but not limited to: abruption of placenta; acute nephritis; cardiac decompensation; documented hydramnios; eclampsia; ectopic pregnancy; insulin dependent diabetes mellitus; missed abortion; nephrosis; placenta previa; Rh sensitization; severe pre-eclampsia; trophoblastic disease; toxemia; immediate postpartum hemorrhage due to uterine atony; retained placenta or uterine rupture occurring within 72 hours of delivery; or, the following conditions occurring within 10 days of delivery: urinary tract infection, mastitis, thrombophlebitis, and endometritis. Common side effects of an otherwise normal pregnancy, conditions not specifically included in this definition, episiotomy repair and birth injuries are not considered complications of pregnancy. Emergency cesarean section will be considered eligible for benefit application, only when provided in the course of treatment for those conditions listed above as a complication of pregnancy.

Billing for Maternity Care

A. Global Maternity Coverage

Normally, a provider should file global maternity care when they provide prenatal care, labor and delivery and post-delivery care.

Policy: Maternity Reimbursement

B. Prenatal, Delivery and/or Postpartum Services Billed Separately

It would be appropriate for the provider to file prenatal, delivery and/or postpartum services separately if:

1. the member's coverage started after the onset of pregnancy,
2. the coverage terminates prior to delivery,
3. the pregnancy does not result in delivery, and
4. the member switches doctors.

C. Multiple Births

Benefits for multiple deliveries will be based on multiple surgery guidelines (100% and 50%) for dates of service effective 10/1/2003.

The correct method of reporting multiple deliveries is as follows:

1. Global maternity care, vaginal delivery

(a) First baby

(i) File 59400 Routine obstetric care including antepartum care, vaginal delivery (with or without episiotomy, and/or forceps) and postpartum care. (100%)

(b) Subsequent baby(s)

(i) File 59409-51 Vaginal delivery only (with or without episiotomy and/or forceps). If more than one subsequent baby is delivered the number should be indicated in the units field. (50%)

(c) If antepartum and/or postpartum care were not provided, then procedure code 59409 should be reported reflecting the appropriate number of deliveries in the units field.

2. Global maternity care, cesarean delivery

(a) First baby

(i) File 59510 Routine obstetric care including antepartum care, cesarean delivery, and postpartum care. (100%)

(b) Subsequent baby(s)

(i) File 59514-51 Cesarean delivery only. If more than one subsequent baby is delivered the number should be indicated in the units field. (50%)

3. Global maternity care after previous cesarean delivery, vaginal delivery

(a) First baby

(i) File 59610 Routine obstetric care including antepartum care, vaginal delivery (with or without episiotomy, and/or forceps) and postpartum care, after previous cesarean delivery.

(b) Subsequent baby(s)

(i) File 59612 Vaginal delivery only, after previous cesarean delivery with or without episiotomy, and/or forceps.

4. Global maternity care after previous cesarean delivery, cesarean delivery

(a) First Baby

(i) File 59618 Routine obstetric care including antepartum care, cesarean delivery, and postpartum care, following attempted vaginal delivery after previous cesarean delivery.

(b) Subsequent Baby(s)

(i) File 59650 Cesarean delivery only, following attempted vaginal delivery after previous cesarean delivery.

D. Referral to Perinatologist

When a member is referred to a perinatologist, that perinatologist office should bill the Evaluate and Management Consult Code (99241-99245) with the diagnosis the member was referred for (not the maternity diagnosis).

Billing/Coding/Physician Documentation Information

This policy may apply to the following codes. Inclusion of a code in this section does not guarantee that it will be reimbursed. For further information on reimbursement guidelines, please see Administrative Policies on the Blue Cross Blue Shield of North Carolina web site at www.bcbsnc.com. They are listed in the Category Search on the Medical Policy search page.

Policy Key Words

Key Words: maternity reimbursement, OB, prenatal care, labor and delivery, labor, delivery, post-delivery, postpartum.

Scientific Background and Reference Sources

Medical Policy Advisory Group—10/200300

Policy Implementation/Update Information

10/03

Original policy issued

10/03

Medical Policy Advisory Group Review: Reaffirm Medical policy is not an authorization, certification, explanation of benefits or a contract. Benefits and eligibility are determined before medical guidelines and payment guidelines are applied. Benefits are determined by the group contract and subscriber certificate that is in effect at the time services are rendered. This document is solely provided for informational purposes only and is based on research of current medical literature and review of common medical practices in the treatment and diagnosis of disease. Medical practices and knowledge are constantly changing and BCBSNC reserves the right to review and revise its medical policies periodically.

BCBSNC may request medical records for determination of medical necessity. When medical records are requested, letters of support and/or explanation are often useful, but are not sufficient documentation unless all specific information needed to make a medical necessity determination is included.

Appendix II

Post-Delivery Care and Stabilization of Mother and Newborn

April 1996

Introduction

The timing of hospital discharge following delivery has become a focus of concern in providing appropriate postpartum care for both mother and infant. Although the trend toward earlier discharge was originally consumer driven during the 1970's as a means of focusing on child birth as a family centered experience, current motives for early discharge are largely driven by changes in the primary function of hospitals and by a perception that insurers will not cover longer stays.

The term "early discharge" reflects the fact that hospital stays used to be considerably longer in previous years. However, it is not meant to imply that longer stays are necessarily better. Early discharge has been defined in various ways in the literature, generally referring to a length of stay between one and two days after delivery. In actual practice, a one day stay may be 13-35 hours, depending on when the mother delivers. A patient who delivers at 11:00 p.m. for example, might be discharged at noon the following day (13 hour stay). A patient who delivers at 1:00 a.m., however, might not be discharged until noon the next day (35 hour stay).

Minnesota statistics demonstrate a trend toward early discharge. In 1985, only 6.2% of infants in the Twin Cities metropolitan area (delivered vaginally without complications) were discharged at one day after delivery, while first quarter 1995 statistics indicate that 42.5% of infants were discharged at one day.

As current healthcare practices require patients to play a more active consumer role in their care, this report attempts to identify the issues surrounding early discharge as they relate to the health and well-being of the mother and infant. Recently, legislation has been passed mandating that insurers pay for a minimum of 48 hours of hospitalization following delivery. In actual practice, however, the optimal time of discharge cannot be established independent of a continuum of care from the prepartum through the postpartum period. This report attempts to identify the medical, physical, social, emotional, and psychological issues related to the appropriate care of mother and baby in the postpartum period, with the objective of reframing the debate from a discussion of discharge timing to a focus on the care that mothers and newborns should receive in the post-delivery period.

Issues

The length of time between delivery and discharge from the hospital is an important issue at this time. Recent legislation mandates insurers to provide coverage for a hospital stay of 48 hours following uncomplicated vaginal delivery. This report addresses the following issues as they relate to timing of discharge:

- Medical and physical issues for the newborn.
- Medical and physical issues for the mother.
- Social, emotional, and psychological issues for the mother and newborn.
- Cost comparison of early *versus* later discharge.

Summary of Literature

Most published studies related to length of stay following delivery describe outcomes of specific programs, each having particular and unique characteristics. Furthermore, socio-economic factors, geography, nationality, ethnicity, birth setting, and other population characteristics vary widely, as do criteria for determining an infant's candidacy for early discharge. As a result, it is often difficult to compare data from different reports or to generalize results from one program to other settings. Most published reports have included only small groups of infants. Because groups are small and adverse outcomes are rare events, a single additional readmission in either early or late discharge groups could, in many cases, affect the overall outcome of the study. In addition, data from the available literature may be outdated and reflect practices that have changes. More research is needed to address this issue. Appendix II provides a summary of articles.

Medical/Physical Issues of the Newborn

1. With discharge within one or two days after delivery, there may not be adequate time for recognition of serious illnesses while the newborn is in the hospital. Although some problems may become evident soon after birth, other problems such as jaundice, heart malfunctions, and intestinal difficulties take longer to become apparent. It is important that discharge programs provide mechanisms to detect and treat problems that do not present until after the patient leaves the hospital.
2. The literature is inconclusive regarding the effect of discharge within one or two days on rehospitalization rates. Most studies do not have a sufficient number of patients to be statistically significant, and results vary depending on the particular

populations studied and the extent of follow-up that is provided. Infants may be readmitted to the hospital for many reasons, including: jaundice, breathing problems, heart irregularities, hypothermia, infection, feeding and circumcision problems.

3. Minnesota requires that all infants be screened for a number of diseases. Screening performed less than two days after delivery may cause some screening test results to be invalid, and those tests will have to be repeated. The expense and difficulty involved in tracking down infants for retesting should be recognized and addressed as barriers to optimal screening. In Minnesota, it is the legal responsibility of either the administrative officer or other person in charge of each institution caring for infants 28 days or less of age or the person required to register the birth of the child to administer these tests and file the required information with the Minnesota Department of Health. Since optimal screening may, in some cases, occur after the baby leaves the hospital, it is important that early discharge plans incorporate screening into their guidelines.
4. In order to care for themselves and their infants, mothers need to be knowledgeable in a number of areas. However, mothers may be least able to assimilate new information in the time immediately following delivery. Early discharge programs should ensure maternal/family readiness to assume responsibility for the newborn through demonstrated skill and ability in feeding techniques, skin and cord care, and the ability to assess infant well-being and seek timely, appropriate treatment.
5. The hospital environment may pose risks to the health of both mother and infant, due to the prevalence of nosocomial infection. When weighing the benefit of increased hospitalization, one must take into account the risk of infection due to hospital-acquired diseases.

Medical/Physical Issues of the Mother

1. Mothers with normal pregnancies and deliveries generally experience a healthy postpartum course regardless of the time of discharge. Although maternal complications are rare, they do occur, and need to be detected promptly so that mothers can return to the hospital for treatment. There are a number of reasons why mothers may be readmitted to the hospital, including inflammation of the uterus and late postpartum hemorrhaging. Less serious maternal problems may be related to perineal bruising, discomfort and hemorrhoids, or breast-related

symptoms. Mothers need to be informed of potential complications and their symptoms so they can seek timely, appropriate treatment.

2. The literature is inconclusive regarding the effect of early discharge on breastfeeding. Earlier discharge does reduce the time available for teaching and support on breastfeeding in the hospital after delivery; some programs compensate for this by providing instruction during the last trimester or in the home environment following the birth. Since the milk supply is generally not established at 24 hours after delivery, and may not be established at 48 hours after delivery, it is important that all mothers receive appropriate education and support for breastfeeding.
3. Regardless of time of discharge, typically, mothers will experience fatigue in the first several days after delivery. Adequate support must be available during this time to assist the mother in caring for her new infant.
4. The hospital environment may pose risks to the health of both mother and infant, due to the prevalence of nosocomial infection. When weighing the benefit of extended hospitalization, one must take into account the risk of infection due to hospital-acquired diseases associated with post-delivery care.

Social, Emotional, and Psychological Issues

1. The literature is inconclusive regarding the relationship between early discharge and postpartum depression.
   Discharge plans need to recognize the potential for postpartum depression among new mothers, and put mechanisms in place to detect it and treat it should it arise.
2. Fatigue will be a factor in the days immediately following delivery regardless of the timing of discharge. In addition to affecting the mother's physical status, fatigue will also impact the mother's emotional and psychological readiness to care for her new baby. Mothers without strong support systems in the home environment may be particularly ill-equipped to deal with the rigors of caring for a newborn. Care plans need to assess the home environment as well as the physical condition of mother and newborn.
3. Many studies mention other aspects of emotional health such as mother-baby bonding, but do not provide data to support or refute a relationship between bonding and time of discharge. However, separation of mother and child in hospitals for medical reasons or discharge of one or the other is viewed as detrimental to bonding.

4. Other issues for which little data exist include the current state of community support systems, such as home care nursing, available routine and emergency transportation, telephone support, support from the family unit (such as father and siblings), and other support systems available to the mother after discharge.

Cost Comparison of Early *Versus* Later Discharge

1. Significant cost savings may be achieved from shorter post-delivery hospital stays. However, this must be weighed against the potential costs associated with readmission and emergency care. In addition, costs of other prenatal and postnatal care (such as home visits or additional office visits) associated with an early discharge must be factored into the analysis, as well as costs generated by the treatment of nosocomial infection. The risks and costs of prolonged hospitalization need to be weighed against the risks and costs associated with early discharge. Further research needs to be done in order to draw any conclusions regarding the cost implications of the timing of discharge.
2. HTAC reviewed the post-delivery care literature for findings from cost effectiveness analysis, which measures the relationship between the cost of care and the benefit that is derived from it. However, data are insufficient to draw conclusions regarding the cost effectiveness of early *versus* later postpartum discharge.

Outstanding Issues

Many issues related to early discharge of mother and infant have yet to be addressed adequately in the literature, including:

- How is health plan coverage interpreted, translated, communicated, and applied in the delivery site? There is an apparent lack of continuity between the discharge criteria of insurers and the actual practice of hospitals. Dialogue between payers and providers may clarify misunderstandings on this issue.
- Where should follow-up after discharge occur (hospital, clinic, home) and how does continuum of care throughout the postpartum period vary with time of discharge?
- How can fail-safe newborn screening take place when infants are discharged early?
- Issues related to rural mothers and infants have not been addressed. For example, response time for medical emergencies after discharge from the hospital, the availability of technologies

and resources in the rural community, and staffing costs in a rural hospital setting are all issues that would have an impact on discharge planning for rural mothers and newborns.

- Is there a relationship between socio-economic status and post-delivery length of stay? This may be of special interest for post-discharge planning where there are fewer resources to assist the mother.
- Patient satisfaction related to early discharge should be explored more thoroughly. What emphasis should be placed on the importance of patient preference?
- Who gets readmitted into the hospital? Are there differences in maternal readmission rates after first *versus* subsequent births?
- The role of hospitals has changed over time. Previously, hospitals served many purposes (treatment, rest, observation, etc.). Currently, hospital stays are used for those requiring intensive evaluation or treatment. Should an intermediate setting for care and services be considered?
- Appropriate education and follow-up services (including screening) are also necessary for families who deliver outside of the hospital setting (i.e., at home).
- The economic ramifications of early discharge need to be addressed in a larger context so as to capture all relevant information.
- Discharge planning for more complicated deliveries, such as cesarian section, should also thoroughly evaluate the individual needs of each mother and infant.

Conclusions

To date, data are inconclusive in demonstrating either a positive or negative correlation between optimal outcome of pregnancies and length of stay following delivery. Local and community-wide research to address many of the concerns related to the timing of discharge are needed.

The birth of each child is unique, with a multitude of factors (e.g., physical status of mother and infant, availability of social support at home and in the community, resources within the hospital) affecting the outcome. To ensure optimal care for both mother and child, the time of discharge should be determined on an individual basis. Care systems need to develop appropriate programs to meet the unique needs of their patients within the context of their communities. Individualized discharge plans can and should be established through medical assessment and community resource assessment.

Care is not adequately measured in terms of hours. The needs of each mother and baby must be assessed on an individual basis, and care delivered in a manner that makes the most sense for each unique birth situation. Therefore, a legislative mandate of any minimum requirement of length of stay cannot assure optimal care. Instead, focus on the continuum of care for the mother and baby, and emphasize the importance of establishing appropriate plans for the post-delivery care and stabilization of mother and newborn is needed.

The guidelines put forth by the American Academy of Pediatrics and the American College of Obstetrics and Gynecology may serve as a basis for meeting the minimum discharge criteria. See the Conclusions section of the full report for the specific discharge criteria recommendations.

TECHNICAL REPORT

Background

Early discharge has been defined in various ways in the literature, generally referring to a length of stay between 24 and 48 hours after delivery. In actual practice, a length of stay may be 13-35 hours, depending on when the mother delivers. A patient who delivers at 11:00 p.m. for example, might be discharged at noon the following day (13 hour stay). A patient who delivers at 12:05 a.m., however, might not be discharged until noon the next day (35-hour stay). The American Academy of Pediatrics defines "early" and "very early" discharge as stays of 48 and 24 hours or less, respectively, after uncomplicated vaginal delivery.

Hospital discharge following delivery has become a focus of concern in providing appropriate postpartum care for both mother and infant. Although the trend toward earlier discharge was originally consumer driven during the 1970's as a means of focusing on child birth as a family centered experience, current motives for early discharge are largely driven by changes in the primary function of hospitals and by a perception that insurers will not cover longer stays.

Minnesota statistics for the 7-county metro area mirror this trend. In 1985, 6.2% of infants delivered vaginally without complications were discharged at one day, 53.5% were discharged at two days, and 33.8% were discharged at three days. In contrast to this, the 1995 first quarter statistics indicate that 42.5% of infants were discharged at one day, 47.5% were discharged at two days, and 7.9% were discharged at three days.

Opinion varies widely regarding the desirability of early-discharge practice. Proponents of early discharge claim that it is safe and may be advantageous from both a medical and psychological standpoint. Opponents, on the other hand, argue that an element of risk may be involved because detection of significant illness may be either missed or delayed outside of the hospital. To further complicate the issue, economic considerations often constitute a driving force behind the trend to earlier discharge.

Still, others argue that appropriate postpartum care is not related to the timing of discharge. Instead, the issue is the patient's condition at discharge and the services available once a mother arrives home with a newborn baby. They further suggest that a decision for early discharge should be individualized and should be a mutual decision between the patient, her family, and obstetrical provider.

As current healthcare practices require patients to play a more active consumer role in their care, this report attempts to identify the issues surrounding early discharge as they relate to the health and well-being of the mother and infant. Recent legislation has been passed mandating that insurers pay for a minimum of 48 hours of hospitalization following delivery. In actual practice, however, the optimal time of discharge cannot be established independently of a continuum of care from the prepartum through the postpartum period. This report attempts to identify the medical, physical, social, emotional, and psychological issues related to the appropriate care of mother and baby in the postpartum period, with the objective of reframing the debate from a discussion of discharge timing to a focus on the care that mothers and newborns should receive in the post-delivery period.

Review of the Evidence: Continuum of Postpartum Care

Summary of Literature: Most published studies on early discharge describe outcomes of specific individual programs, each with its own particular and often unique characteristics. Socio-economic factors, geography, nationality, ethnicity, birth setting, and other population characteristics vary widely, as do criteria for determining an infant's candidacy for early discharge. Varied methods of risk screening and parental education have been utilized, maternal support systems at home differ widely, and mechanisms of follow-up vary from phone calls to home and office visits. The definition of early discharge differs considerably among studies: infants discharged in the "late" group in one study may actually go home at an earlier postnatal age than the "early" group of another. As a result, it is often difficult to compare data from different reports or to generalize results from one program to other settings.

Medical/Physical Issues for the Newborn

Psysiologic Stability: An important advantage to earlier hospital discharge is that nosocomial (hospital-acquired) infection is minimized for both infant and mother. However, this must be weighed against the risk that early discharge may not provide adequate time for routine medical and social assessment of the mother-infant dyad.

The Committee on Fetus and Newborn of the American Academy of Pediatrics recommends that the hospital stay of the mother-infant dyad should be long enough to allow identification of problems and to ensure that the family is able and prepared to care for the baby at home. Many cardiopulmonary problems related to the transition from an intrauterine to an extrauterine environment become apparent during the first 12 hours after birth. However, other problems such as jaundice, ductal-dependent cardiac lesions, and gastrointestinal obstruction may require a longer period of observation by skilled personnel.

Norr and Nacion, in their comparative review, observed that

although infants discharged early are rehospitalized more often than their mothers, their rehospitalization rate is still low. Infant readmission rates vary a great deal from one program to another, in contrast to the relative stability of maternal readmission rates. In the Norr study, almost all of this variability reflected differences in the definition and treatment of hyperbilirubinemia. Other reasons for readmission included: transient tachypnea, bradycardia, and hypothermia.

Other studies reconfirm that treatment of jaundice with phototherapy is the most frequent cause for readmission in some hospitals. Additional reasons for readmission include; respiratory, feeding, bacterial and viral infection, and circumcision problems. In a study by Pittard and Geddes, suspected infectious disease was overwhelmingly the major cause for readmission; while hyperbilirubinemia was rarely the reason for readmission. Maternal age, race, and parental financial status were not predictors of early infant readmission in this study. The high variability in readmission rates for jaundice, historically the most significant reason for readmission, suggests that hospitals can sharply affect their readmission rates for newborns by changing their management of hyperbilirubinemia.

The criteria delineated to measure physiologic stability for infant discharge from the University of Colorado Health Sciences are reported by Conrad. The criteria for early discharge were:

- Apgar scores at 1 and 5 minutes are >7.
- The infant is term (38-42 weeks) and weights 2700 to 4000 grams.
- Minimum stay of 24 hours, transition to normal thermoregulation in an open crib, completion of two successful feedings, evidence of stool and void, completion of neonatal screening for metabolic disease and blood type and Coomb's test (Rh- and O mothers) prior to discharge.
- Vital signs are within normal ranges at discharge:
  - o Axillary temperature: 36.1EC to 37.2EC
  - o Heart rate: 110 to 150 beats per minute
  - o Respirations: 25/min. to 60/min.
- The infant has a normal hospital course and resents no signs or sumptoms that require continuous observation.
  - o Blood dextrose concentration maintained >2.5 mmol/L
  - o Hematocrit 0.45 to 0.65
  - o Infants with ABO-incompatible infants must be held for 48 hours and released only if they do not require therapy for hemolysis.
- Physical examination completed by house officer.

Although infant mortality has not been reported in relationship to early discharge, 1994, Minnesota health statistics indicate that infant mortality rates decrease after the first day of birth. Of 64,277 live births, 296 resulted in neonatal deaths, 189 in first-day deaths (largely associated with low birth weight and congenital anomalies), and 57 in 1-6 day deaths. See Appendix IV for distribution of causes of death.

Screening: Screening programs are designed to prevent morbidity and mortality through early diagnosis of medical problems and congenital disorders that can have serious sequelae. Adequate screening programs require universal participation, prompt diagnosis, and mechanisms for parental notification and education. Common screening tests include: phenylketonuria, galactosemia, maple syrup urine disease, congenital adrenal hyperplasia, and congenital hypothyroidism. Some states also mandate screening for sickle cell disease and various sexually transmissible infections.

The screening samples are generally designed for samples taken on the second or third day of life. Screening performed less than two days after delivery may cause some screening test results to be invalid, and those tests will have to be repeated. If screening is done too soon, not only will it be necessary for infants to be retested, there is the danger that those administering the screening program will assume incorrectly that the results of these screening tests are reliable. If the infant leaves the hospital before all necessary screening tests have been administered, follow-up screening must be completed in a timely fashion, no later than two weeks after birth.

Minnesota Statute 144.125 states that all Minnesota newborns shall be tested for the following diseases: phenylketonuria (PKU), galactosemia, hypothyroidism, hemoglobinopathy (sickle cell disease) and adrenal hyperplasia. Three of the five tests (PKU, hypothyroidism and adrenal hyperplasia) are not reliable if performed less than 48 hours post-delivery.

The statute further states that it is the duty of the (1) administrative officer or other person in charge of each institution caring for infants 28 days or less of age, and (2) the person required to register the birth of the child to administer these tests in accordance with the rules prescribed by the state commissioner of health.

The duties of the responsible party include: informing parents or guardians that their newborns will be screened and providing explanation for the screening and their rights to refuse; collecting a specimen for screening no later than the fifth day after the infant's birth; if samples have been taken prior to 24 hours after birth, notifying the parents or guardians verbally and in writing of the necessity of having the Phenylketonuria test repeated on their newborns no later than the 14th day of life; recording the date the specimen is collected in a permanent record; and sending the specimen card including all required information to the Minnesota Department of Health.

Care of Newborn

The American College of Obstetrics and Gynecology (ACOG) recommends that early or very early discharge with regard to care of the newborn should ensure maternal readiness to assume independent responsibility for her newborn through demonstrated skill and ability in feeding techniques, skin and cord care, measurement of temperature with a thermometer, and ability to assess infant well-being and recognize common neonatal illnesses. Family members who will care for the child should attend prenatal childbirth education or infant care classes, in which problems of the first days after birth are discussed.

Medical/Physical Issues for the Mother

Carty and Bradley observed that regardless of the time of discharge, the women in their study generally experienced a healthy postpartum course. However, serious complications can and do occur. In the study by Norr and Nacion, the majority of maternal readmissions were for late postpartum hemorrhages. Thurston, *et al.* indicated that less severe maternal problems were most commonly related to perineal bruising, discomfort and hemorrhoids, or to breast-related symptoms.

Although large prospective studies are lacking, some studies indicate significant medical problems in 4.3% of early discharge patients with readmission rates as high as 1.8%. These complications suggest the need for a planned program of follow up and the responsibility to teach patients the warning signs and symptoms for potential problems.

The American Academy of Pediatrics and American College of Obstetrics and Gynecology recommend that prior to discharge, the patient should be informed of normal postpartum events, including the changes in the lochial pattern that she should expect in the first few weeks; the range of activities that she may reasonably undertake; the care of the breasts, perineum, and bladder; dietary needs, particularly if she is breastfeeding; the recommended amount of exercise; emotional responses; and observations that she should report to the physician (e.g., temperature elevation, chills, leg pains, or increased vaginal bleeding).

Additionally, the length of convalescence based on the type of delivery should be discussed, and patients should be counselled to avoid abdominal straining. Patients who have abnormal bleeding or signs of infection or fever should not be discharged. It is helpful to reinforce oral discussion with written information.

Breastfeeding: Some researchers suggest that early discharge may foster enhanced breastfeeding. In a Swedish study by Waldenstrom, infants discharged early were breast-fed significantly more often on the third and fourth days postnatally than those staying in the hospital, although no difference in incidence of breastfeeding was observed during the subsequent 10 days. Carty and Bradley reported that a significant difference in breastfeeding was observed between the early discharge group and the traditional stay group. At one month, 87% of the women in the early discharge group and 79% in the traditional group were giving their babies breast milk only.

According to a study by Waldenstrom, however, cited differences in breastfeeding rates may be more related to differences among women studied rather than to the day of discharge.

Social/Emotional/Psychological Issues for Mother and Newborn

The impact of early discharge on the emotional health of the mother is an important area of concern. Emotional health includes such things as postpartum depression, mother-child separation, the mother's confidence in her ability to be a good parent, stress management, and the need for external support.

In a randomized, controlled study, Carty and Bradley compared discharge at 12-24 hours, 25-48 hours, and four days. The mothers discharged 12-24 hours after giving birth reported themselves to be significantly less depressed at one month postpartum than the two later groups. In addition, the earliest group reported higher levels of confidence at one week postpartum than the other two groups. At one month postpartum, however, the three groups did not differ significantly with respect to levels of confidence.

A study by Beck, *et al.* reports that the lack of any significant difference exhibited between two groups of primiparas regarding the incidence of maternity blues and postpartum depression lends support to the notion that early discharge programs are psychologically safe.

Another study by Romito and Zalate also reports, "the results show that there was no difference in the two groups in the postpartum period as regards tiredness or depression. Both groups felt most tired during the days immediately following discharge, whether discharge was 1 or 6 days after birth.

A document commissioned by Maternal and Child Health Bureau reports on an October 1994 consensus meeting in Boston. There, a group of experts with "intimate knowledge of both hospital and community-based care for mothers and newborns" found that "women who are from high-risk social environments and with limited social support structures may not be best served by a one-day stay." In addition, "separation due to the need to observe either the mother or the newborn was deemed unacceptable." Policies that would result in increased rates of separation were viewed by the group as detrimental to mother/infant bonding, infant and maternal health, and threatening to breastfeeding. Clinicians recognized a distinction between 24 hours and 72 hours because mother/infant bonding occurs during this early critical time period.

Although many other studies mention aspects of emotional health such as mother-baby bonding and the mother's support system, they do not provide data. Other issues for which little data exist include the current state of community support systems, such as home healthcare nursing, available transportation, telephone support, and other support systems available to the mother after discharge from the hospital.

Conrad comments that illiteracy, young maternal age, lack of transportation, and inability to defray the cost of prenatal care may serve to limit prenatal child care education and medical care for women in lower socio-economic groups. Single-parent status may limit support at home. Provision of healthcare through several ambulatory systems as well as frequent household moves and a lack of telephone service compromise the establishment of optimal follow-up in the postpartum period. These problems could serve to limit the applicability of early newborn discharge, as outlined by the AAP and ACOG, to large segments of the population that otherwise meet the medical criteria.

Education: Braveman points out, "Early discharge has reduced the time available for in-hospital teaching and support on breastfeeding, infant care, women's health needs, and family planning, and for maternal and family psychological assessment." For this, Beck suggests, "What early discharge programs need to routinely include are teaching sessions during the last trimester, which focus on postpartum discharge instructions for mothers and babies such as episiotomy care and umbilical cord care."

In contrast to this, Harrison suggests that education may be more effective and appropriate in the home environment following the birth: "Compared with the hospital environment, the home may provide more opportunities to include other family members in the teaching program. In addition, parents are often more ready to learn in their home environment, after they have had a chance to assume responsibility for their infant's care."

Cost Comparison

Financial saving and more optimal utilization of healthcare resources are often cited as advantages of early discharge, yet published studies vary in their conclusions with respect to these issues. In a one-year study (1993) of 26 New Hampshire hospitals, the financial impact of early *versus* later discharge was calculated using the mean pediatric charge excluding perinatal condition. In this population based study using 15,000 annual births, approximately 24% of infants qualified for early discharge and were discharged in less than 48 hours after delivery.

In a letter submitted to the Congressional Record regarding the New Hampshire study, Frank reported, "The total charges for those infants who were discharged early and required readmission or ER visits were approximately $183,000. The total charges for one additional day for the mother infant dyad discharged early were approximately $7,466,000. Thus, the saving for the healthcare industry was approximately $7,283,000."

In an article reviewing Frank's study, Seal cautioned that the study is not look at additional costs for prenatal and postnatal care provided by some healthcare facilities to accompany early discharges. For example, St. John's Hospital and Health Center reports that they have incurred some additional nursing costs in order to intensify new mother education.

Yanover, *et al.* compared 44 early discharge mothers with 44 receiving traditional care at Kaiser-Permanente Medical Center, San Francisco. Their observation was "we estimate that the cost of providing our program's services is approximated by the immediate saving derived from early discharge. The expenses include salaries of nurse doctors, paramedical personnel, and medical consultants, as well as automobile expenses and home-care supplies."

Gonzalves and Hardin reported on the cost effectiveness of the Irwin Army Community Hospital early discharge program. Data was collected from a retrospective audit of out-patient records for the period from November 15, 1991 through May 31, 1992. In this trial program they concluded, "Cost effectiveness was demonstrated in bed days saved and the ability to implement other cost-saving initiatives as a result of this program. A total of 788 bed days valued at $705,260 were made available for use by other patients (cost per hospital day is $477.50 per patient). The additional nursery beds were utilized to return premature infants from local tertiary centers to our facility an average of 6 days earlier than before our program was instituted. An approximate cost avoidance of $224,350 was realized as a result of this action."

Recommendations for Postpartum Care

The following are recommendations put forth by various organizations regarding optimal postpartum care.

The American College of obstetricians and Gunecologists: The American College of Obstetricians and Gynecologists (ACOG) believes that changes in practice such as early discharge following obstetrical delivery should be based on sound scientific data that demonstrate good outcomes for mother and infant, as well as being cost effective. As yet, these data do not exist.

ACOG acknowledges that selective, early discharge is safe and desirable for some mothers and babies. However, a decision for early discharge should be individualized and should be a mutual decision between the patient, her family, and the obstetrical provider—taking into account medical risk factors, support systems for the family, and the readiness of the mother to care for herself and her newborn.

ACOG supports legislation addressing insurance coverage for postpartum care that meets the following criteria:

- The appropriateness of individual discharges is left to the discretion of the physician and patient.
- The Guidelines for Perinatal Care provides the basis for required coverage.
- Patients are not provided incentives or disincentives by insurers to access care that is inconsistent with the Guidelines for Perinatal Care.

The American College of Nurse-Midwives: The American College of Nurse-Midwives (ACNM) position is that the timing of discharge after birth is a clinical decision determined by the patient's medical condition and circumstances, the content and quality of prenatal care, the conduct of labor and birth, the newborn's condition, and the availability of qualified personnel to provide early postpartum and newborn assessment. Many women and their newborns are appropriate candidates for early discharge, and payers should be flexible in the decision regarding timing of discharge.

The ACNM will welcome what it and others would embrace as a balanced and broad-reaching Newborns and Mother's Health legislation by which no clinician would be forced to fight for care that is safe, and no mother forced to return home before receiving adequate medical, physical and social support to care for herself and her baby.

Minnesota Medical Association: The Minnesota Medical Association (MMA) passed a resolution at its most recent annual meeting stating that an appropriate postpartum length of stay and any required follow-up care, including nurse home visits, should be determined by the physician and patient and not by an arbitrary time integral. The resolution also indicated that the MMA opposes mandatory reduced hospital stays of one day for vaginal delivery, and three days for cesarean sections (the day of delivery being defined as day 0).

American Medical Association: The American Medical Association (AMA) is concerned that managed care's practice of requiring routine early discharge for newborns and their mothers may be dangerous to the health and well-being of the mother and child. The decision of when to leave the hospital should be left to the physician and patient and not be based solely on the financial considerations of the managed care company, S. 969 would provide reasonable protection for mothers and their babies so that they are not forced to leave the hospital before it is safe to do so.

Minnesota Nurses Association: The Minnesota Nurses Association (MNA) has also passed a resolution regarding postpartum hospital stays. Their position is that legislation mandating 48-hour hospitalization does not address the need for assessment of anticipated problems in the postpartum period and education of parents. The maternal and child health Registered Nurses in the hospital settings have the ability and responsibility to assess for complications and plan necessary education and post-hospital referrals. Discharge timing should be a mutual decision made by the family and their doctors including registered nurses.

Therefore, the MNA supports state and federal policies, which create incentives for the insurance industry to provide adequate coverage for maternal-child healthcare, based upon individual need including a length of stay, as determined by the client with the Registered Nurse, Certified Nurse Midwife, or Physician. In addition, the MNA supports state and federal policies, which would require third party payers to cover a minimum of two home visits by a Public Health or Registered Nurse with expertise in community and maternal child health nursing.

American Academy of Pediatrics: The American Academy of Pediatrics' Committee on Fetus and Newborn have developed minimum criteria for newborn discharge.

American Academy of Family Physicians: The American Academy of Family Physicians (AAFP) adopted a resolution in September 1995 stating that the AAFP reaffirms physician authority for decision-making regarding length of stay of mothers and newborns after delivery. Furthermore, the AAFP endorses reimbursement of both professional and hospital costs for medically-indicated stays determined by the physician.

Council on Scientific Affairs: The Council on Scientific Affairs has stated that in the absence of definitive empirical data, perinatal discharge of mothers and infants should be determined by the clinical judgment of attending physicians and not by economic considerations. This decision should be made based on the criteria of medical stability, delivery of adequate pre-discharge education, need for neonatal screening, and determination that adequate feeding is occurring. A plan should be in place for psychosocial and medical follow-up, as outlined in the Guidelines for Perinatal Care developed by the AAP and ACOG.

Minnesota Policies/Standard of Care

The following are recommendations put forth by Minnesota health insurers regarding the timing of discharge following delivery.

HealthPartners

HealthPartners position statement on discharge states that hospital discharge following normal vaginal delivery is dependent on the medical and physical stability of the mother and her newborn infant; it is not dependent upon a prescribed length of hospital stay. Appendix III of this report identifies HealthPartners' criteria to be met and procedures to be followed when considering discharge within 24 to 36 hours after normal vaginal delivery.

Additionally, HealthPartners states that early discharge is only an option and that the final decision for each patient's length of stay is based on medical necessity and mutual agreement between the patient and her provider.

Blue Cross Blue Shield of Minnesota

Blue Cross Blue Shield of Minnesota's (BCBSM) policy statement for postpartum stays, states that the decision of the length of stay should be based on medical necessity and determined on a case-by-case basis. The decision for an appropriate discharge will be made collaboratively between the attending physician, facility, and the patient.

BCBSM will become involved in the decision if the length of stay exceeds 48 hours for a normal vaginal delivery and 96 hours for a cesarean section. The case will be reviewed for medical necessity using standard criteria.

Medica

Medica provides discharge guidelines, which are to be met prior to discharge following vaginal delivery. Medica discharge criteria are presented in Appendix III of this report.

Outstanding Issues

Many issues related to early discharge of mother and infant have yet to be addressed in the literature. For this reason, the outstanding issues presented below are intended to identify those issues, which should be considered in the early discharge debate but for which little information is currently available:

- How is health plan coverage interpreted, translated, communicated, and applied in the delivery site (hospital)? There is an apparent disconnect between the discharge criteria of insurers and the actual practice of hospitals. The dialogue between payers and providers may clarify misunderstandings needs to be better understood on this issue.
- Where should follow-up after discharge occur (hospital, clinic, home) and how does continuum of care throughout the postpartum period vary with the time of discharge?
- How can fail-safe newborn screening take place when infants are discharged early?
- Issues related to rural mothers and infants have not been addressed. For example, response time for medical emergencies after discharge from the hospital, the availability of technologies and resources in the rural community, and staffing costs in a rural hospital setting are all issues that would have an impact on discharge planning for rural mothers and newborns.
- Is there a relationship between socio-economic status and post-delivery length of stay? This may be of special interest for post-discharge planning, in cases where there are fewer resources to assist the mother. The level of support that is available to women who depend upon economic assistance may not be adequate to address their needs. This issue needs to be studied in greater detail.
- Patient satisfaction related to early discharge should be explored more thoroughly. What emphasis should be placed on the importance of patient preference?
- Are there differences in maternal readmission rates after first *versus* subsequent births? We need a better understanding of who gets readmitted into the hospital.
- The role of hospitals has changed over time. Previously, hospitals served many purposes (treatment, rest, observation, etc.). Currently, hospital stays are used for those requiring intensive evaluation or treatment. Should an intermediate setting for care and services be considered?
- Appropriate education and follow-up services (including

screening) are also necessary for families who deliver outside the hospital setting (i.e. at home).

- The economic ramifications of early discharge need to be addressed in a larger context so as to capture all relevant information.
- Discharge planning for more complicated deliveries, such as cesarian section, should also thoroughly evaluate the individual needs of each mother and infant.

Conclusions

To date, data are inconclusive in demonstrating either a positive or negative correlation between optimal outcome of pregnancies and length of stay following delivery. Local and community-wide research to address many of the concerns related to timing of discharge are needed.

The birth of each child is unique, with a multitude of factors (e.g., physical status of mother and infant, availability of social support at home and in the community, resources within the hospital) affecting the outcome. To ensure optimal care for both mother and child, the time of discharge should be determined on an individual basis. Care systems need to develop appropriate programs to meet the unique needs of their patients within the context of their communities. Individualized discharge plans can and should be established through the utilization of medical assessment and community resource assessment.

Care is not adequately measured in terms of hours. The needs of each mother and baby must be assessed on an individual basis, and care delivered in a manner that makes the most sense for each unique birth situation. Therefore, a legislative mandate can not assure optimal care. Instead, we should focus on the continuum of care for the mother and baby, and emphasize the importance of establishing appropriate plans for the post-delivery care and stabilization of mother and newborn.

Guidelines for Infant Discharge: The guidelines put forth by the American Academy of Pediatrics may serve as a basis for meeting the minimum discharge criteria. See below for specific discharge criteria recommendations:

- The antepartum, intrapartum, and postpartum courses for both mother and baby are uncomplicated.
- Delivery is vaginal.
- The baby is a single birth at 38-42 weeks' gestation and the birth weight is appropriate for gestational age according to appropriate intrauterine growth curves.
- The baby's vital signs are documented as being normal and stable for the 12 hours preceding discharge, including a respiratory rate below 60/min. a heart rate of 100 to 160 beats per minute, an axillary temperature of 36.10C to 37.0C in an open crib with appropriate clothing.

- The baby has urinated and passes at least one stool.
- The baby has completed at least two successful feedings, with documentation that the baby is able to coordinate sucking, swallowing, and breathing while feeding.
- Physical examination reveals no abnormalities that require continued hospitalization.
- There is no evidence of significant jaundice in the first 24 hours of life.
- The mother's knowledge, ability, and confidence to provide adequate care for her baby are documented by the fact that she has received training sessions regarding the following issues:
  - o Breastfeeding or bottlefeeding: The breastfeeding mother-infant dyad should be assessed by trained staff regarding nursing position, latch-on, adequacy of swallowing, and mother's knowledge of urine and stool frequency.
  - o Cord, skin, and infant genital care.
  - o Ability to recognize signs of illness and common infant problems, particularly jaundice.
  - o Proper infant safety (e.g., proper use of a car seat and positioning for sleeping).
- Family members or other support person(s), including doctors, such as the family pediatrician or his/her designees, familiar with newborn care and knowledgeable about lactation and the recognition of jaundice and dehydration are available to the mother and the baby for the first few days after discharge.
- Laboratory data are available and reviewed, including maternal syphilis and hepatitis B surface antigen status, cord or infant blood type and direct Coombs' test result as clinically indicated.
- Screening tests are performed in accordance with state regulations. If the test is performed before 24 hours of milk feeding, a system for repeating the test must be assured during the follow-up visit.
- Initial hepatitis B vaccine is administered or a scheduled appointment for its administration has been made within the first week of life.
- A physician-directed source of continuing medical care for both the mother and the baby is identified. For newborns discharged in less than 48 hours after delivery, a definitive appointment has been made for the baby to be examined within 48 hours of discharge. The follow-up visit can take place in a home or clinic setting, as long as the personnel examining the infant are competent in newborn assessment and the results of the follow-up visit are reported to the infant's physician, or designees, on the day of the visit.
- Family, environmental, and social risk factors should be assessed. These risk factors may include but are not limited to:

(1) untreated parental substance abuse/positive uring toxicology results in the mother or newborn; (2) history of child abuse or neglect; (3) mental illness in a parent who is in the home; (4) lack of social support, particularly for single, first-time mothers; (5) no fixed home; (6) history of untreated domestic violence, particularly during this pregnancy; or (7) teen mother, particularly if other conditions above apply. When these or other risk factors are present, the discharge should be delayed until they are resolved or a plan to safeguard the infant is in place.

It is essential that all infants having a short hospital stay be examined by experienced doctors within 48 hours of discharge. If this cannot be assured, then discharge should be deferred until a mechanism for follow-up evaluation is identified.

The purpose of the follow-up visit is to:

- Assess the infant's general health, hydration, and degree of jaundice; identify any new problems; review feeding pattern and technique, including observation of breastfeeding for adequacy of position, latch-on, and swallowing; and assess historical evidence of adequate stool and urine patterns.
- Assess quality of maternal-infant interaction and details of infant behavior.
- Reinforce maternal or family education in infant care, particularly regarding infant feeding.
- Review the outstanding results of laboratory tests performed before discharge.
- Perform screening tests in accordance with state regulations and other tests that are clinically indicated.
- Identify a plan for healthcare maintenance, including a method for obtaining emergency services, preventive care and immunizations, periodic evaluations and physical examinations, and necessary screening.

In summary, the fact that a short hospital stay (<48 hours of age) for healthy term infants can be accomplished does not mean that it is appropriate for every mother and infant. Each mother/infant dyad should be evaluated individually to determine the optimal time of discharge.

Guidelines for Maternal Discharge

The American Academy of Pediatrics and the American College of Obstetricians and Gynecologists have developed Guidelines for Perinatal Care; an excerpt related to care of the mother is shown below:

Upon discharge, the following points should be reviewed with the mother or, preferably, with both parents:

- Condition of the neonate.
- Immediate needs of the neonate (e.g., feeding, methods and environmental supports).
- Roles of the obstetrician, pediatrician, and other members of the healthcare team concerned with the continuous medical care of the mother and neonate.
- Availability of support systems, including psychosocial support.
- Instructions to follow in the event of a complication or emergency.
- Feeding techniques, skin care, including cord care; temperature assessment and measurement with the thermometer; and assessment of neonatal well-being and recognition of illness.
- Reasonable expectations for the future.
- Importance of maintaining immunization begun with initial dose of hepatitis B vaccine.

When the mother is discharged early, certain criteria should be met:

- The mother should have an uncomplicated vaginal delivery following a normal antepartum course and should have been observed after delivery for a sufficient time to ensure that her condition is stable. Pertinent laboratory data, including a postpartum determination of hemoglobin or menatocrit level and, if not previously obtained, ABO blood group and Rh typing, should have been obtained. If indicated, the appropriate amount of RhIg should have been administered.
- Family members and other support person(s) should be available to the mother for the first few days following discharge.
- The mother should be aware of possible complications and should have been instructed to notify the appropriate doctor, as necessary.
- Procedures for readmission of obstetric patients should be consistent with hospital policy, as well as local and state regulations.

Appendix III

Glossary

The following definitions define terms as they pertain to this report. These definitions do not necessarily apply when these terms are used in specific citations from other sources.

Abdomen

A part of the body from below the ribs to the pelvis. Some call it the stomach.

Anesthesiologist

A doctor who maintains safe pain relief during labor and delivery, prepares patients for surgery, and cares for patients during surgery. The anesthesiologist delivers pain control during labor and appropriate sedation for cesarean deliveries.

Average length of stay

The average number of days spent in the hospital to give birth and recover, includes the time before and after childbirth.

Cesarean section

A surgical procedure to deliver a baby. The doctor makes an incision through the mother's abdomen and uterus. Also referred to as a c-section, cesarean, and cesarean birth.

Complications

Additional problems that develop during the pregnancy, labor, delivery or postpartum period.

Cord blood

The blood that is in the umbilical cord.

Cost Effectiveness Analysis

A technique used to measure the relationship betweeen the cost of care and the benefit that is derived from it.

Doula

A doula is a non-medical person experienced and trained in

childbirth whose role is to comfort and support the mother and family before, during, and after birth. A doula provides the mother with information, support, reassurance, and assistance throughout the birth process including assistance with breast feeding.

Early Discharge

Generally refers to a length of stay between one and two days after an uncomplicated vaginal delivery. A one day stay may be 13-35 hours, depending on when the mother delivers.

Episiotomy

An incision into the perineum to prevent tearing during childbirth.

Fallopian tubes

Fallopian tubes move the egg to the uterus (also called the womb).

Fetus

Unborn baby.

High risk

The chance of having or developing problems is greater due to the patient's current medical condition compared to the rest of the population.

Labor, delivery, recovery (LDR) room

Labor, Delivery, Recovery rooms (LDR) are rooms in which the mother labors, delivers and recovers. Mothers are then transported to a separate postpartum room

Labor, delivery, recovery, postpartum (LDRP) room

Labor, Delivery, Recovery, Postpartum rooms (LDRP) are those rooms in which the mother labors, delivers, and recovers and spend her postpartum period in the same room. She does not move to a separate postpartum area.

Lacerations

A laceration is a tear in the vagina. Third- and fourth-degree lacerations are the most severe types of tears. Third and fourth degree lacerations can result in rectal, vaginal, and urinary problems.

Lactation consultant

Lactation consultants help mothers with breastfeeding skills. Lactation consultants give information and guidance and help prepare pregnant mothers for breastfeeding. Lactation consultants give support to mothers having problems after delivery and after discharge from the hospital.

Length of Stay

The amount of time a mother and infant are hospitalized following delivery. This time does not include the time spent in the hospital preceding delivery.

Level I Nursery Services

Level I hospitals have all the capabilities for normal births and births with minor complications. This type of hospital is designed for newborns that have been carried near the full term and the delivery is expected to be uncomplicated.

Level I Obstetrics Services

Level I hospitals have all the capabilities for normal births and births with minor complications. This type of hospital is for mothers that have carried their babies near the full term and expect an uncomplicated pregnancy and delivery.

Level II Nursery Services

Level II hospitals have additional equipment and staff to handle more complicated deliveries. This level is for newborns with a slight potential for risk during the delivery. In general, Level II hospitals can provide care to newborns delivered at 32 weeks or at 3 pounds 5 ounces or more.

Level II Obstetrics Services

Level II hospitals have additional equipment and staff to handle more complicated deliveries. This type of hospital is for mothers with a slight potential for risk during delivery.

Level III Nursery Services

Level III hospitals have equipment and staff to handle very complicated cases. This type of hospital can care for babies that are fairly premature (babies delivered before 32 weeks and at very low birth weights of less than 3 pounds 5 ounces) or that have serious illnesses or abnormalities requiring intensive care before, during or after delivery. Level III hospitals also provide care for uncomplicated deliveries.

Level III Obstetrics Services

Level III hospitals have equipment and staff to handle very complicated cases. Mothers and or newborns with serious illnesses or abnormalities requiring intensive care before, during and or after delivery may receive care at a Level III hospital. Level III hospitals also provide care for uncomplicated deliveries.

Level III Plus Nursery Services

Level III Plus hospitals can provide care for very complicated cases and they are located near a Level IV hospital to ensure rapid transfer of the newborn if additional care is needed. Level III Plus hospitals provide selected specialty services. Level III Plus hospitals also provide care for uncomplicated deliveries.

Level III Plus Obstetrics Services

Level III Plus hospitals can provide care for very complicated cases and they are located near a Level IV hospital to ensure rapid transfer of the newborn if additional care is needed. Level III Plus hospitals provide selected specialty services. Level III Plus hospitals also provide care for uncomplicated deliveries.

Level IV Nursery Services

Level IV hospitals can care for the most complicated deliveries. Level IV hospitals provide comprehensive critical care for the newborn and have a full range of specialty services. Level IV hospitals also provide care for uncomplicated deliveries.

Level IV Obstetrics Services

Level IV hospitals can care for the most complicated deliveries. Level IV hospitals provide comprehensive critical care for the newborn and have a full range of specialty services. Level IV hospitals also provide care for uncomplicated deliveries.

Level of care

The range of treatment or procedure a patient receives includes the medical level of expertise available.

Midwife

Certified nurse midwives are licensed care doctors educated in both nursing and midwifery. Midwives provide prenatal care, labor and delivery care, care after birth, and newborn care.

Neonatal Intensive Care Unit (NICU)

A neonatal intensive care unit (NICU) is a hospital unit where highly trained medical professionals specialize in the care of babies born prematurely and/or with other special problems. Doctors that care for newborns are specially trained pediatricians called neonatologists. Nurses are specially trained to provide the intensive level of care. Special beds are used to provide warmth, isolation, and handle any special devices used to monitor the baby's heart rate, blood pressure, breathing, special blood and feeding equipment. In Maryland, this term applies to hospitals designated as Level III or above (see definition for Level III)

Neonatologist

A neonatologist treats disorders in newborns from birth and throughout the NICU stay. Neonatology is a pediatric specialty.

Nosocomial Infection

Hospital-acquired infection; the source of infection is directly attributable to the hospital environment.

Obstetrician

A doctor specializing in the care of the pregnant woman and delivery of the baby.

Obstetrics

Care provided in the delivery of babies. Doctors and nurses provide the care.

Out-patient birth

Childbirth that occurs outside the hospital, at the mother's home or in a birthing center.

Perinatologist

A perinatologist cares for the mother and unborn baby that are at high risk for complications. The perinatologist provides care before, during and after delivery. Perinatology is an obstetric specialty.

Perineum

The area between the vagina and anus.

Postpartum

The time after delivery or after childbirth.

Postpartum

The period of time following the delivery of the infant, typically identified as 6 weeks following delivery. This report focuses on the portion of postpartum that relates to discharge time.

Prenatal

The time before delivery or before childbirth.

Primary cesarean section

A woman's first cesarean section birth.

Repeat cesarean section

A woman's second or greater cesarean section birth.

Tubal ligation

A surgical procedure performed to prevent future pregnancy. The fallopian tubes are closed to prevent a fertilized egg from reaching the uterus. Also referred to as tying tubes.

Umbilical cord

A structure for passing blood and nutrients between the mother and unborn baby. The umbilical cord is attached to the placenta.

Umbilical cord blood

The blood that is in the umbilical cord.

Uterus

An organ in a females body where the baby grows. Also called the womb.

Vagina

The birth canal.

VBAC

Vaginal birth after cesarean section. A vaginal delivery after a previous cesarean section birth.

APPPENDIX IV

Summary of Reviewed Articles

The following is a tabulation of the articles reviewed thus far. Observations and summaries of the articles follow this table:

Reference	*Site/Design*	*No. of Patients*	*Discharge time post-delivery*	*Follow-up care*	*Results*
Carty, 1990	Tertiary care maternity hospital in Vancouver. Vaginal deliveries only. Random selection.	Grp.1: 44 Grp 2: 49 Grp. 3: 38	Grp.1: 12-24 hrs. Grp.2: 25-48 hrs. Grp.3: 4 days (traditional stay)	Nurse home visits: Grp. 1: day 1, 2, 3, 4, 5, 10. Grp. 2: day 3, 5, 10. Grp. 3: day 10 only.	No differences found in patient health. ED reported more satisfaction and more confidence in mothering role.
Conrad, 1989	Univ. Of Colorado School of Medicine. Indigent population. Retrospective analysis.	Grp. 1: 1091 Grp. 2: 343 Grp. 3: 563	Grp.1: 24-36 hrs. Grp.2: 36-48 hrs. Grp.3: >48 hrs.	Mandatory outpatient visit within 48 hrs. of discharge.	Group 1 had more readmissions than group 3.
Arborelius, 1989	Motala Hospital, Sweden. Voluntary early discharge.	ED: 26 Ctrl: 22	ED: 0-2 days Ctrl: 5-6 days	Daily home visits by midwife and/or nurse. Examination at hospital 6-7 days after birth.	No difference regarding psychological factors or breastfeeding.
Pittard, 1988	Medical Univ. of South Carolina. Retrospective analysis. Economically diverse grp.	ED: 1714 Ctrl: 622	ED: 31+5 hrs. Ctrl: 92+44 hrs.	Not mentioned.	No difference in infant readmissions within 6 weeks of birth.
Thurston, 1985	Large general hospital, Calgary. Voluntary participation.	ED: 376 Ctrl: None	Within 48 hrs.	Home visits on 3rd, 4th, 5th postpartum day.	Hospital stay deemed appropriate by 86% of participants, too short by 7%, and too long by 7%.
Yanover, 1976	Kaiser-Permanente Medical Center, San Francisco. Random selection. Low risk patients.	ED: 44 Ctrl: 44	ED: 12-48 hrs. Ctrl: >48 hrs.	Daily home visits through 4th postpartum day, additional visits as needed. Nurse available during first 2 weeks.	No differences in number and types of morbidity for mothers or infants in first six weeks after delivery. The cost of providing the program was approximated by the immediate savings from early discharge.

Key: ED = Early Discharge group, Ctrl = control group.

Observations from the Trials

Most reports published until now are either retrospective studies or studies done with voluntary early discharge, decided before delivery.

Britton observes that most published reports have included only small groups of infants, and consequently sufficient statistical power is lacking. Because groups are small, a single additional readmission in either early or late discharge groups could, in many cases, affect the overall outcome of the study.

Assuming a minimum incidence of problems requiring re-admission in the population to be 1%, 38,211 infants would be needed in each group to detect a difference in outcome of 25%. It is unlikely that a study of this magnitude could be performed at a single center, and a multi-center effort would be needed.

Summary of Articles Reviewed

Carty, 1990

The study took place at a tertiary care maternity hospital in Vancouver. All women expecting a vaginal birth were eligible to participate. Women who agreed to be randomly assigned to one of three discharge times were visited at home by a project nurse at approximately 38 weeks' gestation who explained the study in greater detail, obtained written consent, and assigned time of discharge. The final sample consisted of 131 women. The discharge schedules were as follows:

Early discharge: Group 1-12 to 24 hrs. (n=44)
Group 2-25 to 48 hrs. (n=49)
Traditional stay: Group 3-4 days (n=38).

Five project nurses made home visits to the women under their care according to the following schedules : group 1 on days 1, 2, 3, 5, and 10 after delivery; group 2 on days 3, 5, and 10; group 3 on day 10 only. At each visit the nurses provided similar nursing care to that received by women in hospital. They conducted a physical assessment of the mother and baby, dealt with the immediate concerns of the parents, assisted them with getting to know their baby, and dealt with the many facets of incorporating a new member into the family. Questionnaires were left with the participants to be completed at four time periods : 37 weeks' gestation, during hospital stay, 1 week postpartum, and 1 month postpartum.

Results

The demographic characteristics of the women in the three groups did not differ significantly after randomization. Over 95% of the women were Caucasian, 93% were married or living with their partner, 65% had completed junior college or university, and 58% had a combined family income over $40,000. Fifty-three percent were primiparas and 47% multiparas.

Maternal and infant health

Regardless of the time of discharge, the women experienced a generally healthy postpartum course. The frequency of maternal problems requiring physician referral in the first 10 days postpartum was 5.3% (n=5) in the early discharge groups and 7.9% (n=3) in the traditional stay group. One instance of each problem was reported, by group, as follows: group 1—urinary tract infection and episiotomy infection; group 2—mastitis, episiotomy infection, and sub-involution; and group 3—endometritis, episiotomy infection, and sub-involution. Of women referred to a physician, two (1.5% were hospitalized within the first month postpartum : one from the earliest discharge group for a urinary tract infection, and the other, from the traditional stay group for endometritis.

During the first 10 days postpartum, the frequency of problems in infants requiring physician referral was 4.3% in groups 1 and 2, and 2.6% in group 3. Reasons were hyperbilirubunemia, cord infection, ABO incompatibility, diaper rash, and respiratory difficulties.

Breastfeeding

On discharge from hospital, 98% of all women in the study were breastfeeding. At one month, 87% of the women in the early discharge groups and 79% in the traditional group were giving their babies breast milk only. The one-month questionnaires were returned by mail with a rate of return of 75%.

Psychological functioning

The responses of the women in the three groups did not differ significantly with respect to levels of trait anxiety, or state anxiety assessed prenatally, in hospital at one week, or at one month postpartum.

Women in the three groups did not differ on their prenatal scores on the Beck Depression Index. Those who stayed in hospital for 4 days scored significantly higher on that index at the 1-month follow-up ($P<0.05$) than did women who were discharged 12 to 24 hours postpartum.

At one week, women who were discharged within 24 hours scored significantly higher than those in the two other groups on the sub-scale assessing confidence regarding the mothering role ($P<0.03$). There were no significant differences among the groups with respect to scores on this sub-scale completed at one month postpartum. This finding suggests that women who have complete responsibility for their baby earlier feel more confident initially than those who do not. It could also mean that the nursing visits enhanced women's feelings of confidence regarding their mothering role.

Patient satisfaction

All the women were satisfied with their care, as demonstrated by their responses on the patient satisfaction questionnaire. However, women who were discharged earliest reported being significantly more satisfied than those discharged later (P<0.0009) they were also significantly more satisfied with nursing care.

In summary, this study shows favorable results for early discharge. However, it is appropriate to point out that since participants were healthy, well-educated women and living in a stable relationship with their husbands or partners, the findings cannot be generalized to a high-risk population. Moreover, since participation was voluntary, it studied only a particular type of woman, who is willing to experience postpartum care that ranges from going home within 12 to 24 hours after birth to a hospital stay of 4 days. As for satisfaction, since the nurses providing home visits were specially chosen, one can only conjecture that some of the findings related to satisfaction, depression, and confidence in the mothering role might have been different if the study nurses had also provided in-hospital care for group 3.

Conrad, 1989

This is a retrospective review of newborn hospital and out-patient medical record of 2000 consecutively born infants admitted into the transitional nursery for level I care at University of Colorado Health Sciences Center, Denver. Infants who initially required a higher intensity of care (i.e., direct admissions in level II or III nursery units) were excluded from this study. The data collected included the following : sex, gestational age, birth weight, length of hospital stay, neonatal complications, need to transfer into level II or III units, reason for the hospital stay to exceed 36 hours, documentation of out-patient follow-up within 48 hours of initial discharge, and readmission to the hospital within seven days of initial discharge.

Results

Review of the financial status of mothers demonstrated that 77% were in a lower income bracket (23% were eligible for Medicaid assistance, and the remaining 54% had an average income for a family of four <$17,000 per year). The maternal age in this group was 23.2+5.1 years.

The newborn medical records from the 2000 infants born during the study period were divided into three groups. Group 1 consisted of infants discharged within 24 to 36 hours of birth (n=1091), group 2 infants were discharged 36 to 48 hours after birth (n=343), and group 3 infants were discharged more than 48 hours after birth (n=563). Although no significant differences in birth weight and gestational age were found among any of the discharge groups, there was a trend in group 3 toward greater numbers of infants of 37 weeks' gestation or less and 42 weeks' gestation or longer, as well as greater number of infants small or large for gestational age.

The reasons hospital stay exceeded 36 hours for group 2 and 3 infants included:

- Maternal problems that included recovery from cesarean section, postpartum tubal ligation, and recovery from pregnancy-induced hypertension and genital injuries (lacerations and contusions of the maternal genitalia).

- Infant problems—low birth weight was the most frequent neonatal cause for the newborn hospitalization to exceed 36 hours (10.3%). The 51 infants who stayed for social reasons included all infants born to mothers with psychiatric disease and substance abuse.

All infants in group 1 had a mandatory outpatient follow-up visit within 48 hours of discharge. Successful visits were accomplished in 91.1% of the cases. Reasons for the 8.9% unsuccessful visits were : no documentation 3.8%, could not locate 4.1%, refused by parent 0.6%, child adopted 0.3%.

The overall readmission rate for the entire population studied was 1.8%. Significantly greater number of readmissions came from infants in group 1 (2.3%) than from group 3 (0.895, P<.05). Treatment of jaundice with phototherapy was the most frequent cause for readmission, 65% of these came from group 1. The second most common reason for readmission was physical signs suggesting bacteremia or viremia.

The authors comment that illiteracy, young maternal age, lack of transportation, and inability to defray the cost of prenatal care may serve to limit prenatal child care education and medical care for women in lower socio-economic groups. Single-parent status may limit support at home. Provision of healthcare through several ambulatory systems as well as frequent household moves and a lack of telephone service compromise the establishment of optimal follow-up in the postpartum period. These problems could serve to limit the applicability of early newborn discharge, as outlined by the AAP and ACOG, to large segments of the population that otherwise meet the medical criteria.

Arborelius, 1989

This study was carried out from October 1984 to September 1985 in Motala Hospital, Motala, Sweden. Early discharge was a voluntary alternative for subjects of this study. All pregnant women living in the central parts of Motala were informed by their midwives at the end of the pregnancy. They were told that no decision had to be made before the delivery, and that they could return to the hospital if things did not work out.

Early discharge was defined as hospital stay of 0-2 days after birth, and late discharge as 5-6 days after birth. The families who chose early discharge got daily home visits by a midwife and/or a pediatric nurse. The patients were also free to call the hospital at any time. At the hospital a pediatric examination of the child was done 6-7 days after birth; if necessary an obstetrical examination of the mother was also done.

Altogether 44 women (7 primiparae and 37 multiparae) participated in this study, 22 in the early discharge group and 22 in the controls. There were no differences between the early discharge group and the control group regarding demographic variables such as age, living conditions, education, social class, marital status and nationality. The fathers were also interviewed. There were no differences between the groups regarding the number of days the fathers had been at home during the first month after birth.

Results

Both the early discharge group and the control group were very satisfied with their choice of length of stay.

Breastfeeding

A full month after birth 18/22 mothers in the early discharge group were breastfeeding and 21/22 in the control group. Half a year after birth the corresponding numbers were 12/19 and 14/19. The differences were not significant.

Pittard, 1988

This study is a review of the hospital charts for all infants admitted to the well-baby nursery is the Medical University of South Carolina between January 1 and December 31, 1985. Because of the need for obstetric beds, the practice at the MUSC was to discharge newborn infants after 24 hours but before 48 hours after delivery. To assess neonatal well-being after this moderately early discharge, the number of infants readmitted to the hospital within 6 weeks of birth was evaluated.

The early discharge group comprised 1714 infants who had no maternal or newborn clinical problem identified within the first 24 hours of life. These neonates remained in the hospital for 31 + 5 hours after delivery. The 622 infants in the control group were those who had no neonatal problems identified during the first 24 hours of life and were assigned to an extended hospitalization (92 + 44 hours) solely as a result of maternal concerns. All neonates with extended hospitalization because of neonatal problems were not included in the study.

Results

Of the 1714 babies discharged moderately early, 52 (3.0%) were readmitted within 6 weeks of birth. Of the 622 control cohort infants, 17 (2.7%) were readmitted by 6 weeks of age. Of the 69 total readmissions, 50 (72%) resulted from suspected infectious disease. Six infants had sepsis, with blood or spinal fluid cultures positive for bacterial growth. Five infants were readmitted for jaundice in the first week after discharge. None of these infants required an exchange transfusion, and the serum bilirubin concentration declined with phototherapy in each case.

Of the total study population, 3.3% of the indigent, 3.1% of the

Medicaid babies, and 1.5% of the private service babies were readmitted within 6 weeks of birth. Of the babies delivered by cesarean section 2.7% were readmitted by age 6 weeks. This incidence did not differ significantly from the readmission incidence of either the remaining control infants or the experimental infant group.

Of the infants discharged moderately early, 2.6% of black infants and 4.0% of white infants were readmitted within 6 weeks of birth. These rates did not differ significantly from each other, nor from the readmission rates among the extended hospitalization group.

In conclusion, therefore, suspected infectious disease was overwhelmingly the major cause for readmission; hyperbilirubinemia was rare. Maternal age, race, and parental financial status were not predictors of early infant readmission.

Thurston, 1985

This is an evaluation of safety and satisfaction of patients discharged early after delivery. Participation in the early discharge program by both mothers and physicians was voluntary. Discharge was proposed within 48 hours postpartum.

Mothers electing early discharge were assessed by their physicians for suitability. Routine home visits were made on the third, fourth and fifth postpartum days by a select group of specially trained Community Health Nurses who had received additional recent theoretical content and clinical experience in obstetrics. This was followed by a further at about two or three weeks post-delivery, a visit which was already being made to all new mothers. Nurses followed established protocol on each of these visits, providing routine patient care, postnatal teaching, and assessment of the physical and emotional status of the mother and physical condition of the baby. A total of 376 women participated in this program.

Results

A high percentage of mothers (78%) breast fed their babies at discharge from the hospital and 75% had continued breastfeeding at five days postpartum. Nursing records indicated maternal problems were most commonly related to perineal bruising, discomfort and hemorrhoids or to breast-related symptoms. For babies, the most frequently noted problems were associated with a "jaundiced" coloring or to difficulties with skin care such as diaper rash.

Three mothers and three babies had developed a more serious complication during the first few weeks post-delivery. Two infants were discharged with bilirubin readings on the second day exceeding that stated in the criteria, and, for one baby, it is unclear whether discharge occurred before the level was known. Both were readmitted to hospital with high bilirubin levels, and were treated with phototherapy. Another baby was seen and readmitted for respiratory illness at 32 days after discharge.

Two mothers had late postpartum hemorrhages owing to retained placenta and were readmitted for dilation and curettage.

The hospital stay was deemed appropriate in length by 86% of respondents, too short by 7%, and too long by the remaining 7%. Altogether, 97% of participants would suggest the program to friends, and 93% would participate again. Reasons cited were that the program was basically good, that they were more relaxed at home, that bonding improved, and that a home support system was available to them. Only 5% of patients would not participate again, stating that they required more rest, additional help at home, or did not want early discharge.

Yanover, 1976

A total of 88 low-risk patients were randomly assigned to either the early discharge group (n = 44) or control group (n = 44), at Kaiser-Permanente Medical Center, San Francisco. There were no statistically significant differences between the two groups in age, race, father's occupation, planned pregnancy, duration of marriage, length of time to conceive, mother's and father's education, presence of another child in the home, or mother's preference regarding enrolment in prenatal education classes, natural childbirth, or breastfeeding.

Patients in the control group were discharged not earlier than 48 hours with a pediatric visit at two weeks, and obstetric visit at six weeks. Patients in the study group stayed for 12-24 hours postpartum, and the perinatal nurse doctor made daily home visits for health surveillance and teaching of parent craft through the fourth postpartum day, with additional visits as needed. The perinatal nurse doctor who was assigned to a family was available to that family during the first two weeks postpartum.

Results

No significant differences or trends were observed in the numbers and types of morbidity occurring during hospitalization or during the first six weeks after delivery in mothers or infants of the study and control groups. The 13 cases of infant morbidity are:

The mother's complications included precipitous or prolonged labor, midforceps delivery, obstetric laceration, postpartum infection, and postpartum hemorrhage.

The authors estimate that the cost of providing the program's services was approximated by the immediate saving derived from early discharge.

Type of Morbidity	*Number of Cases*	
	Study	*Control*
Apgar score < 7 at 5 min.	0	2
Total bilirubin > 15 mg/dl	2	2
Superficial skin infections	2	3
Pneumonia		
Aspiration	0	1
Intrauterine	0	1
Total	4	9

Appendix V

Health Plan Policies

HealthPartners

In its position statement for maternity lengths of stay, HealthPartners outlines the following criteria for discharge occurring within 24-36 hours of delivery:

1. Maternal Criteria

1. Vaginal term delivery without extensive lacerations or tears.
2. Absence of postpartum hemorrhage.
3. Afebrile and other vital signs within patient's normal limits.
4. Ambulatory without assistance.
5. Voiding without difficulty and in sufficient amounts.
6. Tolerating fluids or light diet.
7. Review and documentation of maternal knowledge and comfort level regarding the following:
    1. Self-care including perineal care, breast care, use of medications, and
    2. Infant care including feeding, handling/positioning, normal newborn behavior, cord care, circumcision care (if applicable).
8. Adequate support available in home setting.
9. Absence of medical contraindications to discharge and mother is physically and psychologically/emotionally ready for discharge.

2. Newborn Criteria

1. Gestational age at least 36 weeks.
2. Birth weight at least 2500 grams.
3. Vital signs stable.
4. Normal glucose or chemstrip.
5. Routine newborn screening done.
6. Tolerated at least two feedings.
7. Newborn examination by family doctor, pediatrician, or pediatric nurse-doctor supports plan for discharge.

3. *Other Factors for Consideration (List includes but is not limited to the following):*

1. Assessment of emotional, behavioral, psychological and/or social issues.
2. Indications of substance abuse.
3. Previous perinatal loss.
4. Maternal fatigue or exhaustion.
5. Multiple gestation.

Discharge Procedures

6. Mother and, if possible, her support person are informed of abnormal signs or symptoms to watch for in the first several days following discharge and given written instructions on how to receive assistance if questions or emergencies arise.
7. A home or office visit to assess newborn status is scheduled within 2 to 5 days following discharge. If the patient declines, cancels, or fails the visit, a phone call is made within this time frame to ascertain the well-being of both mother and infant.
8. Routine pediatric (well child) care commences within 2 weeks and a postpartum visit is scheduled within 4 to 8 weeks.

Expectations

9. Expectations of hospitals:
   1. Policies, procedures and or protocols are in place to support appropriate postpartum monitoring and assessment.
   2. Review and reassurance are provided for safe transition of care to home.
10. Expectations of obstetric providers:
    1. Facilitate the inclusion of newborn care into prenatal education.
    2. Discharge planning is initiated prior to hospitalization.
    3. Timing of discharge is coordinated with assessments of maternal medical and physical stability, newborn status, and patient concurrence.
11. Expectations of doctors who provide newborn care:
    1. Provision of appropriate home nursing visits or office visit within 2 days of discharge.
    2. Office or phone availability for questions by either home nurse or parents.
12. Expectations of HealthPartners:
    1. Ongoing monitoring of patient outcomes and satisfaction.
13. Expectations of patients:
    1. Assume an active role in planning for the birth process and the transition of care from hospital to home.

2. Identify the doctor selected to provide newborn care prior to hospitalization.

Childbirth Complications

Childbirth used to be a very dangerous process, resulting in the deaths of many mothers and babies. Thanks to modern medicine, it is now remarkably safe. The rate of death for newborn babies is quite low, and for mothers even lower. Nevertheless, certain conditions, known as complications, may occur before, during, or immediately after birth. These require special medical attention to prevent death or lasting harm. Complications that may affect the baby's health include premature delivery, premature rupture of membranes (PROM), abnormal fetal presentation, cord prolapse and cord compression, asphyxia, breathing problems, birth injuries, and persistent fetal circulation. Complications in childbirth that can affect the mother include cephalopelvic disproportion, postpartum bleeding and cesarean section.

Premature Delivery

One of the greatest dangers a baby can encounter is to be born too early, before the body systems are mature enough to ensure survival. The lungs, for example, may not be able to breathe air, the body may not generate enough heat to keep warm, and the digestive system may not be able to transform food into nourishment. Whenever possible, drugs and other measures prevent or stop premature labor before it results in birth. If these fail, intensive care can keep many premature babies alive.

As a fetus approaches birth, it should move into position with its head down. Just before birth, the fetus turns and faces the mother's back, but if there is premature rupture of the membranes, the birth process begins before the fetus has reached the correct position.

Premature Rupture of Membranes (PROM)

Normally the membranes surrounding the baby in the uterus break and release amniotic fluid (known as the "water breaking") either during labor or right before it. Sometimes, however, the membranes rupture prematurely, and labor does not immediately follow. Without the protection of the membrane sac, the baby runs a high risk of infection.

If the baby is mature enough to be born, the usual remedy is either chemically induced labor or surgical delivery (cesarean section). If the baby is still immature, antibiotics and other means are used to prevent infection and hold-off labor.

Abnormal Fetal Presentation

Most babies, by the time they are ready to be born, are positioned head down in the uterus and facing the mother's back. This is the safest and easiest presentation for birth. Other positions, such as a breech presentation, with the head up and the legs or buttocks down, cause difficulties with delivery and may require a cesarean section.

Cephalopelvic Disproportion

The largest part of a baby is the head. Sometimes the head (cephalos in Greek) is too big to pass through the ring of the mother's pelvic bones. If the disproportion is severe enough, a cesarean delivery may be necessary.

Cord Prolapse and Cord Compression

Until a baby is born and breathing air, the hollow umbilical cord between the placenta and the baby's navel is a vital lifeline for the delivery of oxygen. Without a steady supply of oxygen, the baby will suffer dangerous asphyxia. Before or during labor circulation through the cord may become reduced or cut-off. The cord may be compressed if it gets tightly wrapped around the baby's body. Or it may slip forward (prolapse) into the birth canal during labor and then get trapped between the baby and the canal. The cord can sometimes be freed during ordinary delivery, but an emergency cesarean may be necessary.

Asphyxia

Before birth the oxygen a baby needs must be supplied by the mother, carried in blood that is transferred through the placenta and the umbilical cord. At birth this source is cut-off, and oxygen must be absorbed from the baby's own lungs.

In either case, if the oxygen supply is interrupted, the baby quickly suffers oxygen deprivation, or asphyxia which may cause death or permanent damage. For example, asphyxia is thought to trigger bleeding into the brain which in turn is believed to be a major cause of cerebral palsy, epilepsy, and hydrocephalus. Before birth asphyxia may result from several conditions, ranging from pre-eclampsia to prolonged labor. The main solution is to deliver the baby as soon as possible, by cesarean section if necessary.

Birth Injuries

A baby's passage through the birth canal is often a tight squeeze, and injuries are not uncommon. Most of them, such asbruises and swellings on the head, are minor and soon disappear. Others, such as a broken collarbone or damaged nerves in the neck, may require treatment with a supporting splint or even surgery.

Breathing Problems

For any of several reasons a newborn may have trouble breathing properly and may risk asphyxia. The baby might have wet lung syndrome, for example: The lungs fail to become entirely free of the fluid that filled them before birth and as a result cannot absorb enough oxygen. Or the lung surfaces may be clogged with meconium (mee-KOH-nee-um), a waste material released prematurely from the baby's bowel. Or the normal flow of nervous impulses that control breathing may be impaired, causing temporary apnea, or "non-breathing."

A variety of resuscitation measures are used to stimulate breathing and to ensure a supply of oxygen to the lungs. These range from simply massaging the chest to administering stimulative drugs and providing oxygen through a mechanical respirator.

Persistent Fetal Circulation

At birth there is normally a shift in the baby's heart and major blood vessels, so that more blood is diverted to the now active lungs. Occasionally this shift fails to take place as soon as it should. Without a sufficient blood supply, the lungs cannot deliver enough oxygen to the rest of the body, and the baby may suffer from asphyxia. The standard treatment is to direct extra oxygen to the lungs until the shift takes place.

Postpartum Bleeding

After delivery natural contractions of the mother's uterus should squeeze shut the blood vessels that formerly supplied it, so that bleeding is kept to a minimum. Massage and a hormone that encourages contractions are often used to help the process along. But sometimes dangerously heavy bleeding does occur. It is treated with drugs to encourage clotting and, in rare instances, with surgery to close the blood vessels. Occasionally the placenta will not release and can cause some bleeding by not allowing the uterus to contract. Sometimes a gentle tug on the umbilical cord is all that is needed; however, sometimes manual extraction must take place. Pain medication will be given to allow your doctor to slip a hand into the uterus to help separate the placenta.

Cesarean Section

A cesarean section or cesarean birth is the birth of a fetus through an incision in the lower abdominal cavity and uterus. This is considered a surgical operation and requires a trained surgical team and Anesthesiologist (A doctor who specializes in giving medications that will make patients be in an altered state without pain.). This procedure has dramatically increased over the years, and currently one out of every four births will be cesarean. In most cases cesarean sections are performed as a medical emergency to save the life of the mother or fetus. About 20% of C-Sections are performed because of the following: complications with the umbilical cord or placenta, the mother has an active case of genital herpes, the mother's pelvis is too small for the baby to fit through, or the baby is lying transversely in the uterus. The other 80% of C-Sections are related to the mother's failure to progress with labor, breech presentation, fetal distress, or a repeat cesarean.

Two types of surgical incisions can be performed; classic or lower segment cesarean. The classic incision involves making a vertical cut through the abdomen and a vertical cut through the uterus. This procedure was always used in the past but has lost popularity today. This incision is much more painful for the mother because it involves a great number of abdominal muscles and a great amount of healing. Also, this incision has been found to create a greater amount of blood loss, infection, and uterine rupture with following pregnancies. If a woman had a cesarean with the classic incision, she would also have to have a cesarean with the following pregnancies. The lower segment cesarean is used very widely today. This surgical procedure involves a horizontal, and much smaller cut, along the pubic hairline of the woman. The surgeon can then decide to make a vertical or horizontal incision in the uterus. This procedure is associated with faster abdominal muscle healing, less blood loss, and less infections. The woman can also then decide to have a vaginal birth after cesarean (VBAC) with future pregnancies..

Cesarean Sections include added risks because they are a surgical procedure. Maternal complications occur in 25 to 50% of all cesarean births and include wound infection, hemorrhage, life threatening clots that travel to the lungs, urinary tract infections, injuries to internal organs (bladder or bowel), and complications with anesthesia. Fetal injuries can also occur during the cutting of the uterus. The mother will need a great amount of time for healing and may have considerable pain. In addition, the mother can also have feelings of disappointment with her birth experience. Therefore, the mother should be allowed to bond with her child as soon as possible after the procedure is over.

Appendix VI

Adolescent Deliveries Managed at KK Hospital, Singapore

S. Nadarajah, N.K.Y. Leong

Introduction

Adolescent pregnancy is really a problem of children having children, when they are on the threshold of adulthood. Adolescent girls who are pregnant are physically as well as socially disadvantaged when compared to their older counterparts. The aim of this study was to analyse the adolescent pregnancies managed at KK Hospital especially with regards to antenatal complications, mode of delivery and birthweights of the babies.

Materials and Methods

The period of study was from January 1997 to December 1997. All deliveries of girls aged 17 and below were retrospectively analysed. The gestation at booking, number of antenatal visits, antenatal complications, mode of delivery, birthweights of the babies and postnatal complications were studied.

Results

There was a total of 108 deliveries by girls aged 17 and below. This accounted for 0.7% of all deliveries in KK Hospital for 1997. For 84.3% of the girls, it was their first pregnancy. For 5 in the 16-year age group and 12 in the 17-year age group, it was their second pregnancy. This accounts for 15.7% of all deliveries. Ninety-five percent (88%) of the girls had some form of antenatal care while 13 (12%) were unbooked, i.e. had no prior antenatal care. Among the girls who sought antenatal care, 51.9% had their first visit in their third trimester, with 30.5% and 5.6% having theirs in the second and first trimesters respectively. The average number of antenatal visits was 3.9 per pregnancy. Twenty-four (22%) of the girls were unsure of their last menstrual period. Anaemia and pre-term labour were the most common antenatal complications, each affecting 19 (17.6%) of the girls. Anaemia is defined as a haemoglobin level of less than 10 gm% and pre-term labour as the onset of labour before 37 weeks of gestation. Pre-labour rupture of membranes affected 6 (5.6%) of the pregnancies. There was a single case each of gestational diabetes, syphilis, and intrauterine growth retardation. Two girls admitted to having abused drugs during their pregnancies. Of the 108 pregnancies, 100 had normal vaginal deliveries, 3 (2.7%) delivered via lower segment Caesarean section, and 5 had forceps assisted vaginal delivery. Two girls developed peripartum and postpartum pregnancy induced hypertension, and 1 girl developed postpartum haemorrhage.

Discussion

While 18 and 19-year old girls are by definition teenagers, the medical and social disadvantages of childbearing is apparently less in these girls when compared to girls who are 17 and below. Therefore, this study was confined to the latter group of girls. While the Malay population forms only 23% of the population in Singapore, they formed 58.3% of teenage pregnancies in KKH. The same trend is seen in the general population with pregnancies of Malay girls aged 19 and below accounting for 42.3% of all teenage pregnancies in Singapore. This may in part be explained by the fact that Malay women in general marry at a younger age. However, it is questionable whether it alone accounts for the high proportion of teenage pregnancies in this racial group.

Most of the medical problems of teenage pregnancies are directly or indirectly related to psycho-social factors. Late or non-existant prenatal care is a feature in most pregnancies. While 53.3% of these patients had their first visit in their third trimester, 12.1% were completely unbooked, having their first contact with any form of obstetric care only when they went into labour. It is well documented that there are more complications in pregnancies when patients receive any prenatal care until they are into their third trimester.

Anaemia is one of the most common antenatal complications in teenage pregnancies. It was found to be twice as common in pregnant teenagers when compared to pregnant women who were more than 20 years of age. This is usually due to poor nutrition secondary to financial reasons or to poor dietary habits of teenagers who do not have the benefit of nutritional advise. This is further compounded by late booking where they do not have the benefit of supplemental vitamins.

Pre-term labour was as common as anaemia, affecting 17.6% of the pregnancies. The incidence of preterm labour in the general population in a developed country such as Australia is 6.7%. The higher incidence seen in teenage pregnancies is thought to be due to lifestyle factors such as smoking, drug abuse and the presence of genital tract infection in these teenagers, rather than to their age *per se.*

There were 4 girls with pregnancy-induced hypertension. It is well documented that pregnant teenagers have a higher risk of developing pregnancy-induced hypertension. There was a single case of syphilis. While all pregnant women are routinely screened for syphilis as part of the antenatal check up, they are not routinely checked for other sexually transmitted diseases like chlamydia, gonorrhoea and AIDS. Therefore, the incidence of sexually transmitted disease may in reality be higher. Only two girls admitted to abusing drugs, but as drug abuse is a serious crime in Singapore, requiring mandatory detention and rehabilitation, most girls would have been reluctant to volunteer this information.

Adolescents, because of their smaller physical build, have always been thought to have a higher risk for cephalopelvic disproportion and subsequent Caesarean section. However, this has been refuted by several studies. In this study, the Caesarean section rate was only 2.7%. The reason for this may have been due to the high incidence of low birthweight among the babies born with 21.2% weighing less than 2.5 kg. Several studies have attributed the higher rates of low birthweight babies among adolescent pregnancies to unfavourable socio-demographic and healthcare factors such as substance abuse, low income, single parent status, low educational level and delayed or absence of prenatal care. However, in countries where teenage childbearing is not concentrated in the lower socio-economic classes, adolescents still have disproportionately high rates of low birthweight infants. In Saudi Arabia, where early marriage and teenage pregnancy is common in all socio-economic groups as a result of religious beliefs, the incidence of low birthweight infants born to mothers 17 years of age or less has been reported to be 23%. Therefore, it is likely that a combination of factors are responsible for adolescents having low birth weight babies.

The repeat pregnancy rate was 15.7%. Of these, 10.2% had a termination of pregnancy in their first pregnancy and 5.5% delivered a live baby. It has been found that women who bear only one child during their adolescence seem to have the best chance of educational and economic

Distribution of Pregnancy by Race and Age

	Age			
Race	14	15	16	17
Malay (63) 58.3%	2	2	22	37
Chinese (38) 35.2%	1	6	12	19
Indian (7) 6.5%	0	0	1	6
	3 (2.8)	8 (7.4%)	35 (32.4%)	62 (57.4%)

Distribution of Birth Weight according to Material Age

Age	ELBW (1 1000)	*Birth weight* VLBW (1 1.5 kg)	LBW (1 2.5 kg)
14	0	0	1
15	0	0	1
16	0	0	8
17	1	1	11

19.4% of the babies had LBW with 1 baby each with VLBW and ELBW.

achievement if they receive adequate support after birth of their first child. The birth of a second child during adolescence predicts a negative outcome. They are less able to achieve an education, independence and financial security. The high rate of repeat pregnancy at such a young age is probably a reflection of inadequate counseling by healthcare workers with regards to contraception and the benefits of spacing subsequent pregnancies.

Conclusion

Fortunately adolescent pregnancy does not pose a major problem in Singapore as it does in some other countries. However, it must be recognised as a high risk pregnancy and managed accordingly. In addition, greater efforts must be directed towards reducing the high number of repeat pregnancies in a group that is ill-equipped to handle even just one pregnancy. (S. Nadarajah, MBBS, MRCOG, Registrar).

Appendix VII
International Council on Management of Population Programmes

The ICPD Programme of Action suggests a move from the narrowly defined MCH-FP to comprehensive reproductive health services programmes defined as follows:

Reproductive health is a state of complete physical, mental and social well-being and not merely the absence of disease or infirmity, in all matters relating to the reproductive system and to its functions and processes. Reproductive health therefore implies that people are able to have a satisfying and safe sex life and that they have the capability to reproduce and the freedom to decide if, when and how often to do so. Implicit in this last condition are the rights of men and women to be informed and have access to safe, effective, affordable and acceptable methods of family planning of their choice, as well as other methods of their choice for regulation of fertility, which are not against the law, and the right of access to appropriate healthcare services that will enable women to go through pregnancy and childbirth and provide couples with the best chance of having a healthy infant. In line with the above definition of reproductive health, reproductive healthcare is defined as the constellation of methods, techniques and services that contribute to reproductive health and well-being by preventing and solving reproductive health problems. It also includes sexual health, the purpose of which is the enhancement of life and personal relations, and not merely counselling and care related to reproduction and sexually transmitted diseases. (para 7.2, ICPD Programme of Action)

Thus, the Programme of Action recognizes the rights of men and women to undertake sexual activity safely, without fear of unwanted pregnancy and of contracting diseases; if pregnancy is desired, women should be able to carry the pregnancy to term safely, to deliver a healthy child and to be able to nurture it. It also recognizes the need to provide services to adolescent females and males.[1]

The Platform of Action at the Beijing Conference builds on the ICPD, "human right of women include their right to have control over and decide freely and responsibly on matters related to their sexuality, including sexual

---

1. World Bank, 1993, investing in Health, World Development Report, New York: Oxford University Press.

and reproductive health, free of coercion, discrimination and violence."

Furthermore, it should be recognized that reproductive health does not only depend on health services; it is closely linked to the socio-economic conditions and cultural practices, particularly women's status and gender relations. Therefore, a broader reproductive health programme would take into account the latter issues as well as incorporate provision of reproductive health services in order to achieve comprehensive healthcare for women and men of all ages, including adolescents.

Reproductive Health

Reproductive Health Status

In the Asian countries, about one-third of the total disease burden in women between 15 and 44 years of age is linked to health problems related to pregnancy, childbirth, abortion, human immunodeficiency virus (HIV) and reproductive tract infections (RTIs). Problems such as female genital mutilation, malnutrition and anaemia, unwanted pregnancy, reproductive tract infections including sexually transmitted diseases and HIV/AIDS, infertility, sexual and gender violence, unregulated fertility, maternal mortality and morbidity, reproductive tract cancers, osteoporosis and prolapse contributes to women's ill-health throughout their lifecycle.[2]

Components of Reproductive Health Services

Although the priority for specific reproductive health services will differ from country to country, the following services should generally be included:

- family planning counselling, information, education and services,
- prevention and treatment of RTIs and STDs,
- prevention, clinical assessment and referral of HIV/AIDS cases,
- education and services for prenatal care, delivery and postnatal care including breastfeeding, and infant and women's healthcare,
- prevention and appropriate treatment of infertility,
- prevention of abortion and management of the consequences of abortion, and abortion services where legal,
- services for women's gynaecological problems, and
- active discouragement of harmful practices such as female genital mutilation.

The constellation of services reflects a need to considerably broaden

2. Dr. Tomris Turmen, Reproductive Health: WHO's Role in a Global Strategy. Paper presented at the Meeting on the Development and Delivery of Reproductive Health in the context of Primary Healthcare, Geneva, 23-24 March-1 August.

the range of services provided by most of the current MCH-FP programmes. They need to respond to the needs of individuals, couples and families. The quality of care improves as programmes become client-centred. Clients are able not only to meet their contraceptive needs but could also seek services for other reproductive health needs. If the services they seek are not available at the first point of contact, clients should have access to other facilities. Quality implies sufficient information and choice of contraceptive methods. Clients could also expect to participate in the design, implementation and evaluation of the services. The transition from MCH-FP to reproductive health programmes has many managerial implications, and these are discussed in the following section.

Managerial Implications

Paradigm Shift

The transition from MCH-FP programmes to comprehensive reproductive health programmes requires not only the addition of services but a paradigm shift.

Managerial Implications

The paradigm shift has many managerial implications: (1) reorientation and restructuring of programmes; (2) addressing gender concerns; (3) establishing mechanisms for partnership and building linkages; and (4) strengthening leadership.

Reorientation and restructuring of programmes

A reproductive health approach requires that clients are guaranteed quality services that meet their needs, given informed choices, and treated with respect and dignity. Since quality of care is the yardstick for measuring success of reproductive health services, there needs to be changes in monitoring and performance appraisal reflecting quality and not quantity. In addition to MCH-FP services, other components of reproductive health services need to be included in the existing programmes.

With the expansion of services, redefinition of roles and training/retraining of providers and staff cannot be avoided. Many existing programmes have female providers and if men's reproductive health needs are to be met, however, male providers must be recruited and trained. At the same time, providers working with adolescents need to be trained to enable them to effectively reach adolescents. The development of competencies must be accompanied by adequate supply and equipment.

Gender concerns

Reproductive health services should respond to the needs, concerns, views and expectations of women as well as those of men. However, because women suffer more from reproductive health problems, special attention should be given to them and their needs.

Furthermore, women's low social, political, economic and cultural status in most cultures has excluded them from making decisions concerning their health and lives. In order to meet their needs, women who are often ignored in decision-making must be actively involved in the design, implementation and evaluation of programmes.

Many have argued that the disadvantaged position and discrimination suffered by women from birth to adulthood are strong factors contributing to women's poor health. Since childhood, women have been conditioned to accept ill-health and consequently do not demand services. The culture of silence must be broken if women's health is to improve. Empowering women, particularly grassroots women, and creating a supportive environment are powerful tools to break the silence.

Establish mechanism for partnership and building linkages

The interdependence of the various components of reproductive health call for partnerships with government, NGOs, and international agencies. Partnership should be built on trust, respect and flexibility. There may also be a need for a body to coordinate the various efforts by the partners. The private sector can play a significant role and the government should encourage their participation by developing supportive policies and including this sector in the overall programme strategy.

Reproductive health programmes also require building linkages with agencies or facilities offering various services. Such linkages are particularly important for referrals as not all programmes are able to provide all the services related to reproductive health.

Strengthening leadership

To successfully move towards a reproductive health programme, strong leadership is needed at both the top and the middle management levels. Top level managers need to create and sustain national commitment, establish partnerships and linkages, create values among staff and in society conducive to reproductive health services, and finally strengthen programme implementation. Middle management is required, amongst others, to improve programme management, ensure quality of services, build support for reproductive health services, and establish networks with the community and community resources. To effectively perform their roles, managers must develop these skills, either through long-term technical and management training or through short management courses.[3]

What can be Done?

There are no comprehensive reproductive health programmes yet.

3. Rushikesh Maru, Management Perspectives on Manpower Development in Health and Family Planning Program. In *Managing a New Generation of Population Programmes: Challenges of the Nineties*, Edited by Satia, J., Schonmeyr, C., and Tahir, S., 1994.

However, despite the problems described above, numerous agencies particularly NGOs have successfully implemented innovative projects in addressing specific issues of reproductive health. This issue of Innovations presents four case studies highlighting innovative approaches as well as shedding some light on how problems were overcome and issues addressed.

Male Responsibility

Myths that men are not willing to take an active role in fertility regulation and be responsible for the reproductive health of their spouses and the health of their families abound. The few experiences of male motivation and service provision projects, however, have indicated otherwise. These experiences show that men are willing to be responsible provided that they are well-informed and that services meet their needs. Unfortunately, efforts to educate men and provide services to meet their needs have been largely ignored.

Although there have been calls for male responsibility and involvement, the strategies for motivating them and for service provision remain unclear.

PRO-PATER: Meeting Men's Reproductive Health Needs

This case study proves that men are willing to play a role in reproductive health and family planning if quality services that meet their needs are accessible. While clients are given services at a number of clinics, various approaches including TV and radio campaigns and outreach activities were mobilized to inform men and the community about services offered by PRO-PATER.

RTIS, STD and HIV/AIDS

STDs and HIV/AIDS can no longer be associated with high risk groups only. Statistics show that each year 250 million men and women are infected with some form of STDs. In Thailand, the nationwide average rates of HIV infection among women attending antenatal clinics between 1990-93 grew from 0.4 per cent to 1.8 per cent.[4] A study in two rural villages in India found that among 650 women, an alarming 92 per cent suffered from one or more gynaecological or sexual diseases[5]. The average number of these diseases per woman was 3.6. In Bangladesh, 25 per cent of almost

4. Sittitrai, W., Brown, T., and Carl, G., Incorporation of STD and HIV/AIDS within FPIMCH Programmes in Thailand. Paper presented at the Consultative Group Meeting on STDs and AIDS Prevention in the Indian Family Welfare Programme, Surajkund, India, 1994.
5. Commentary on a Community-based Approach to Reproductive Healthcare, Rani Bang and Abhay Bang and SEARCH Team, *International Journal of Gynaecology and Obstetrics*, 1989, Supple. 3:125-129.

3,000 women surveyed reported symptoms of a reproductive tract infection and two-thirds of these had clinical or laboratory evidence of an infection.[6] In rural Egypt, 52 per cent of 509 non-pregnant women had a RTI, 56 per cent had uterine prolapse, 14 per cent had a urinary tract infection, 11 per cent had an abnormal pap smear and 63 per cent were anemic.[7]

Advocacy for the integration of RTIs, STD and HIV/AIDS in MCHFP programmes is strong and is making an impact. However, progress in implementation is rather slow. While integration is one of the best approaches to addressing the problem, starting an integrated approach has numerous managerial and financial implications and may not be an effective solution in many settings. An integrated programme has to deal with training and/or retraining of staff, provision of adequate supplies, development of relevant IEC materials, etc. With these activities to be implemented, in addition to existing MCH-FP programmes, the cost will increase.

Responding to STDs and HIV/AIDS in Kenya

Through improving quality of services and motivating staff to treat clients with respect, this pilot project shows how an STD clinic can be a friendly service outlet and attract the general population to utilize the services provided. The project also strengthened its linkages with primary health centres and other development programmes, which inform the public about the services offered at the STD clinic.

Family Welfare Services: The Tata Steel Experience in India

What can the private sector do to enhance the health and quality of life of its employees? The case study of the Tata Iron and Steel Company is a classic example of how commitment at the highest level allows employees and their families to enjoy health services as well as other development efforts.

Youth Sexuality and Reproductive Health

A growing number of young people are engaging in sexual activities. This development is compounded by societal stigma against teenage sexuality and social constraints against providing contraceptive services to unmarried couples, resulting in a significant increase in teenage pregnancy and induced abortion. 15 million children are born to teenage mothers annually, thus putting the health of these mothers as well as that of their babies at risk. As many as 5 million abortions involving young girls take place annually, of which thousands die under clandestine, dangerous and unhygienic circumstances. While there are health implications with teenage pregnancy, it is also a social problem.

---

6. Reproductive Health Problems Common in Asian Countries Women Outlook, 1994 August; 12 (2) 3.
7. *Ibid.*

Another issue related to youth sexuality is the prevalence of STDs including HIV infection. Statistics show that STDs are highest amongst young people between the ages of 20-24 followed by 15-19 year age groups. Worldwide, between 20-25 per cent of HIV infections are estimated to occur among young people.[8]

Many are in agreement that youth sexuality and reproductive health need to be addressed urgently. However, they differ in what actions to be taken. Numerous NGOs and some international agencies have taken the lead in implementing small scale projects. While the majority of these projects focus on educational activities and almost no services, the issues addressed vary from biology to STD and HIV/AIDS to relationships, depending on the environment where the projects are being implemented. Unfortunately, most governments have yet to take action. The sensitivity of the subject coupled with the lack of capacity and widely accepted programme models are reasons for inaction on the part of most governments.

Youth Helping Youth in Tanzania

The UMATI youth programme is based on the experiences of similar programmes carried out in Sweden. In the programme, a core group of youth are trained to reach out to their peers. Linkages with health clinics were established so that medical services are available to youth in need of such services.

8. The Health of Young People: A Challenge and a Promise, World Health Organization.

Appendix VIII

Women's Health in India: Whither Women's Health

RECENT trends in public policy and awareness about women's health needs, and actual access by women to the services to address those concerns show complex and contradictory tendencies according to Gita Sen in her paper entitled 'Whither Women's Health', which was presented at a seminar on women's health. This paper identifies these tendencies and argues that a critical absence of focused attention to their implications underlies the weak progress made in improving women's health in the country.

The decade of the 1990s highlighted a number of policy shifts and changes with direct and indirect implications for women's health. These include: (i) the overarching economic reforms agenda with its emphasis on liberalizing controls in different industries, and controlling the fiscal deficit through real expenditure cuts; (ii) a contested paradigm shift in national population policy in line with the new ICPD ethos of meeting the reproductive and sexual health needs of individuals and couples; (iii) growing concern over HIV/AIDS and its increasing 'feminisation' as it spreads from high-risk groups into the general population; and (iv) growing recognition after the 1993 Vienna Conference on Human Rights and the Fourth World Conference on Women of Beijing (1995) of violence against women as a major health and human rights problem.

Were women's health needs taken seriously prior to the 1990s? Although women became central targets of the family planning programme from the late 1960s on, it is well known that their reproductive health needs were neither acknowledged as a policy concern nor set within an overall integrated approach to their health. The field of women's health in India was full of resounding policy and research silences, misdirected and partial approaches, and insufficient attention to critical issues such as co-morbidity or the reversal of the traditional gender paradox in health. In many ways these problems in India mirrored a global lack of attention to gender equity in health. But the acute nature of gender bias and son preference in the country made their consequences even more severe.

Problems of irregular bleeding and amenorrhea were left unaddressed despite growing evidence of the prevalence of malnutrition and iron-deficiency anemia among girls and women. The cross-linkages between anemia and vulnerability to malaria continued to be ignored by policy and programme. So also did the prevalence of violence against women and its connections to sexual health and rights. In a country where abortion had been legal since the early 1970s, it continued to be unsafe for an overwhelming majority of those who needed the service. It is true that awareness of the problem of declining sex-ratios and gender bias within households in favour of boys' and men's nutrition and healthcare had grown. But many other problems, such as those above, were only weakly recognized. And if the field of reproductive health was weak during this period, this was true of areas such as occupational, environmental or mental health. Nor was much attention given to gender concerns in the handling of infectious diseases.

Undoubtedly the weak policy and funding support that bedevilled women's health in this period was experienced most seriously by the poor and by women especially among the poor. Official statistics on illness in the latter half of the 1980s shows higher untreated illness rates for women. That is, the access gap for poor women was even greater than for poor men. Over 70 per cent of out-patient care was provided by the private sector. However, partly because of greater cost differentials, only 40 per cent of in-patient care was handled by the private sector.

It wasn't until the conferences of the 1990s (Vienna, Cairo, and Beijing) that major changes in policy thinking occurred. The recognition in Vienna of women's rights as human rights and of violence against women as a violation of those rights, the paradigm shift of ICPD from top-down demographic control to population policies focused on meeting reproductive and sexual health and reproductive rights, and the reinforcement of these forward shifts at the Beijing conference had a major impact on policy thinking. The direct impact was the repudiation of targets in the family planning programme, and the attempt to introduce an approach to service delivery based on community needs assessment. A new programme on Reproductive and Child Health (RCH-1) was introduced with major donor funding and with significant new programme elements included. Although neither the target-free approach nor RCH-1 were as effective as the intention behind them, the policy direction appeared definitely to be changing. However, the RCH programme depends for its effectiveness on the public health infrastructure of sub-centres, PHCs and hospitals, as well as staffing, logistics and management inputs from the public health system. This system went through major negative changes during this period. During this entire period, the health sector was undergoing the direct and indirect effects of structural reforms in the overall economy. Real expenditures on public health stagnated, accompanied by infrastructural decline and rising user charges. Perhaps the most significant increases in health costs came from the rapid liberalization of the pharmaceutical industry resulting in sharp increases in drug costs. Recent detailed micro-studies of poverty in 12 villages of Rajasthan and 20 villages of Gujarat show health costs as the single most important reason for households falling into poverty in the last 25 years. Barring PHC use, the use of public and private hospitals, nursing homes and health facilities run by charitable institutions are all now tilted strongly towards the better-off economic groups. This is true for both women and men. This means that not only the private sector health services, but even public health services are more utilized by the better-off. How and whether this changes under RCH-2 remains to be seen. While the paradigm shift towards the ICPD approach appeared to be gaining ground during the 1990s, this seems to have become more shaky recently. But politicians in some states and especially, at the Centre, have now begun to jump on the population control bandwagon. One of the fallouts of the forced sterilizations during the Sanjay Gandhi period was that no politician wanted to be associated with the family planning programme, which was, as a result, left in the hands of the bureaucrats. The renewed debates set-off by ICPD have made population once more a 'touchable' issue for the political class.

Thus, focusing on incentives or disincentives on family size will have very little impact on the growth of population. If we are indeed concerned to bring down the growth rate of population, we would do better by improving the quality of family planning services, empowering women to make reproductive decisions, and lowering the effect of population momentum by raising the effective age at marriage.

Although the first HIV case in the country was detected only as late as 1986 in Chennai, a decade of silent but deadly spread of the disease now leaves us with approximately four million official cases (and perhaps 10 million actual cases). After South Africa, India now has the largest number of HIV-infected persons. Over 85 per cent of transmission is sexual, and a growing proportion is heterosexual. Almost 90 per cent of reported cases are in the age 18-49, i.e., the most sexually active and reproductive population. Women currently account for about a quarter of the infections, but given the rate at which the infection appears to be spreading from the so-called 'high risk' groups to the general population, this ratio is very likely to increase in the near future. The window of opportunity for controlling the epidemic in the country may be closing rapidly. The most alarming aspect of the current situation is the combination of heterosexual transmission and the weakness of sexual rights for women in the country. The right to say 'no' to sex within marriage, and the ability to negotiate condom use with male partners are capacities that very few women have. Family planning practices in even a more socially advanced state such as Kerala see couples typically using no family planning methods after marriage until the desired two children have been had. At this point the woman undergoes sterilization. Spacing and condom use are still relatively low. Rising concerns about HIV/AIDS have certainly generated greater willingness to tackle awareness about sexuality, adult and adolescent sexual behaviour, and complex issues of medical ethics. All the dilemmas faced by women's health at this time point in the direction of approaches that reinforce women's rights. The responsibility to ensure these rights lies with families, communities and the government at both state and central level. Ensuring effective and equitable access to affordable health services is the job of the state. An effective public health infrastructure can act as a floor for health access, and is a crucial ingredient of poverty reduction. Providing this on a priority basis will both improve health status and also support the paradigm changes of the 1990s. But women's health as we know is not only a matter of access to services; it also requires a change in mindsets and power equations. Without these changes, no real paradigm change is possible.

Reproductive Health

Reproductive health has been defined as ". . . a state of complete physical, mental, and social well-being and not merely the absence of disease or infirmity, in all matters related to the reproductive system and to its functions and processes." Given its broad definition, many factors influence reproductive health, including access to professional maternity care and other reproductive health services, the ability of women to participate in health decision-making, and domestic violence. In India, maternity-related complications are leading causes of death and disability among women during their reproductive years. WHO and UNICEF estimate that women face a 1 in 37 risk of dying from pregnancy or childbirth during their lifetime. By contrast, European women have a 1 in 1,400 risk of dying from these causes. Globally, one out of four women who dies from maternity-related complications resides in India. The vast majority of these deaths are preventable.

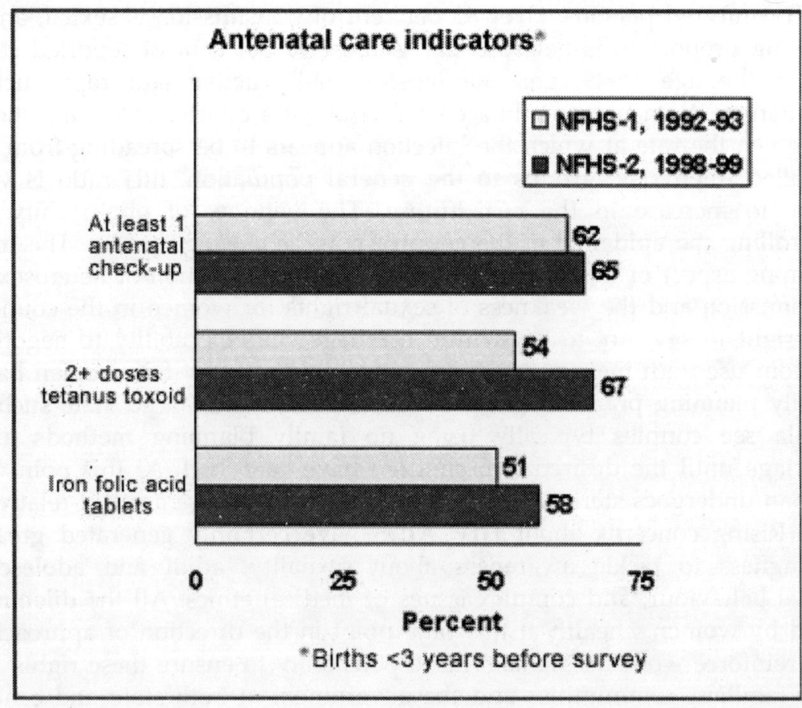

Use of recommended antenatal care is low, but some progress has been made. Only 20 percent of mothers receive all of the recommended types of antenatal care. Coverage ranges from 65 percent in Kerala to 4 percent in Uttar Pradesh. Other poorly performing states include Bihar, Rajasthan, and Nagaland. Since the early 1990s, coverage for different antenatal services has increased

Mothers and families still need to be better informed about the benefits of antenatal check-ups. Among those who did not receive check-ups, most said that they did not consider antenatal check-ups to be necessary. Among those who received antenatal check-ups, three-quarters had their abdomens examined. Only two-thirds or fewer received any of the other recommended checks or advice. Relatively few women—36 percent—were told about signs and symptoms of a risky pregnancy. Access to professional delivery care improves, with some states close to meeting the National Population Policy goals for 2010. Some states are close to meeting the National Population Policy goal of having a health professional attend all births by 2010: Tamil Nadu (84 percent), Goa (91 percent), and Kerala (94 percent). One of the most important ways of preventing maternal deaths is to ensure that women give birth with the help of an obstetrician.

Other states still perform well below average: 30 percent or fewer women receive professional delivery care in Meghalaya, Assam, Uttar Pradesh, Bihar, and Madhya Pradesh. Nearly two-thirds of births are delivered at home. Most women who give birth at home receive no postpartum care (83 percent). Nearly half of women have no say regarding their own healthcare. The proportion of women involved in decision-making regarding their own healthcare ranges from 37 percent in Madhya Pradesh to 81 percent in Himachal Pradesh.

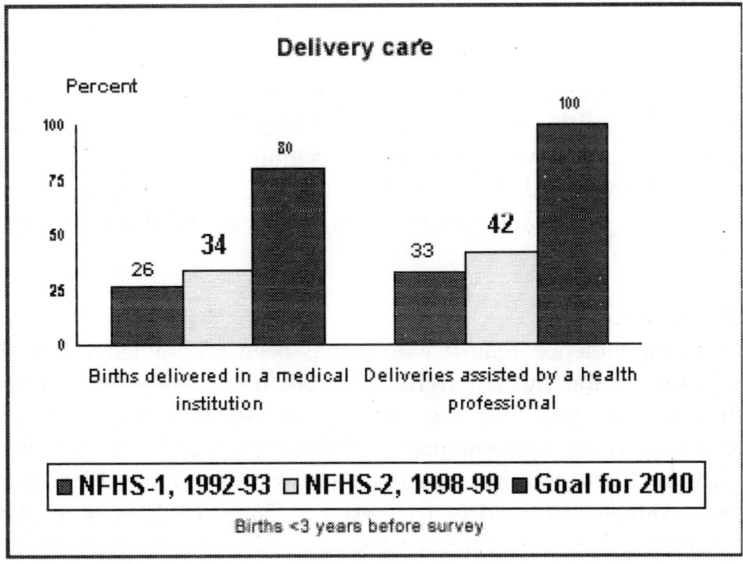

Reproductive Health Problems

Many women experience reproductive health problems; most endure the symptoms without seeking healthcare. Nearly four out of ten currently married women report at least one reproductive health problem that could be symptomatic of a more serious reproductive tract infection. If left untreated, reproductive tract infections can cause pregnancy-related complications, congenital infections, infertility, and chronic pain. They are also risk factors for pelvic inflammatory disease and HIV. In all but five states, at least one-third of women report one or more reproductive health problems. The percentage of currently married women with any reproductive health problem varies from 19 percent in Karnataka to 67 percent in Meghalaya. The consistently high self-reported prevalence suggests that reproductive health problems are widespread among all groups of women and in almost all states.

Currently married women with any reproductive health problem	
15-20%:	Karnataka
20-29%:	Orissa, Tamil Nadu, Punjab, Gujarat
30-39%:	Himachal Pradesh, Delhi, Uttar Pradesh, Haryana
39%:	India
40-49%:	Maharashtra, Goa, Arunachal Pradesh, Kerala, Rajasthan, Bihar, Madhya Pradesh, West Bengal, Nagaland, Andhra Pradesh, Sikkim
50%+:	Assam, Mizoram, Manipur, Jammu & Kashmir, Meghalaya

Among women who report any reproductive health problem, two-thirds have not seen anyone for advice or treatment. An important objective of the Reproductive and Child Health Programme, however, is the identification and management of reproductive tract infections. Women who seek advice or treatment for reproductive health problems do not usually go to government health professionals. This highlights the need to educate women regarding the symptoms and consequences of reproductive health problems and the need to expand counseling and reproductive health services in both rural and urban areas, particularly through the public sector.

Domestic Violence

Domestic violence against women has been acknowledged worldwide as a violation of the human rights of women. An increasing amount of research also indicates that the acceptance and experience of domestic violence has adverse consequences for women's health and the health of their children. Many women accept wife-beating as justified under certain conditions. Almost three out of five women (56 percent) believe that wife-beating is justified for at least one of six specific reasons. Women are most

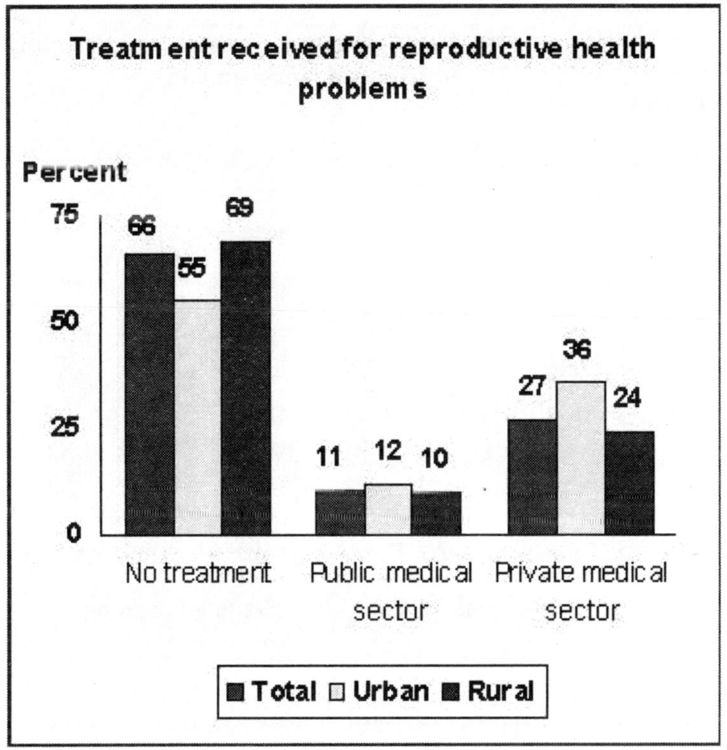
Treatment received for reproductive health problems
Percent
75
50
25
0
66
55
69
11
12
10
27
36
24
No treatment
Public medical sector
Private medical sector
Total
Urban
Rural

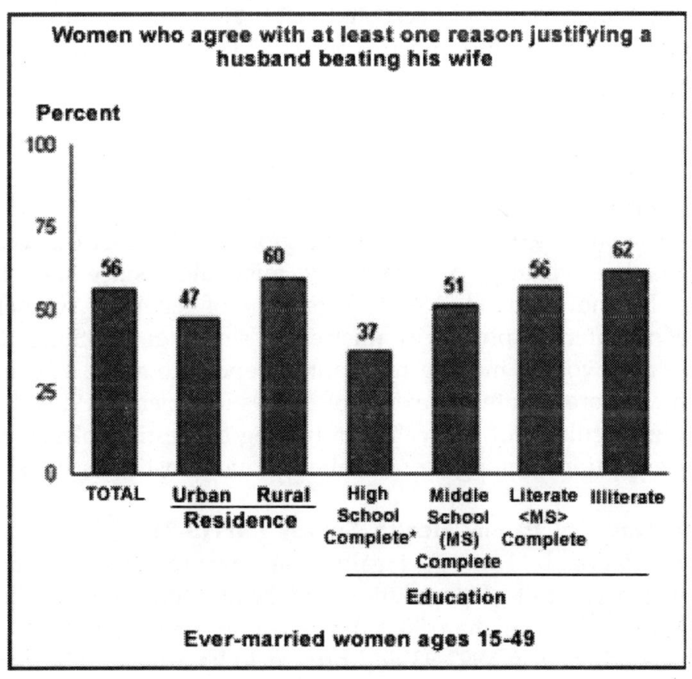
Women who agree with at least one reason justifying a husband beating his wife
Percent
100
75
50
25
0
56
47
60
37
51
56
62
TOTAL
Urban
Rural
Residence
High School Complete*
Middle School (MS) Complete
Literate <MS> Complete
Illiterate
Education
Ever-married women ages 15-49

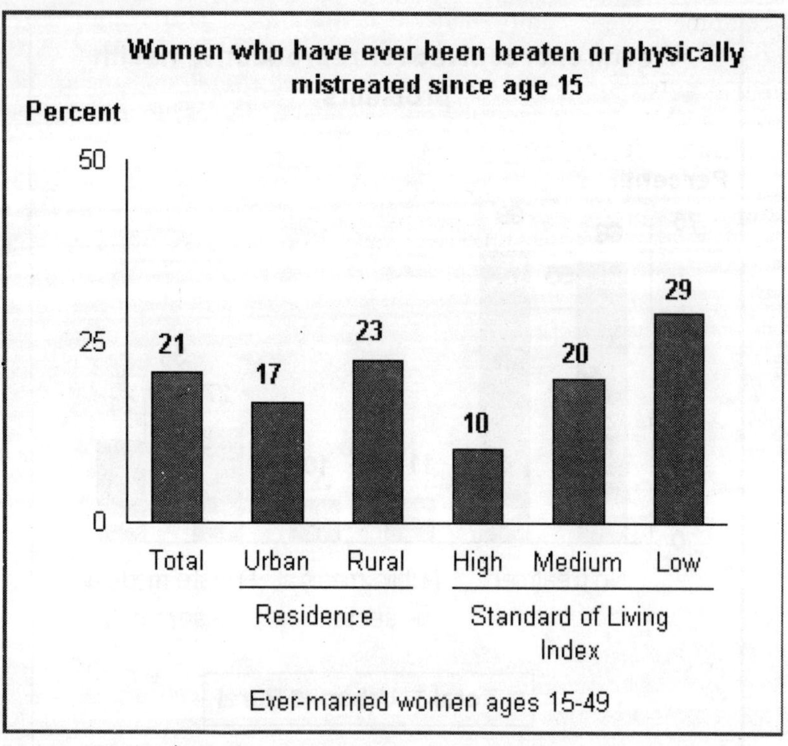

likely to agree that neglecting the house or children (40 percent) justifies wife-beating. Other commonly accepted justifications include the wife going out without telling the husband (37 percent); the wife showing disrespect for in-laws (34 percent); and the husband suspecting his wife is unfaithful (33 percent).

Less acceptable reasons include the wife not cooking the food properly (25 percent) and the parental family not giving expected dowery or other items (7 percent).

Many women experience domestic violence. At least one out of five women has been beaten or physically mistreated since age 15, most commonly by the husband. Nearly three out of ten poor women report having been beaten or physically mistreated since age 15. Since this topic is sensitive and women may be reluctant to report domestic violence, these results may underestimate the extent of domestic violence. Possible reasons why include a "culture of silence" surrounding domestic violence, fear, and different perceptions among women about what constitutes violence.

About the National Family Health Survey (NFHS-2)

The National Family Health Survey (NFHS-2) provides a comprehensive portrait of population and health conditions in India. The NFHS-2 surveyed more than 90,000 women in 1998 and 1999. The first NFHS was conducted in 1992-93 and proved to be a major landmark in the development of a comprehensive demographic and health database for India. The second National Family Health Survey further expands the database, providing information on trends over time and meeting emerging needs in new areas of population and health. The International Institute for Population Sciences (IIPS, Mumbai) served as the nodal agency for both the NFHS-1 and NFHS 2. Project funding was provided by the United States Agency for International Development, with additional funds for nutrition data collection in the NFHS-2 from UNICEF. Technical guidance was provided by ORC Macro and the East-West Center. Thirteen organizations were responsible for data collection, including five Population Research Centres and eight research companies. (Victoria A. Velkoff and Arjun Adlakha).

Appendix IX

Report of U.S. Department of Commerce, Economics and Statistics Administration, Bureau of the Census, Issued December 1998) : India

India is one of the few countries in the world where women and men have nearly the same life expectancy at birth. The fact that the typical female advantage in life expectancy is not seen in India suggests there are systematic problems with women's health. Indian women have high mortality rates, particularly during childhood and in their reproductive years. The health of Indian women is intrinsically linked to their status in society. Research on women's status has found that the contributions Indian women make to families often are overlooked, and instead they are viewed as economic burdens. There is a strong son preference in India, as sons are expected to care for parents as they age. This son preference, along with high dowry costs for daughters, sometimes results in the mistreatment of daughters. Further, Indian women have low levels of both education and formal labor force participation. They typically have little autonomy, living under the control of first their fathers, then their husbands, and finally their sons. While women in India face many serious health concerns, this profile focuses on only five key issues: reproductive health, violence against women, nutritional status, unequal treatment of girls and boys, and HIV/AIDS. Because of the wide variation in cultures, religions, and levels of development among India's 25 states and 7 union territories, it is not surprising that women's health also varies greatly from state to state. To give a more detailed picture, data for the major states will be presented (Chatterjee, 1990; Desai, 1994; Horowitz and Kishwar, 1985; The World Bank, 1996). All of these factors exert a negative impact on the health status of Indian women. Poor health has repercussions not only for women but also their families. Women in poor health are more likely to give birth to low-weight infants. They also are less likely to be able to provide food and adequate care for their children. Finally, a woman's health affects the household economic well-being, as a woman in poor health will be less productive in the labor force. According to International Institute for Population Sciences, 1995, the following is the Percent Distribution of Contraceptive Users by Method: Female sterilization 67%, Condom 6%, Traditional 11%, IUD 5%, Male sterilization 9%, Pill 3%.

Many of the health problems of Indian women are related to or exacerbated by high levels of fertility. Overall, fertility has been declining in India; by 1992-93 the total fertility rate was 3.4 (International Institute for

Population Science (IIPS), 1995). However, there are large differences in fertility levels by state, education, religion, caste and place of residence. Utter Pradesh, the most populous state in India, has a total fertility rate of over 5 children per woman. On the other hand, Kerala, which has relatively high levels of female education and autonomy, has a total fertility rate under 2. High levels of infant mortality combined with the strong son preference motivate women to bear high numbers of children in an attempt to have a son or two survive to adulthood. Research has shown that numerous pregnancies and closely spaced births erode a mother's nutritional status, which can negatively affect the pregnancy outcome (e.g., premature births, low birth-weight babies) and also increase the health risk for mothers (Jejeebhoy and Rao, 1995). Unwanted pregnancies terminated by unsafe abortions also have negative consequences for women's health. Reducing fertility is an important element in improving the overall health of Indian women. Increasing the use of contraceptives is one way to reduce fertility. While the knowledge of family planning is nearly universal in India, only 36 percent of married women aged 13 to 49 currently use modern contraception (IIPS, 1995). Female sterilization is the main form of contraception; over two-thirds of the married women using contraception have been sterilized. Place of residence, education, and religion are strongly related to both fertility and contraceptive use. More than half of married women with a high school education or above use contraceptives, compared to only one-third of illiterate women. Not surprisingly, the total fertility rates for these two groups are significantly different: 4.0 children for illiterate women compared to 2.2 children for women with a high school education or above. Differentials among the religious groups also are pronounced, e.g., Muslims have the highest total fertility rate and the lowest contraceptive use (IIPS, 1995). Despite a large increase in the number of women using contraceptives and limiting their fertility, there is still unmet need for contraceptives in India.

Nearly 20 percent women who either do not want any more children or want to wait 2 or more years before having another child, but are not currently using contraception, are said to have an unmet need for family planning. The total fertility rate is the number of children a woman could expect to bear in her lifetime given the prevailing age-specific fertility rates of married women in India either want to delay their next birth or have no more children (IIPS, 1995). Most of the unmet need among younger women is for spacing births rather than limiting them. This implies that methods other than female sterilization, the method strongly promoted by India's family planning program, need to be considered. Over 100,000 Indian Women Die Each Year From Pregnancy-Related Causes. Maternal mortality and morbidity are two health concerns that are related to high levels of fertility.

India has a high maternal mortality ratio-approximately 453 deaths per 100,000 births in 1993. This ratio is 57 times the ratio in the United States. The World Health Organization (WHO) and United Nations

Children's Fund (UNICEF) estimate that India's maternal mortality ratio is lower than ratios for Bangladesh and Nepal but higher than those for Pakistan and Sri Lanka (WHO, 1996). The level of maternal mortality varies greatly by state, with Kerala having the lowest ratio (87) and two states (Madhya Pradesh and Orissa) having ratios over 700 (UNICEF, 1995). This differential maternal mortality is most likely related to differences in the socio-economic status of women and access to healthcare services among the states. The high levels of maternal mortality are especially distressing because the majority of these deaths could be prevented if women had adequate health services (either proper prenatal care or referral to appropriate healthcare facilities) (Jejeebhoy and Rao, 1995). In fact, the leading contributor to high maternal mortality ratios in India is lack of access to healthcare (The World Bank, 1996). Few Pregnant Women Receive Prenatal Care. The most recent National Family Health Survey (NFHS) was conducted in 1992-93; it found that in the 4 years preceding the survey, 37 percent of all pregnant women in India received no prenatal care during their pregnancies (IIPS, 1995). The proportion receiving no care varied greatly by educational level and place of residence. Nearly half of illiterate women received no care compared to just 13 percent of literate women. Women in rural areas were much less likely to receive prenatal care than women in urban areas (42 percent and 18 percent, respectively). Most women who did not receive healthcare during pregnancy said they did not because they thought it was unnecessary (IIPS, 1995). Thus, there is a definite need to educate women about the importance of healthcare for ensuring healthy pregnancies and safe childbirths. Another reason for the low levels of prenatal care is lack of adequate healthcare centers. It is currently estimated that 16 percent of the population in rural areas lives more than 10 kilometers away from any medical facility (Bhalla, 1995). Majority of Births in India Take Place at Home. Place of birth and type of assistance during birth have an impact on maternal health and mortality. Births that take place in non-hygienic conditions or births that are not attended by trained medical personnel are more likely to have negative outcomes for both the mother and the child. The NFHS survey found that nearly three-quarters of all births took place at home and two-thirds of all births were not attended by trained medical personnel. While healthcare is important, there are several other factors that influence maternal mortality and health. Medical research shows that early age at first birth and high numbers of total pregnancies take their toll on a woman's health. Although fertility has been declining in India, as noted earlier, many areas of the country still have high levels. In 1993, five states had total fertility rates of over 4 children per woman (India Registrar General (IRG), 1996a). In general, high maternal mortality ratios are related to high fertility rates. One in Five Maternal Deaths Related to Easily Treated Problem Anemia, which can be treated relatively simply and inexpensively with iron tablets, is another factor related to maternal health and mortality. Studies have found that between 50 and 90 percent of all pregnant women in India suffer from anemia. Severe anemia accounts for 20 percent of all maternal deaths in India (The World Bank, 1996). Severe anemia also increases the chance of dying from a hemorrhage during labor. Every 5 minutes, a violent crime against a woman is reported. Research by Heise (1994) has shown that violence against women is a health problem that is often ignored by authorities who view such behavior as beyond their purview. Likewise, many donor agencies do not want to work on this problem as they consider it culturally sensitive. In certain societies, violence, such as wife beating, is perceived as "normal" or as a husband's right. However, as Heise concludes, violence against women is detrimental to economic development because it deprives women of the ability to participate fully in the economy by depleting both their emotional and physical strength. Violence against women also can have negative consequences for the children of the victims. While violence is a serious health issue for Indian women, it is difficult to say how widespread it is because data are limited. The data that are available show an increase in the reported level of violent crime against women. However, such statistics do not reflect the actual levels of these crimes because many incidents, particularly domestic violence, go unreported (Kelkar, 1992). The data that are available show that much of the violence to which women are subjected occurs in the home and/or is carried out by relatives. For instance, the majority of reported rapes are committed by family members. Many of the victims are young women; 30 percent of all reported rapes happened to girls who were age 16 or younger (National Crime Records Bureau (NCRB), 1995). In the past few years, there has been an increase in the reported incidence of torture—cruelty by the husband and the husband's relatives. The reported number of incidents of torture increased 93 percent between 1990 and 1994. The crime rate for torture was 5.9 cases per 100,000 females in 1994. Often women are tortured by other women such as a mother-in-law. The most media-sensationalized type of violence against women in India is dowry death. When a woman marries, her family provides the husband's family with gifts (e.g., clothes, household goods, cash). In many instances, the demand for these gifts does not end with the marriage but continues, as the husband's family persists in making additional dowry demands for years after the wedding. A dowry death is defined as the unnatural death of a woman caused by burns or bodily injury occurring within the first 7 years of marriage, if it can be shown that the woman was subjected to cruelty by her husband or her husband's relatives shortly before death in connection with a demand for dowry (Johnson, 1996; Prasad, 1996). Nearly 5,000 women were reported to have suffered this type of death in 1994, about 1 dowry death for every 100,000 women (NCRB, 1995). The actual number is certainly larger, as there are many deaths that should be reported as a dowry death and are not. While studies have shown that dowry-related violence against women occurs among all sub-groups of the population, the rates are higher among the poor and the lower castes. Alcoholism is also associated with increases in violence against women (Rao and Bloch, 1993). Unfortunately, because many crimes against women are domestic, women have limited recourse. Many women who suffer from domestic violence have little or no education, are not likely to be able to support themselves, and are unlikely to be able to turn to their parents if they leave their husbands because their parents either will not (because of the social stigma) or cannot (because of economics) take them in. Generally, the police have not been helpful to women in domestic violence cases, and there are few community support programs available to these women (Johnson *et al.*, 1996; Kelkar, 1992). Thus, many victims of domestic violence remain in abusive situations. More than half of Indian children are malnourished. Numerous studies indicate that malnutrition is another serious health concern that Indian women face (Chatterjee, 1990; Desai, 1994; The World Bank, 1996). It threatens their survival as well as that of their children. The negative effects of malnutrition among women are compounded by heavy work demands, by poverty, by childbearing and rearing, and by special nutritional needs of women, resulting in increased susceptibility to illness and consequent higher mortality. While malnutrition in India is prevalent among all segments of the population, poor nutrition among women begins in infancy and continues throughout their lifetimes (Chatterjee, 1990; Desai, 1994). Women and girls are typically the last to eat in a family; thus, if there is not enough food they are the ones to suffer most (Horowitz and Kishwar, 1985). According to the NFHS, Indian children have among the highest proportions of malnourishment in the world. More than half (53 percent) of all girls and boys under 4 years of age were malnourished, and a similar proportion (52 percent) were stunted (i.e., too short for their age). Other studies show that many women never achieve full physical development (The World Bank, 1996). This incomplete physical development poses a considerable risk for women by increasing the danger of obstructed deliveries.

Mother's education, according to the NFHS, is highly correlated with the level of malnutrition among children. Children of illiterate mothers are twice as likely to be undernourished or stunted as children whose mothers have completed at least high school. The differentials are even larger when severely undernourished children are considered. Children of illiterate mothers are three times as likely to be severely undernourished as children of mothers with at least a high school education. Nutritional status of children also differs by state. Bihar and Uttar Pradesh have the highest proportion of undernourished children and Kerala has the lowest, consistent with the different levels of socio-economic development in these states.

Several studies have found that one of the reasons for the poor health of Indian women is the discriminatory treatment girls and women receive compared to boys and men (Das Gupta, 1994; Desai, 1994). The most chilling evidence of this is the large number of "missing women" (i.e., girls and women who have apparently died as a result of past and present discrimination). Recent estimates place this number at approximately 35 million (The World Bank, 1996). In other words, there is a deficit of 35 million girls/women who should be part of the population but are not. This deficit of females is due to higher female than male mortality rates for every age group up (IRG, 1996a). Differential treatment of girls and boys in terms of feeding practices and access to healthcare is among the factors responsible for higher female mortality. As a consequence of their lower status overall, women experience discrimination in the allocation of household resources including food and access to health services. Boys are breast-fed longer than girls; 25.3 months *versus* 23.6 months on average (IIPS, 1995). Boys who are ill are more likely to be taken for medical treatment than are girls (Bhalla, 1995; Jejeebhoy and Rao, 1995). Causes of death for children aged 1 to 4 show girls dying at a higher rate than boys from accidents and injuries, fever, and digestive disorders—all causes that are related to living conditions and negligence (Government of India, 1995). As with other indicators of health status, differential treatment of boys and girls varies by state. The infant mortality rate by sex can be used as a proxy for differential treatment. In the vast majority of countries worldwide, males have higher mortality in infancy than do females. Higher female rates are therefore considered likely to signal discrimination against girls. Only 7 of the 15 major states in India have higher male infant mortality. In the remaining states, equal or higher female rates suggest that girls suffer greater neglect.

One of the most extreme manifestations of son preference is sex-selective abortion. The use of medical technology to determine the sex of a fetus is on the rise in India, and over 90 percent of fetuses that are aborted are female (The World Bank, 1996). In all countries, more boys are born than girls, with a sex ratio at birth around 105 boys per 100 girls. Data on hospital births from various parts of India show that sex-selective abortion has increased the sex ratio at birth to 112 boys per 100 girls (Das Gupta, 1994). The HIV/AIDS epidemic in India is spreading rapidly and increasingly will affect women's health in coming years. A recent study estimated that between 2 and 5 million Indians are currently infected with HIV (AIDS Control and Prevention Project of Family Health International *et al.*, 1996). High rates of infection are found in population groups with certain high-risk behaviors (i.e., sex workers, intravenous drug users, and sexually transmitted disease patients). However, infection also is increasing in the general population. For example, HIV sero-prevalence among pregnant women in the state of Tamil Nadu quadrupled between 1989 and 1991 from 0.2 to 0.8 percent (U.S. Bureau of the Census, 1995). The epidemic is fueled by both married and unmarried men visiting sex workers who have high rates of infection. Migrant workers and truck drivers are important components of the spread of HIV. Surveys in some areas show 5 to 10 percent of truck drivers in the country are HIV infected (AIDS Analysis, 1996). Despite the alarming growth of the epidemic, most women in India have very little knowledge of AIDS. The NFHS found that a large majority of Indian women had never heard of AIDS. Even among those who had heard of the disease, there were many misconceptions about modes of transmission.

APPENDIX X

A Norway Study on Women's Health

1. Introduction

We have collected knowledge about women's health and living conditions at the end of a millennium in one of the countries in the world where health and life expectancy are reasonably good. In the course of this century, there have been rapid and dramatic changes in women's education, participation in employment, birth patterns, marriage patterns and gender equality. There are groups of women living in Norway today whose life experience and expectations vary considerably simply because they were born at different times during this era of rapid change.

Women's health in Norway can first and foremost be described in positive terms. Norwegian women live longer than most other women in the world and longer than any male population in the world. Many women in Norway can expect to enjoy good health. Norway offers well-developed health services and fairly good maternity care and conditions for child care. Why then do we need a report on women's health? Some people will say that a special public report on women's health is unnecessary, provided that we ensure the best possible health service for all inhabitants—as well as good facilities for the things that only women are involved with: pregnancy and childbirth.

However, at the same time, women do have a different anatomy and biology from men. Women experience different symptoms than men. Women talk about illness in a different way. Women have less power and influence in society in general and in the health services in particular. Women have some illnesses that men do not suffer from. Many illnesses take on a different character for men and women. Women give birth and still have the main responsibility for caring for the children they bring into the world. Women use the health services in a different way from men and often say that the health services do not take them seriously. And, partly because there are more of them among the elderly in Norway, women also suffer from more chronic illnesses than men.

In some respects, women live rather different lives from men in modern Norway, but there are also great variations between women. Throughout this report, we will, therefore, look at women's health from a comparative gender perspective, while taking care to avoid over-simplified presentations of "the Norwegian Woman."

2. Use of concepts—gender perspective of health and illness

The report starts with a discussion of central concepts and definitions that form the foundation for the work of the Committee. Illness and health are concepts that are defined in many different ways. On the one hand, the Committee has chosen a practical approach, based on the diseases and ailments that are relevant to women's health. On the other hand, the Committee has given importance to showing how the medical profession, institutions and tradition sometimes base descriptions of sickness and health on particular female images—or absence of female images—which has consequences for women's health.

What any individual person experiences as good health is affected both by social conditions and by that individual's history and life situation. Everyone meets health challenges. A central perspective is to uncover and support the individual's resources and ability to cope with health problems.

Gender is biology and as such obviously relevant to the understanding of sickness and health. But gender is also identity (how we see ourselves as men or women), cultural symbols (how we associate certain qualities and expressions with femininity and masculinity) and structure (how the distribution of power, resources, work, etc. are systematically linked with gender). We will show how all of these dimensions of gender increase the understanding of women's health and of how medical science, health services and welfare schemes meet female patients and users.

A recurring theme in many of the sub-sections of the report is the way in which basic knowledge, regulations and practice are often based on an unexpressed male norm. Medical research often excludes women in data collection; welfare benefits are often based on the stable, full-time employee, and occupational health measures focus more often on hazardous substances and loud noise than on heavy lifting and emotional stress in the care section. In this way, the report reveals a general lack of gender-specific knowledge and gender perspective.

The evaluations and recommendations of the Committee are based on certain fundamental value choices. Firstly, health policy must strive for fairness between the sexes on equal terms; women must thus be given equally good treatment and other benefits as men for the same type of complaints. Secondly, special premises must be recognised; good knowledge about and facilities for special women's health complaints or burdens must be obtained, whether these are biologically or socially dependent. Thirdly, definitions of health and disease, preventive measures, treatment and welfare facilities must be evaluated from a gender perspective—so that fundamental premises do not systematically discriminate against women or groups of the population that are predominantly female. Fourthly, a user perspective is probably even more important for women than it is for men, since what little knowledge there is about women's health is not so well integrated in the health services. Fifthly, quality assurance from a gender perspective must not depend on the enthusiasm and efforts of the individual. Knowledge, awareness and institutional practices that ensure that women's health is taken care of must be given active priority and some fixed terms of reference.

3. Women's health from an international perspective

Between 1992 and 1996, six major international conferences were arranged under the auspices of the United Nations. These resulted in increasingly strong support for women's rights in the consensus documents signed by the participating states. The use of the legal system to protect women's health has thus become the object of greater attention in the course of the nineties.

Under the action plan adopted by the UN's Fourth International Women's Conference in Beijing in 1995, the participating governments are committed to ensuring that all policy-making reflects integration of the perspective of gender. This presumes, among other things, that the authorities will carry out a prior evaluation of all decisions, measures and programmes to see what bearing they have on women and men. Norwegian experience contributed to provide pointers for the formulation of this document.

The action plan contains many concrete proposals for what countries have to continue to work on with regard to health issues, aiming particularly at countries where health services are weakly built up or where rights are poorly developed. At a time of major change in population structure and basic values, increasing cultural and religious diversity and a widening gap between the poor and the rich, the action plan is relevant to and important for the work of integrating gender perspective in every country's health policy.

The international debate on women's health focuses particularly on sexual and reproductive health. Reproductive rights are a concretisation of previously adopted human rights in the field of reproductive health and imply the right for a woman to decide herself if and when she wants to have a child and to avoid unwanted sexual relations. This includes the right not to have to endanger her life and health for the sake of reproduction and the right to enjoy the benefits of scientific progress.

The reason why the work on human rights focuses on sexual and reproductive health is that this aspect of women's health is the most strongly politicised, and existing practice is closely linked with norms for sexual behaviour, relationships between the sexes, child upbringing and women's roles. Collaboration between countries and the comparison of experience in different countries have proved useful in dispelling prejudices and myths.

A statistical connection has been found between general prosperity and low fertility. A common denominator for the poor countries is the setting aside of women's own wishes and priorities, either by forcing them to use contraception they do not want or by refusing contraception to women who want it. Pregnancy, childbirth and abortion still represent a risk in the lives of poor women in Asian countries and this is largely due to the fact that the health services have not been able to provide adequate facilities for these women.

Poor countries have poor health and disease statistics and mortality is much easier to measure than morbidity. Data for morbidity is, therefore, far more uncertain than data for mortality. We know enough, however, to be able to say that there are three prominent areas where there are major differences between women and men. These are sexual and reproductive health, infections and nutrition.

The health of women in poor countries shows the same sickness patterns today as were seen in Norway a hundred years ago, when reproduction, infections and deficiency diseases constituted a serious risk to women's life and health. Recent years have brought an increasing recognition of how women are subjected to health risks, for biological, social, cultural and not least financial reasons. Yet it seems as if the situation may be getting worse and worse. The feminisation of poverty, i.e. the fact that an increasing proportion of the world's poor are women, is a very serious matter in view of how this affects health. Finding out how quality can be maintained in the health service with the tight economic frameworks that exist in many countries also presents a major challenge.

Norway has to follow-up the commitments that are inherent in the Beijing action plan, both nationally and internationally, and cooperate actively with international organisations and voluntary organisations in order to achieve the objectives set out in the plan.

The lives of European women have changed a great deal in the past thirty years. There are still differences in living conditions between women and men both in and between the EU countries. The differences are least noticeable in basic health issues and education, but are clearer when it comes to distribution of income and economic and political representation. By and large, European women enjoy good health, but there are a number of health challenges linked with lifestyle factors and living conditions which give grounds for concern. The ever-increasing proportion of elderly has a predominant share of women, and the health of older women is in focus. The general picture for morbidity and mortality agrees to a large extent with what we find in Norway, although there are variations between the countries. Chapter 4 also contains a general presentation of Norwegian women's health.

The action plan from the Beijing conference underlined the need for knowledge about interaction between the sexes, about economic and social processes and about women's health in different cultures and situations. The acquisition of a minimum of relevant, research-based knowledge about women's health will require gender-specific data about living conditions, burden of disease and access to services at the national level.

Many of the instruments that are used to rank countries with reference to social and economic indicators are not able to pick up factors that are significant to women's health. The pictures of the situation that are created in this way are altered when data collection focuses on gender differences and women's lives. The fact that the picture becomes altered when gender-sensitive measuring instruments are used, reveals a definite need to make a critical evaluation of frequently applied health targets from a gender perspective.

4. Changes in women's lives—illnesses and living conditions

It is difficult to understand major health issues without taking living conditions into consideration. One important way of looking at this question is how living conditions create different bases for individuals to find meaning and coherence in their lives and a chance to influence and control their own lives. The living conditions of women in Norway vary considerably, not only because they have grown up at different times in a century characterised by rapid change, but also because there are marked differences today in women's education, workplace and income, cultural background, family situation, social network and place of residence. We know a great deal about how women live in Norway. In order to link this up with their state of health, however, we have had to piece together many fragments of knowledge. We lack links between the understanding of health and the understanding of living conditions and these relationships have been very poorly elucidated from a gender perspective.

During the post-war period there has been important changes in circumstances for women as regards birth patterns and marriage, equal opportunity policy and education, with particular emphasis on participation in employment and occupational health. Most women in Norway have greater rights to manage their own affairs and greater opportunities than ever before. At the same time, large groups struggle with badly paid and strenuous work, often in combination with extensive, unpaid carer responsibilities. On the one hand, there is a noticeable gender split in the labour market, while, on the other hand, knowledge, regulations and occupational health measures are characteristically based on male workers and workplaces where men are in the majority. There is an urgent need for new knowledge and gender perspective in this field.

An important question is whether the increased participation of women in a number of arenas is beneficial or detrimental to their health. One Norwegian study shows a positive relationship between important goals for health and participation in marriage, motherhood and employment. Married women with children and a full-time job have the fewest health problems. This is probably due both to the fact that participation has a favourable effect on health (causal relationship) and to the fact that selection takes place, i.e. it is the women with good health who manage to participate. These are tendencies which are based on major statistics. The exceptions are important. For most women paid work is a good thing; for some the workplace is detrimental to health. For many, having a family is beneficial to health; for some, where abuse is involved, marriage is a direct hazard to health.

Women's participation in employment depends more than men's on good welfare schemes: nursery school places, right to leave of absence and public care for close relatives. Many women's jobs represent health hazards due to strenuous work, low pay and subordinate positions. These will be very important policy areas in the prevention of women's health disorders. At the same time, it is vital to health that also those who are not covered by the system are guaranteed a life that is worth living.

5. Femininity—healthy or dangerous

The report describes some important ways in which femininity is understood and formed in Norway today. This leads on to a discussion of what is potentially good and what is potentially bad for health in different arenas in women's lives: in private relationships (family, lover, friends, children), in relation to their own bodies, food, alcohol, drugs and leisure time. Three important dimensions in many women's lives are given focus:

- Orientation towards relations: Girls are taught to a greater extent than boys to be attentive and caring towards other people and to understand themselves in relation to other people. Health benefits can be found in good close relationships and networks; health hazards in ignoring one's own limits and needs.
- Self-reflection: Research in a number of different areas describes women as having a greater tendency than men to understand events and situations in the light of their own actions and abilities—reactions are turned inward rather than outward to external circumstances. This tendency can increase their possibility of coping, but can also lead to a strong feeling of guilt when something goes wrong.
- Beauty and aesthetics are important projects for many women, and these aspects of femininity are given enormous attention in our culture. Great health benefits lie inherent in caring for oneself and looking after one's appearance. However, excessive focus on physical appearance can lead to self-contempt, exaggerated slimming and exercise, eating disorders and risky surgery.

Women still take the main responsibility at home, both as regards caregiving and housework. Women with children also have a greater responsibility for bridging the gap between private and public spheres: making sure that the tasks and functions of private life are organised so that family members get to nursery school, school or work at the right time, reasonably clean, fed and rested. This requires effort and coordination. Always keeping an eye on other people's needs and time schedules can lead to a state of physical readiness which, without adequate rest and recreation, will represent a threat to health, particularly as regards chronic pain and other stress symptoms.

Women's diets are generally good and somewhat healthier than men's, but they vary according to their socio-economic status and lifestyle. At the same time, both obesity and eating disorders are growing health problems which have to be understood in the light of both lifestyle and women's self-image. The prevalence of eating disorders in our cultural circle reflects general attitudes to the body and to food and, in view of its strongly gendered nature, can be interpreted as a statement about the conditions for girls' and women's socialisation. Eating disorders are most prevalent in environments where there is a strong emphasis on body aesthetics and coping. Greater expertise is needed in the primary health service.

The use of alcohol among women increased from 1970 until the eighties, but is still lower than among men. The same pattern largely applies to the use of drugs. Many women with an alcohol or drug problem have a difficult family situation, weak relationships to girlfriends and their mothers and have experienced being abused. In women, problems involving substance misuse often develop more quickly than in men, both physiologically and socially. At the same time, women put-off treatment longer, both because they may feel more ashamed and because they are afraid of attracting the attention of the child welfare service. We need more women-oriented treatment measures, measures which can identify clients at an early stage and base treatment on knowledge about and adaptation to women's lives.

One worrying aspect of women's health behaviour is the fact that women now smoke as much as men and smoking among young girls is on the increase. While it was women with a high education, position and power who broke the female norm of not smoking earlier this century, the majority of smokers is now to be found among disadvantaged women. The most important motivation for starting to smoke is friends' and parents' smoking habits, low educational ambition and regarding oneself as a loser at school. For girls, preoccupation with weight and body image is also important. A general improvement in the school environment and the possibility of pupil influence can be more effective than special anti-smoking measures among young people. In spite of extensive research into smoking behaviour, there has been little study of gender differences. More attention should be given to women's fear of putting on weight and psycho-social factors such as stress and a poor network.

Exercise is extremely important in the prevention of health problems and half an hour's brisk walk each day is enough to gain most of the health benefit. Women are less competitive than men. They do not find sport so entertaining, but they exercise more for the sake of their health and to lose weight. Among parents of small children, there are far more women than men who stop taking regular exercise, and neither organised sport nor commercial health studios seem to have facilities that appeal to mature women or to mothers and families along with children. A major health gain could be achieved by developing facilities for women at different stages of their lives.

Many women experience mental strain or problems in their lives. Sufficient allowance is not made in psychiatry and psychology in Norway for gender differences in mental health, either in the understanding of how problems arise or in their treatment. In some counties, more than three-quarters of the persons receiving medication for mental problems are women, and no fundamental questions have been raised about why or whether this should be the case. It is necessary to develop better services and to strengthen the primary health service's gender-specific knowledge about mental health.

Violence and fear of violence constitute a serious threat to many women's health. Men are exposed to violence outside the home and most often as isolated incidents. Women are injured at home and the abuser is usually known to them. This chapter describes women's fear of and vulnerability to outdoor violence, battering, rape and child abuse. The women's movement and women's shelters have put domestic violence on the agenda since the seventies. Statistics vary and are, understandably, unreliable, but the problem is an extensive one and the consequences are serious. The Committee finds reason to point out in particular the lack of expertise in and cooperation between the health service, the judicial system and the child welfare service.

6. Many women's lives—different health conditions

Some groups face enormous challenges when it comes to health and the opportunity to participate in important social arenas. We have chosen to throw light on health challenges faced by immigrant women, disabled women, especially vulnerable single mothers and older women. Of course, many of these women manage remarkably well and are in good health, but here the focus in on challenges and problems.

Many immigrant women meet a very alien culture, find themselves cut-off from their accustomed social set-up and still have the main responsibility for looking after the close relationships in their own families. Some have been the victims of abuse and torture in their home countries. Language problems can be aggravated by illness and life crises. Understanding the health of immigrants represents a major challenge for Norwegian healthcare workers.

As members of a minority, Sami women will also face challenges. We know very little about how cultural challenges affect Sami women's general state of health. There are huge gaps when it comes to systematic knowledge about Sami women's health and circumstances of life, and it is necessary to bring this knowledge to light with the help of the Sami women and their organisations.

Women who live with a disability often find that they are the losers on many fronts. Women are poorer than men and disabled women find that they both have limited access to resources and limited access to facilitation for participation in society.

Single mothers who have given birth at a young age, who have a low standard of education, weak ties with the labour market and little contact with the child(ren)'s father, are in particular danger of finding themselves in financial trouble, of being disregarded for a long time by the labour market and wearing themselves out because they have been left alone with carer responsibilities. Many of them feel distaste at being dependent on benefits from the social welfare service. This kind of situation entails a health risk for both mother and children.

The fact that women live for a long time means that Norway has a large number of elderly women. Age often brings with it chronic suffering, pain and functional impairment. Many older women are, moreover, single and receive too small a share of the benefits of the welfare state.

7. Reproductive health

Compared with the international situation, Norwegian women enjoy good reproductive health. Maternal mortality has virtually been eliminated now and infant mortality which was just over 150 per 1000 births around 1860, is now almost the lowest in the world. We are a little concerned today about the low birth rate in relation to the ageing population. However, reproductive health is an important positive health concept which embraces relational components (sexuality), birth, pregnancy, abortion, contraception, as well as sexually-transmitted infections, cancer and infertility.

The age of women giving birth for the first time has become steadily higher during the past decade. More are stopping after one child, but at the same time we are seeing an increase in third child births. Postponing giving birth means that many of today's young women will have small children far into their forties, unlike the generations immediately before them.

There is no doubt that better education, higher status for women and a greater degree of self-determination in a health context, including the possibility for women to manage on their own, increases freedom of choice with regard to reproduction. This applies to the possibility of refusing unsafe sex and having the financial and personal ability to obtain the necessary health service, including family planning or abortion if this is necessary or desirable.

However, we must not forget that the role of childbearer is only one of the dimensions of being a woman. Reproductive health is not just about women. Men's need to reproduce the distribution of power between women and men in different cultures and men's sexual behaviour are also part of determining reproduction and the role of women in relation to this. It is important to bring men's responsibility into all aspects of reproductive health. It is particularly important to raise awareness of the fact that consideration for women's reproductive health is stressed, not because it benefits children and men or because women administer most of the carer values, but because women and men are equal citizens in society.

In Norway, a woman's right to make decisions concerning her own body is a major, guiding principle, made visible through the Abortion on

Demand Act, good access to contraception, right to free health services during pregnancy and childbirth, and the limited possibility to implement control measures against expectant mothers. A feature found in girls who do not protect themselves against either infection or conception is that they claim to have problems enjoying their own sexuality. These girls drink alcohol more often prior to sexual intercourse which is in turn directly connected with not using contraception. In this light, it is important to encourage young girls to get to know and accept their own sexual and emotional needs. This includes access to good information and individual guidance. Support must be given to attempts to increase the availability of contraception to young sexually active women and men in Norway. Nonetheless, it is important that the safety of using contraceptives is continuously subjected to quality evaluations.

Maternity care and health services in connection with childbirth are generally good in Norway, but nevertheless face important challenges. Health services in the field of reproductive health must not be incomprehensible transfers of technology from experts to users, where a woman's body becomes the object of interventions she does not understand, possibly with side-effects she experiences but is unable to communicate. The educational element in primary health information is important with regard to giving women room for control and understanding of the factors that influence their own health. There are strong indications that such aspects are best looked after in programmes where women take part in planning, policy formulation and practical healthcare at all levels. Even in Norway, women doctors and midwives show better following up of women in maternity care.

Internationally, the tendency is now to look critically at the content of routine medical check-ups of expectant mothers and to reduce the number of recommended check-ups. The reason for this is that frequent check-ups of expectant mothers are unlikely to increase the health gain; the danger of over-medicalisation may be greater. All in all, we can say that the routines and organisation of the health services for expectant mothers in particular are the subject of continuous discussion with the users, and changes are taking place. At the same time, we see an ever-decreasing tolerance regarding unforeseen complications and law suits in the wake of deaths and births of sick children which in turn scares the staff into increasing routine monitoring, intervention and technology—in spite of the fact that the level of medical expertise in the field of obstetrics is already very high. A dilemma may arise between the quality of care in maternity care and the increasing number of technological investments and this must be discussed continuously and in collaboration with the users.

The Committee believes that efforts should be made to ensure that the perspective of user and layman is always taken into account in reaching decisions concerning women's reproductive health in administrative and top level medical contexts. Further work should be done to structure and try out different forms of user participation—including laymen conferences—in various contexts where women's reproductive health is the subject.

8. Illnesses

We have devoted a large part to reviewing what we know about women and illness. Here, we have entered the world of medicine and asked experts to give a general outline of gender differences in diseases. Female and male biology differ quite considerably in fundamental areas and this can have major effects on how pathogenic factors work at both cell level and in the body as a whole. We have attached particular importance to diseases that almost exclusively affect women, or affect women more often or earlier than men (examples are anorexia, osteoporosis, rheumatoid arthritis and breast cancer), diseases that affect both sexes, but where the prevalence, course, outcome or consequences are different for men and women (heart disease, diabetes and the consequences of violence) and the diseases that statistically affect many women, although they also affect many men (lung cancer and other forms of cancer, serious mental illnesses). We have also attached importance to conditions which society regards as problematic (depression and anxiety, chronic musculo-skeletal disorders and pain).

The main conclusion is that there is reason for concern about some features of the development of illness in women. The increase in lung cancer is one such feature; the relatively bad prognosis for breast cancer is another. Women in Norway top the European statistics for bone fractures, and many women are either not treated, or else treated only with medication, for mental disorders. Research into illness in women must take into account new understanding of women's biology and at the same time integrate to a greater extent knowledge about women as individuals in society. There is a great need for more basic research into gender differences in the prevalence of disease and the courses diseases take. We have an acute need to set-up good core communities in all the medical faculties which can be the prime movers in getting this type of research started. We also believe that clearer directions should be given to bodies that allocate money to research to include gender differences as an significant dimension in all research projects relating to health.

9. Gender perspective of health service facilities and their use

One main issue is whether men and women have equal access to good health services and to what degree health services are able to meet women's needs when it comes to investigating, treating and coping with health problems. The user's sex may possibly have significance for:

- how the user perceives and interprets body signals,
- how the user evaluates the need to go to the health services, how the user presents problems and needs when he/she goes to the health service, and

- how the user is interpreted, investigated, diagnosed, referred, treated or given advice and guidance.

Two things stand out very clearly in descriptions of women's use of the health services. In the first place, women have more contact with the health service than men. In the second place, women's meetings with the health service are often described as problematic, full of conflict or not very constructive. In this chapter, we will therefore, give a quantitative description of women's contacts with the different sections of the health service, compared with men's. This is followed by a description of different aspects of women's "problematic or conflict-filled meetings." Finally, we outline and discuss some examples of and criteria for what women regard as good services and meetings.

Women's more frequent contact with the health service applies in the first instance to consultations with general medical doctors, in old people's homes and rehabilitation institutions. If we look at consultations in hospitals' out-patient departments, the gender difference is almost eliminated and the same applies to admission to hospital, if we exclude admission due to childbirth and pregnancy.

About 60% of patients contacts in general practice are women. Consultations concerning women's reproductive functions explain some of this over-representation. The hypothesis that women have a lower threshold for visiting the doctor has not been confirmed. Most women have few visits to the doctor each year, while a small minority have many. This small group of women (5-8%), who report more than eleven contacts with the doctor each year, probably includes a large number of pregnant women, but also many women whose problems are difficult to study closely and help—because the doctor does not find out what is wrong with them. This group may also include women with chronic diseases who need close, special monitoring.

The same type of treatment has been found to give different results in women and men, but the availability of various forms of treatment has also been found to differ, as regards both gender and class. Since advanced surgical, medical or other specialised treatment is initiated or takes place in hospital, the most important thing here is probably more thorough studies of treatment results. Developing and applying gender-specific knowledge about treatment is a major challenge, in addition to looking more closely at differences in availability of different forms of treatment—in both the general and the specialist health services.

Many of the chronic and complex ailments that groups of older women suffer from have a low status in the hierarchy of diseases. This applies to musculo-skeletal disorders, mental disorders and geriatric complaints. In these fields it is difficult both to recruit specialists and to obtain enough of other types of resources. Many individual women and groups of women (as well as men) probably have an "under-consumption" of health services. This is a problem that requires its own strategies and solutions.

In other words, the needs of men and women for health services and the availability of these services should be defined and investigated more closely in the light of health status, preferences and documented effect of the treatment given. Women live longer than men, but a longer life is associated with greater lifetime risks of functional disabilities and chronic disease, including cancer, cardiovascular disease and dementia, and a greater need for long-term care.

In the case of the non-specific complaints and chronic pain—which strike women more often than men—it is difficult for the health service to offer good facilities. In this chapter, we look more closely at how women are met by the health service when they complain of indeterminate chronic ailments, mental disorders and injuries from abuse. For all of these groups, the following has been revealed:

- low prestige within the medical community,
- poorly developed and badly integrated research-based knowledge,
- too little expertise among general doctors—with subsequent inadequate identification of the problem, help and referral,
- communication with and interpretation of the women characterised misconceptions and prejudices,
- conflict in relation to the traditional ideal that the doctor will 'sort things out': make a diagnosis and prescribe treatment,
- inability to understand complaints in the light of the individual woman's life situation, resources and ability to cope, and
- too little capacity and expertise in the specialist health services.

The women concerned constitute a minority of all women who make use of the health services in Norway, but they are women with serious, long-term ailments. They challenge and make heavy demands on resources, and they often find they get little help. These are good reasons for investigating and developing new approaches.

The Committee would like to suggest two particular approaches to alternative forms of treatment. The first is for general medical doctors and other healthcare workers to develop and acquire communication techniques which allow them to identify and make use of an individual woman's own health resources and ability to cope. The second is to organise treatment as a holistic service for specific groups of patients, rather than various specialists dealing with isolated symptoms, organs or functions. This is particularly relevant for women with a combination of complaints and problems, and good experience has been gained from a number of inter-disciplinary resource centres.

Continuity of contact is an important part of the service for women. We are looking forward to more women being able to anchor their health services with one regular doctor, but we also point out certain problems with regard to how this regular doctor scheme is to be organised.

10. Women and welfare benefits

The intention of the National Insurance Act is to safeguard us, among other things, against loss of income or major expenses incurred through illness. Through the social security and welfare schemes, a distribution—and a redistribution—takes place. The very purpose of some of the social security schemes is to distribute funds from the healthy to the sick or to persons with impaired health. Special attention is therefore, given to benefits aiming to safeguard income in the event of illness. The distribution systems also have an effect on gender relations in the labour market, in the family and elsewhere. For example, the scope of rights during pregnancy and childbirth and services linked with child care will affect women's participation in employment and how employers regard women as employees.

A number of schemes are described as formally gender-neutral—in ways which systematically place women in a poorer position. The National Insurance Act is a so-called gender-neutral Act. The requirement of being employed means that working women have the same possibilities as men to earn rights, but no consideration is given to the fact that the actual possibilities of taking paid work have been and still are different for women and men—and this is due to a large degree to women's unpaid work. At least until 1992, the work of caring for others was not rewarded in the same way with pension points or additional pension rights. Equal rights or formal gender equality thus gives women less than they are entitled to.

Many welfare state researchers have been concerned about the way in which the welfare state contributes to freeing paid employees from dependency on the market—at least from the worst effects of the market, by providing support during unemployment or sickness. In the case of women, it is important that this liberation also includes liberation from dependency on marriage or being supported. In other words, the welfare state becomes a safety net for women so that they can choose whether to marry or not (to remain married or not), regardless of their financial situation. This can be achieved by adopting two strategies: by building up schemes which provide support for women who have the sole responsibility for children or by making it possible for women to participate in the labour market on an equal footing with men.

Social security benefits were originally introduced to give men compensation for loss of income resulting from unemployment, illness, disability, occupational injury, etc. The benefits that were developed for women were based on loss of support and provided compensation for loss of a family supporter or for lack of support. Now many women are employed themselves. We also have a far larger variety of forms of family than we used to; couple relationships are less stable; the number of households with one adult has grown, and women are less dependent on men as family supporters. Family status is still an important requirement for a number of benefits and many new problems have cropped up.

The work approach in welfare policy means that instruments and welfare schemes are formulated individually and collectively to promote the government's aim of employment for everyone. The benefit schemes are intended to motivate people to work. The goal of high employment also includes people who are poorly qualified to compete on the labour market, but it is also based on the existence of good welfare schemes for individuals to fall back on if they can no longer work for health-related or other reasons. The work approach leads to a major dilemma in welfare policy. On the one hand, social security benefits are intended as a safety net for people who lose their income from employment, but they must be designed to ensure that employment is the first choice.

The work approach has had tremendous influence on the forming of our welfare benefits since it was introduced. However, little consideration has been given to it as a problem with regard to whether it will have a different effect for women and men. In the first place, women who have few ties with the workplace and a low education may find it more difficult to return to work or to retrain for employment. In the second place, all jobs will not necessarily lead to self-respect, integration and financial independence. Many workplaces for women pay badly, have poor working conditions and provide little right for self-determination.

If the work approach is to have the desired effect, it is also very important that all parts of it function. The fact that a number of women have had their claims for a disability pension refused and have been referred to the social welfare office or private support shows that the work approach does not work as intended. They have not been returned to work and they have not been granted social security. If the work approach is to succeed, these women must be given a concrete offer of training, qualifying or suitable work. If such work is not available and there are no opportunities for them, then social security must be an alternative for these women as it is for other people.

Social security rights depend on the definition of the concept of illness in the regulations and in social security service practice. The tightening up at the beginning of the nineties led to criticism of the concept of illness as practised under the national insurance scheme, because the tightening-up had a limiting effect on women's rights in particular. In the main, the national insurance scheme's concept of illness is defined in accordance with the way "medical science and practice formulate the term illness at any given time and the practice that has developed in this area." Specific requirements are often made of the illness with regard to diagnosis, type of symptoms or consequences. When women's illnesses are given less priority than typical men's illnesses, this may be reflected in who is entitled to social security benefits and the understanding one is met within the social security system. The Committee therefore, questions whether the current concept of illness is suitable as the basis for assessing social security rights, and proposes that more weight should instead be given to assessing the individual applicant's functional ability in relation to the work tasks involved.

The Committee would also point out that the work approach must be implemented from a user perspective, focusing on the user's needs and including them in the process of creating participation or motivation.

11. Measures

The report reveals a lack of knowledge, in some cases a serious lack of knowledge, especially when it comes to giving a gender perspective to existing fields of research. At the same time each subject treated in this report shows that we possess sufficient knowledge to initiate measures to prevent women's health problems, to improve treatment and other benefits and to strengthen the ability to cope and to improve quality of life. It is, therefore, communication and integration of knowledge that is lacking.

Several specific measures thus aim to create structures, routines and tools that can ensure the integration of gender perspectives in research and other acquisition of knowledge, in policy-making, preventive work, health services and welfare schemes. Both user perspectives and inter-disciplinary teamwork play a central role.

The Committee was given very wide terms of reference. We have given priority to developing overriding perspectives, and measures which can open the way for the application of these perspectives in healthcare policy and practice. There are a number of fields where it has not been possible for us to give details of the measures in more concrete form. The measures are arranged under the following headings: decision-making processes, development and distribution of knowledge, healthcare practice, violence and abuse, welfare schemes and the workplace, other measures and general equality between the sexes.

Decision-making processes

- Develop criteria for the documentation of gender perspective in research, production of statistics and investigations.
- Review indicators and sets of questions in health-related statistics and decision-making systems, with regard to whether they identify gender differences and aspects of women's lives.
- Ensure that persons with expertise about women and gender perspectives are heard or involved in relevant planning and decision-making processes.
- Hold open hearings or laymen conferences in health policy investigations and decision-making processes.
- Organisations which receive grants from public funds should be encouraged to ensure that the gender perspective is taken into account in deciding priorities and work and that tools and guidance routines are developed to help the organisations in this work.

Development and distribution of knowledge

- Establish separate subject areas for women's health and illness at the medical faculties, initially with three new professorships and a network secretariat.
- Make it a requirement for Norwegian research that women are included in clinical studies unless there is a convincing reason for excluding them.
- The gender perspective of health must be taken into account in medical, healthcare and social welfare education. Here the new subject areas at the medical faculties and the project for development of criteria to document gender perspectives (see above) will have a particular responsibility.
- Establish a debate forum to ensure distribution and discussion of knowledge between different groups of specialists and between clinicians and research scientists with regard to the most important women's health challenges.

Specific needs for information

- Knowledge about gender differences in the prevalence of disease, course of diseases and biological differences which can explain gender differences in health. The Committee proposes that NOK 50 million be granted to the Research Council of Norway over a five-year period for such purposes.
- Research with a gender perspective into the side effects of the use of medication, with particular focus on elderly people.
- Studies based on samples which follow patients through the treatment system, and a special evaluation of when women benefit from a different treatment than men.
- The Committee recommends research and development programmes in which geriatric specialists in hospitals and in local primary health services co-operate with a view to spreading mutual expertise, evaluating treatment programmes and developing models for co-operation.
- Systematic review of gender-specific lack of knowledge in the fields of social security and social welfare. Support for research should require that the gender perspective is taken into account.
- The initiation of a three-year research and investigation programme to work on living conditions, health and equal status issues for women with functional disabilities. The prevalence of abuse, possibilities of preventing and surveying abuse and the way government departments deal with abuse must be included.
- There is a need for systematic accumulation of knowledge about both Sami and immigrant women's health and illnesses, and conditions of life related to these.

- An investigation into how understanding of cultural differences can be integrated in education and continuing education of healthcare workers.
- An independent evaluation should be made of breast cancer screening for all women between the ages of 50 and 69. Norway should take part in the international survey of the effect of screening of women between 40 and 50 years of age. The mental strain of incorrect diagnoses must be included in the survey.
- There is a great need for knowledge about occupational health and work environments which take gender differences into consideration.

Healthcare practice

- It is important in the case of persons with chronic or complex complaints that the local authorities are empowered to obtain a list of the people concerned, that responsibility is allocated clearly, and that holistic, inter-disciplinary services are developed for a number of groups.
- In mental healthcare, gender-specific expertise and facilities must be improved, and the facilities made more easily accessible.
- Expansion and development of inter-disciplinary and holistic resource and treatment centres for a number of different groups of patients.
- Immigrants must be recruited as healthcare workers, and the approval of education taken in other countries must be carried out efficiently and rationally.
- Initiation of a national action plan to combat osteoporosis and bone fractures.
- All women must have the same access to good health services for the treatment of breast cancer.
- The Committee recommends that the question of freezing eggs from women who are receiving treatment that can impair their fertility be looked into and reassessed with a view to amending the law.
- Gender-specific measures should be developed and tried out to prevent smoking. Tighter control of tobacco sales to young people is needed.
- Woman-oriented treatment facilities for women with alcohol/drug problems must be further developed, measures both for early intervention and for more advanced addicts.
- Co-operation models for secondary suicide prevention work should be evaluated from a gender perspective and expanded on a national basis.

- Keep-fit facilities must be adapted to the different stages of a woman's life and family situation. Physical activity that is recommended for women must be based on research and projects in which women themselves are participants.

Violence and abuse

The Committee regards violence and abuse of women and children as a major health problem for women and proposes a long list of measures in a variety of fields and at a variety of levels. Among the most important, we can mention:

- The Committee proposes that a committee be set-up to bring violence against women to light, collect knowledge and propose measures to combat violence against women. A holistic perspective of this kind will make it possible to build up more effective ways of protecting women against violence, in which the health service, police, voluntary organisations and legal expertise are represented. Measures to prevent violence against women should be wide-ranging both in the definition of this type of violence and in the use of measures and priority areas. Work to prevent violence and abuse in the home, prevention of rape, work to combat prostitution and efforts to prevent sexual harassment are all areas of work in areas which should come under the definition of violence against women.
- The financial situation and organisation of women's shelters must be improved. Closer forms of co-operation with the social welfare services, housing support and employment support authorities, etc. should be considered.
- Consideration should be given to how women's shelters and co-operating institutions can improve the help available to women with a different ethnic background.
- Healthcare workers and others who encounter victims of violence and abuse in the course of their work must be given systematic training.
- The help available to and research into men who commit abuse must be expanded. Consideration must be given to more serious or long-term sanctions for repetitive abusers.
- The facilities for taking care of victims of violence and abuse must be expanded and quality-assured.
- Follow-up in police investigations and the legal apparatus must be quality-assured and co-ordinated with the child welfare service and treatment facilities.
- The advertising industry must be called on to draw up ethical standards for sexualisation, particularly of children and young people, on the pattern of those drawn up by the press.
- A general confidence-building programme should be developed for girls of school age.

Welfare schemes and the workplace

- Knowledge about women and health must be integrated throughout the national insurance service and in particular among consultant physicians and chief medical officers. A suitable tool should be prepared for executive officers and decision-makers. Advisers with expertise in social security medicine, women's health and gender perspective should be appointed and given responsibility for training and liaison work.
- The consequences of proposals for changes, planning and budgeting work and priorities must be studied from a gender perspective.
- A model for the organisation of the employment services, national insurance service and social welfare office as one unit should be tried out to achieve the objective of co-operation and facilitation based on a holistic consideration of the user's needs. The users must be involved to a greater degree in the decision-making process.
- More importance must be attached to the function and situation of applicants for social security in relation to medical diagnoses. The question of who is to make these assessments must be investigated.
- A more general condition for illness should be introduced which does not discriminate against strain injuries in the assessment of entitlement to occupational injury compensation.
- Gender-specific knowledge about occupational health and work environment must form the basis for monitoring systems, formulation of health, safety and environment tasks and planning and organisation of work.
- There is a particular need to focus on the nursing and care sector, and to develop internal control systems that are suitable for these professions.
- The introduction of occupational health services for the nursing and care sector must be considered without delay. Expertise, tasks and responsibilities must be formulated to meet the challenges, burdens and needs that are typical for the sector, with the emphasis on prevention and rehabilitation.
- No illness should by definition be excluded from acceptance as an occupational illness. This proposal requires an amendment in legislation.
- The Committee requests that the gender perspective be taken into account in the ongoing investigation into the possibility of equating certain strain injuries with occupational injuries.

General equality between the sexes

The Committee believes that, to be successful, the work on women's health and health services must be anchored, in terms of values, in equal status and at the same time give recognition to differences and equality both between women and men and between different women.

12. Economic and administrative consequences

The Committee was asked to propose measures and offer recommendations for how input and activities should be given priority and co-ordinated in services, in health, safety and environment measures and in research, in order to improve women's health and assure the quality of preventive work, treatment and rehabilitation.

One of the main prerequisites for being able to achieve quality improvements is the inclusion of the gender perspective in the generation of knowledge, in decision-making processes and in practice by making it relevant and ensuring that this perspective is applied to practical work at all levels. The responsibility for initiating processes to integrate gender perspective and make the people who are to administer this at local level responsible must be placed centrally in health and social welfare administration and in the field of research and education. The responsibility for following the process must also be placed here and resources must be allocated for this purpose.

If the chosen angle of approach emphasises administrative consequences, this will—in the case of some of the proposals—entail an evaluation of how they should be researched or how work should be done in a different way. Local limits and assumptions will determine to what extent this will lead to administrative consequences. If the emphasis is on economic consequences, it will be possible to integrate a number of the proposals in ongoing processes, for example, state-initiated and funded action plans, programmes and reform processes which are already underway or are being planned and which will have to be evaluated with a view to taking the gender perspective into account. Costs and resource requirements will have to be considered in relation to the content of the plans, programmes and processes and the possibility of altering priorities within the existing resource limits. When measures cannot be integrated in ongoing plans and processes, the consequences in terms of cost may take on other proportions. This will have to be evaluated for each individual measure.

Several of the measures indicate placing the administrative responsibility for initiation and follow-up with underlying government departments and institutions, particularly under the Ministry of Health and Social Affairs, but also under the Ministry of Education, Research and Church Affairs, the Ministry of Local and Regional Government, the Ministry of Justice and the Ministry of Children and Family Affairs. Inter-departmental teamwork will be essential.

The Committee gives priority to measures in six 'main areas'. These are the areas where there seems to be the greatest need for input. These areas are described as decision-making processes, accumulation and communication of knowledge, health practice, violence and sexual abuse, social welfare schemes and the workplace, and gender equality policy.

Measures entailing special costs are the establishment of subject areas for women's health at the universities and grants for research, including NOK 50 million over a five-year period to the Research Council of Norway. (*The Scientist* 15[15]:20, Jul. 23, 2001)

Appendix XI

AYURVEDIC POINT OF VIEW OF HEALTH AND DISEASES IN WOMEN

As has been repeatedly mentioned, any imbalance in the three doshas leads to ailments—at least 80 specific types in case of imbalanced vata, 40 for an imbalanced pitta and another 20 in case of kapha being out of balance. The following chart will give some indications of the problems that one is likely to face in each case:

Vata Ailments	*Pitta Ailments*	*Kapha Ailments*
Pain in the feet	Burning	Anorexia nervosa
Stiffness of the ankle	Acid excreation	Drowsiness
Cramps in the calf	Burning sensation in the chest	Lack of sleep
Sciatica	Burning sensation in the body	Heaviness of the body
Paraplegia	Foul odour of the body	Excess mucus production
Rectal prolapse	Urticaria	Indigestion
Stiffness of the back	Genital herpes	Mucus in the throat
Chest pain	Jaundice	Atheroscleroses or narrowing of the arteries
Gripping abnormal pain	Excessive Thirst	Goiter
Stiff neck	Pharyngitis	Obesity
Toothache	Conjunctivitis	
Cataract	Inflammation of the penis	
Headache	Skin warts	
Dandruff		
Facial paralysis		
Monoplegia		
Violent muscular convulsion		
Giddiness		
Hiccup		
Weakness		
Mental instability		

Women's monthly dread

Many women dread each menstrual period, because they experience pain, flooding and/or poor cycle timing. In many instances they have suffered from these conditions since the time of puberty. A large number of them believe this is a pattern they must put up with throughout their life. This is not the truth because the "dreaded" monthly cycle can be altered and the feeling of fear for the coming cycle can change to one of indifference, after learning how to control the situation.

Discomfort and pain generally starts early in life, with many women, and continues on in one form or another until late in life. This, as we've said, need not be. A young girl that has been fed properly and has lived in a healthy environment with emphasis on exercise, fresh air and sunshine can generally go through life without the discomforts so many suffer. Some of the problems (menstrual suffering) come from the lack of hormone and estrogen balance in the body, and this is often because of poor diet habits, especially the use of processed and overcooked foods. Fruits, vegetables, grains, nuts and seeds in their "wholesome" state carry with them the values (minerals, etc.) brought out of the earth during the growth period as nature intended! They and especially the grains, provide the hormones and estrogens needed throughout a person's life span. When these foods are processed, many of the needed substances and minerals are discarded, or lost. When such foods are eaten in their natural state the vitamins, minerals, hormones and estrogens, etc., are easily assimilated. When one eats good "wholesome" food, the reproductive organs can be kept in a good healthy condition, barring accident of course. Take the automobile, for example--the right kind of fuel, oil and care keeps the car running a long period of time with ease, barring accidents. Without the proper "fuel" and care from the beginning, a girl will be suffering malnutrition and will not have adequate hormones and estrogens for the reproductive organs.

Improperly working bowels are the cause of over 90% of all disease on the face of the earth. Here is a good example of how this principle works. If a woman has suffered a lot during her life with painful menstrual periods, all she has to do is to look back over the past and remember that when she was badly constipated during her menstrual cycle she was in far more pain and discomfort than if she was having free bowel movements. It is good, we feel, to start the subject of "relieving menstrual pain and cramps" with first teaching the proper principle of keeping the bowels in a good clean condition.

There are two ways of working on the bowel in order to clean it up. One is to use purging or strong laxatives to force the issue. This procedure is a habit-forming one and not well accepted by the body itself. This principle will work to give temporary relief by removing some of the compacted and congested fecal matter that is causing griping and pain. By using this procedure, we are only working on the effect and it can give only temporary relief—because we are not going to the cause. Another procedure is to use regular enemas to give relief, and these can also become habit forming. Our program is to go to the cause and rebuild the areas of the body that are not functioning properly and let the body do its own job of its own free will. The organs that are not doing a good efficient job are usually the liver, gall bladder and the peristaltic muscles of the small and large bowel, which muscles are supposed to keep the food particles and the fecal matter moving on their own. In order to get the organs back into a smooth working and healthy condition we have combined a number of herbs (food) that do the job and do it well. This Lower Bowel Formula consists of the following herbs: Barberry bark (Berberis vulgaris), Cascara sagrada bark (Rhamnus purshianus), Cayenne (Capsicum minimum), Ginger (Zingiber officinale), Lobelia herb and/or seed (Lobelia inflata), Red raspberry leaves (Rubus idaeus), Turkey rhubarb (Rheum palmatum), Fennel seed (Foeniculum vulgaris), Golden seal root (Hydrastis canadensis).

As there are no two people alike in age, size or physical construction (and the bowel itself will differ in persons as much as do the fingerprints), most cases will start with two #0 capsules three times a day, and then regulate the dosage from there on. If the stool seems too loose, then cut down; but if it is difficult to get a bowel movement and the stool is hard and takes much effort, then increase the amount accordingly. In order to reach the condition of a free-easy flowing movement in very difficult cases, one could take up to even 40 or more of these capsules a day, for these herbs are only FOOD and can do no damage. Then after the hard material has broken loose and is eliminating, it will gradually decrease (these are hard incrustations of fecal matter that have been "stored" in the bowel for many years that are breaking loose and soaking up intestinal liquids). Do not taper-off the lower bowel tonic dosage so much at this point that you loose this advantageous momentum and continuity of elimination. In most cases, the improper diet has caused the peristaltic muscles to quit working, and it will take six to nine months with the aid of the lower bowel tonics for the average individual to clean out the fecal matter and to rebuild the bowel structure sufficiently in order to have the peristaltic muscles work entirely on their own.

Most people have pounds of old dried fecal matter that is stored in the colon, which is toxifying the system and keeping the food from being assimilated and because of this putrefied condition, most people engorge themselves with many times more food than the actual body requirements. In the process they wear out their bodies trying to get nourishment and yet are still always hungry. On the other hand, when the bowel has been cleaned, the food is readily assimilated and a person can sustain herself on about one-third the quantity of her former food consumption and have some four or five times more power, vitality and life. Now the clean body is able to normally assimilate the simple food values through the cell structure in the colon, instead of it being trapped in a maze of waste, and inhibited by the hard fecal casing on the intestinal wall. For then, or earlier, the largest part of the nutritional substance had been pushed on and eliminated before it could do much good. When the body is completely clean, these herbal aids will no longer be necessary. As long as you stay on the program properly, this should only be used when needed after the bowel is once cleaned.

Let the blood stream be in a good clean condition

When the blood stream is flowing "clean and doing an efficient job by feeding the system properly and carrying-off the wastes, the whole body benefits. The reproductive organs are also being fed and cleansed (fed if the materials are there to deliver). When a "good clean blood-purifying program" is being used, we will see that the toxic poisons are being removed and boils, acne and other skin diseases will start clearing up. The blood stream is life itself and it is our job to keep it clean and pure so that we can have a good circulatory system for delivering food to the body properly, and in addition, to carry-off all waste materials. A good blood purifier in teamwork with a bowel cleansing and rebuilding formula makes a wonderful combination. These two along with a good mucusless diet, can renew and add "healthy years" to a life. This herbal blood rebuilder or formula is made up of some herbs that are cleansers, and also herbs that have astringency, others aid in removing cholesterol, some kill infection, or build elasticity in the veins and arteries to strengthen their walls. It consists of red clover blossoms, chaparral, licorice root, poke root, peach bark, Oregon grape root, stillingia, prickly ash bark, burdock root and buckthorn bark. Use this tea (or two capsules) three times a day, six days a week and week after week to help bring health and give more pep and energy. Now with the bowels operating properly, and the blood stream flowing properly, we now need to see that the basic food (fuel) being carried by the blood stream is the right type. This is the time to be sure to use the mucusless diet, which is "wholesome." Fruits, vegetables, grains, nuts and seeds—as explained in the booklet "Dr. Christopher's Three Day Cleansing Program and Mucusless Diet."

There are so many young people today who have grown up on highly processed foods or a "junk-food" diet! Take wheat for example: it is fashionable to discard the outer layers (bran) and the "germ", which bear the hormones and estrogens, vitamins and minerals needed in our bodies. The human system craves and demands these missing items and so through the stress brought on by the difficulty in trying to get "something for nothing" one can expect troubles in this human mechanism ranging from irritability and other emotional problems to actual "disease." To correct this situation we have, over the years, collected a choice group of herbs that replace these missing items. It is a hormone estrogen herbal combination called Hormonal Changease Formula, consisting of: black cohosh, sarsaparilla, ginseng, blessed thistle herb, licorice root, false unicorn root and squaw vine. These are natural herbal foods that are needed by both men and women of all ages. Since they are natural, the body can accept, assimilate and use those materials that are needed to produce estrogens and other hormones naturally. This formula will assist in rebuilding the weak malfunctioning areas and help keep the organs healthy so they can supply the proper amounts of hormones and estrogens themselves. Herbs are a natural food, so they do not have "side effects" and "after effects" as are so evident in man-made and synthetic drugs. The recommended dosage is a cup of the tea (one teaspoon of tea to cup of hot water) or two #0 capsules, both a.m. and p.m. (or more often if needed) six days a week as long as necessary to get the desired results. This herbal combination is a great blessing during puberty; and again a boon to womankind right after a baby is born in order to replace the estrogens and hormones used during pregnancy.

Female Reproductive formula

One of the most important and helpful formulas for the female reproductive organs is one we have mixed and used over our years of practice and have called it the Female Reproductive formula. This was developed to aid women with weak organs, or ones not fully mature, or do not produce their own hormone and estrogens, or when the organs are not working efficiently and are causing discomfort and/or pain. This female corrective formula can be used from puberty or throughout life as needed. It is merely a combination of herbs in a food formula to feed this specific area of the body. It is comprised of the following herbs: three parts golden seal root and one part of each of the following: blessed thistle, cayenne, cramp bark, false unicorn root, ginger, red raspberry leaves, squaw vine and uva ursi. This is an amazing combination of herbs to aid in rebuilding a malfunctioning system (uterus, ovaries, fallopian tubes, etc.). Over the years herbalists and patients have seen painful menstruations, heavy flowing, cramps, irregularity, etc., that have been helped, and then the patient now has a painless menstrual period, good menstrual timing and a new outlook on life by using these aids to readjust the poorly operating reproductive system.

Recommended dosage is one cup or two capsules or tablets morning and evening or three times a day if needed, six days a week for as long as required to get the desired results. We have seen many severe cases who have had many years of suffering cleared up in ninety to 120 days. Some get relief sooner, some take longer, no two cases are alike. This is a food to rebuild the malfunctioning organs. We have recommended additional helps to cause a more rapid healing of the reproductive organs to help in the more severe cases. One of these is called "the vaginal and/or rectal bolus—VB Herbal Bolus." This is an excellent aid for the women (or rectal bolus for the men) who have problems in the reproductive areas. Boluses are made with healing herbs that (1) draw out the toxins and poisons, (2) aid (with herbal foods) in making the malfunctioning area healthy, so that cysts, tumors, and cancerous conditions will not have waste materials to "live in", because they are scavengers. Herbalists have found that some will come out through the orifices and others disperse into the blood stream and will be eliminated if the program is followed faithfully, (3) the bolus spreads its herbal influences widely from the vagina or bowel through the entire urinary and genital organs. The formula consists of one part of each: squaw vine herb, slippery elm bark, yellow dock root, comfrey root, marshmallow root, chickweed herb, golden seal root, mullein leaves. These herbs are all in powder form. Coconut butter should be melted down so that it will mix well with the herb powder. Mix a small quantity of this powder, and wet to pie dough consistency with coconut butter (which can be purchased from the drug store, health food store, or herb shop). Next, roll this mass between hands until you have a pencil-like bolus approximately the size of the middle finger and in about inch-long pieces. Cool and harden in a refrigerator. Then these are to be inserted into the vagina and/or rectum. It will be necessary to wear a sanitary napkin in order to hold the bolus in the vagina (or rectum). Insert upon retiring and leave in all night, six nights a week. The coconut butter melts at body temperature, leaving only the herbs, and these are easy to wash out with a douche the following morning.

The slant board combination: Here is a further aid in rebuilding the muscle tone and organ tissue in not only the reproductive organs (uterus, etc.) but also for a prolapsed bowel and other organs. Make a concentrated tea (simmer finished tea down to half its amount) of six parts oak bark, three parts mullein herb, four parts yellow dock, three parts walnut bark or leaves, six parts comfrey root, one part lobelia and three parts marshmallow root. Then inject this tea with a syringe into the vagina while on a slant board (head down, of course), or use one cup or so into the rectum. This is to be used to flush out the vaginal/rectal bolus inserted the night before and to give nourishment to the cell structure within the area that can use this excellent herbal food for prolapses and/or hemorrhoid problems. Leave this liquid in the area as long as possible before voiding. Also, while lying on the slant board, knead and massage the pelvic and abdominal area to exercise the muscles, so the herbal tea (food) will be assimilated more readily.

The tea we have just given is one we have called our "yellow dock combination" and should be used orally as well. Drink one-fourth of the concentrated tea in three-fourths cup of steam distilled water—three times a day. To take the teas or capsules and to insert the boluses, then the next morning to flush them out, sounds like a lot of fussing and extra work, doesn't it? Is it worth it? Many of my patients, over the years, have told of continual suffering from menstrual problems throughout their youth as well as adult lives. Why should some enjoy perfect health with problems during this cycle time, while others have lain in excruciating pain a week or more each month. Let's just suppose the discomfort and pain is only for three days each month, ranging from hardly noticeable, to uncomfortable, to severe. Three days is, one-tenth of a month. One tenth of each month for thirty years is three years of suffering in the life of a "still young" woman. Instead of so much suffering and discomfort, why not use a few minutes each day for ninety to one hundred and twenty days. The average patient sees such an amazing and happy change in life, in this short period, that they are astounded.

By having a weakened reproductive system many things can happen to the body in retaliation. This is caused from weakened tissue inviting disease, cysts, tumors, etc., into the body. These are scavengers and must have toxic, low type cells and tissue, weak and dying organs to feed on. All this is the result of malnutrition! We must reverse the condition, strengthen the cells and tissues, making them so healthy they are to "rich" for scavenger diseases to live on. Herpes simplex, yeast infection, leucorrhea, flooding, cramps, swollen and painful breasts, miscarriages, inability to conceive, etc., etc., stem from the reproductive organs or systems being in an unhealthy condition.

Straight Talk About Women's Health

50% of the causes of all 10 leading killers in women—including heart disease, cancer, stroke and lung disease—are related to behavior. Adoption of healthy behaviors during the formative college years can be crucial for young women. The leading causes of death for young women ages 18 to 24 are unintentional injuries, homicide, cancer, and heart disease.

Illnesses and Diseases

Cancer

- Prevention and early detection are the first important steps to reducing your risk for developing cancer, the No. 2 killer of women in the United States.
- Lung cancer is the top cancer killer among American women—75% of all lung cancer deaths would be preventable if women did not smoke. Breast cancer strikes 1 in 8 women and is the second leading cancer killer among women. Women ages 20 through 40 should have a clinical breast examination every three years.
- Cervical cancer strikes up to 2 women of every 100. All women 18 and over should have an annual Pap test and pelvic examination.

Eating Disorders

- Adolescent and young adult women comprise 90% of the millions of Americans afflicted with eating disorders.
- Eating disorders, such as anorexia nervosa and bulimia, affect 1 in 5 women, mostly young women.
- Eating disorders kill up to 10 percent of their victims and are a form of mental illness.
- Eating disorders can result in severe health complications, including stomach rupture, heart failure and digestive disorders, osteoporosis, teeth erosion and even death.

Heart Disease

- Heart disease is the #1 killer of women.
- Although heart disease is a gradual process that usually sets in later in life, young women need to practice healthy lifestyles during these formative years.
- Lifestyle factors associated with heart disease include smoking, lack of exercise, high cholesterol and excess weight.

HIV/AIDS

- HIV infection is one of the top 10 causes of death among 15 to 24 year olds, and the fourth leading cause of death among women ages 25 to 44.
- It's estimated that one in four new HIV infections in the United States occurs among people under the age of 21. That means every day up to 54 people under the age of 21 are infected with HIV—or more than two young people every hour.
- Women are the fastest growing group to be infected by HIV.

Mental Health Illnesses

- Approximately 7% of American women will suffer from a major depression during their lifetime compared to 2.6% men.
- Suicide is the third leading killer of young people between the ages of 15 and 24. Over 90% of all suicides are by those suffering mental or addictive disorders.
- One in 10 women will suffer a mood disorder during her lifetime, with depression being the most prevalent negative mood among women.

Osteoporosis

- Osteoporosis is a debilitating bone disease that strikes women in their later years, but the risk can be reduced in their reproductive years through good nutrition, adequate calcium intake and exercise.
- Women have up to 25 percent less bone mass than men, and most of the body's bone density is determined by age 35. Therefore, calcium plays an important role early in a woman's life. Doctors recommend girls and women between the ages of 11 and 24 take 1,500 mg of calcium daily.

Sexually Transmitted Diseases (STDs) and Contraception

- Women suffer more frequent and severe long-term consequences of STDs than men because they are more susceptible to infection and less likely to experience symptoms.

- 86 percent of diagnosed STDs occur in 15 to 29-year olds.
- 82 percent of pregnancies among women 15 to 19 are unintended and 61% of pregnancies among women 20 to 24 are unintended.
- The most common STDs for young women are chlamydia, genital warts, gonorrhea, herpes, HIV, pelvic inflammatory disease and syphilis.

Lifestyle Risk Factors

By changing poor lifestyle behaviors—such as smoking, drinking and inactivity—young women could lower their risk of premature death and disability by as much as 50%.

Alcohol: Contributes to Heart Disease, Accidents, Diabetes and Infection

- In the United States, more than 800,000 young women aged 18 to 25 engage in heavy alcohol use, which is defined as five or more drinks on at least five occasions per month.
- Drinking has both long-term effects, such as stomach problems, liver or pancreatic damage, heart ailments and memory loss, and short-term effects, such as depressive changes, sleep disturbances, hangovers, excess caloric intake and bad breath.
- 60 percent of college-aged women who contract STDs have had sex under the influence of alcohol.

Nutrition/Exercise

Contributes to Heart Disease, Cancer, Stroke, Pneumonia, Influenza, Diabetes, Infection and Hardening of the Arteries—

- A balanced diet and regular exercise can directly influence a young women's risk for several diseases and disabling conditions, such as heart disease, cancer and stroke, the top three killers of women in the United States.
- The three principles for nutrition and exercise are balance, variety and moderation.
- Exercise not only burns calories and fat, but it also helps maintain a healthy heart, lungs, muscles and bones, and make you feel more energetic and optimistic.

Smoking

Contributes to Heart Disease, Cancer, Stroke, Chronic Lung Disease, Pneumonia, Influenza, Infection and Hardening of the Arteries

- Twenty-three percent of women ages 18 to 24 smoke.
- One in five adolescent girls in the United States smokes, or at least 1.5 million girls.
- 19% of girls ages 12 to 18 smoke.
- 80-90% of young people begin to smoke before age 20. One-third of these people will die of this addiction.
- Tobacco use puts women at special risk for reproductive problems, including reduced fertility, early menopause and pregnancy complications.

Substance Abuse

Contributes to Pneumonia, Influenza, Accidents, Kidney Disease and Infection

- Young women can have special risk factors for drug abuse and dependency, such as low self-esteem, little self-confidence and feelings of powerlessness.
- The primary drugs commonly abused by young women are cocaine, marijuana and hallucinogens.
- Studies suggest that marijuana poses special health risks to women, including reproductive problems, infertility, and higher levels of testosterone, which results in increased body hair and acne.

Bronchitis and Asthma

In Ayurveda, Bronchial Asthma—an allergic condition resulting from the reaction of the body to one or more allergens and is one of the most fatal respiratory diseases—is named 'tamaka shvasa' and its seat of manifestation is the lungs.

Symptoms

During an attack of Bronchial Asthma you have to literally gasp for every breath—breathing out being more difficult than breathing in, since the air cannot be properly driven out of the lungs before you have to take another breath. For chronic patients these frequent attacks, specially in the night or early morning, are often preceded by nasal congestion and sneezing.

Root Causes

Either allergy inducing factors as weather conditions, dust, food, drugs, perfumes, pollution, etc. or psychological factors as deep-seated emotional insecurity, an intense need for parental love, etc. or hereditary/genetic factors.

Healing Options

Herbs	• Tulsi (Ocimum sanctum) • Vasak (Adhatoda vasika)
Ayurvedic Suppliments	• Vasavaleh • Kanakasav • Talisadi Churna • Kantakaryavaleha
Diet	• A limited quantity of carbohydrates, fats and proteins • A liberal amount of alkali-forming foods—fresh fruits, green vegetables, sprouted seeds and grains. • Avoid foods, which tend to produce phlegm—rice, sugar, lentils and curd • Avoid difficult-to-digest foods—strong tea, coffee, alcoholic beverages, condiments, pickles, sauces and all refined and processed foods
Lifestyle	• Avoid excess humidity • Avoid exposure to dust, fumes and pollen grains • Check your allergens
Yoga	• Half Wheel (Ardha Chakrasana) • Bow (Dhanura Asana)

Common Cough and Cold

It is a catarrhal and inflammatory condition of upper respiratory tract due to viral, allergic or mixed infection. In Ayurveda it is known as PRATISHYAYA mainly due to vitiation of Kapha.

Symptoms and Causes

Due to vitiation of Kapha upper Respiratory tract is inflamed and congested. Sneezing, coughing, running nose, heaviness of head followed by inflammation of mucus membrane of nose, body aches, chill and loss of appetite. Allergens, Virus, Bacteria are the common causative factors of this disease. A cough may be caused by the inflammation of the larynx or the pharynx, and develop in the chest due to change in weather. The real cause of this disorder is clogging of the bronchial tubes with waste matters. The reason for higher incident of cough during winter than other seasons due to intake of catarrh—forming foods such as white bread, meat, sugar, porridge, puddings, and pies. Hay fever, flu, sinusitis, etc. are the associated causes of this disease. According to Ayurveda Pratishyaya is classified into VATAJ, PITTAJ, KAPHAJ and TRIDOSHAJ types. In Vataj type there is pain in sinus cavity with sneezing, pittaj type is with fever and in kaphaj type there are whitish secretion and dull headache.

Healing Options

Herbs	• Vasaka • Garlic • Ginger • Basil
Ayurvedic Supplements	• Chyawanprash Special • Kantarayavaleha • Eladi Bati • Kas Bati • Kasamrit (Herbal) • Sitopaladi Churna • Talisadi Churna • Kaphkuthar Ras • Laxmivilas Ras (Kas) • Prawal Pishti
Diet	• In case of severe cold and cough and when fever is present the patient should abstain from all solid foods and only drink food and vegetable juices diluted with water. After this the patient should adopt an all fruit diet for two to three days. Taking three meals a day of fresh juicy fruits such as apple, pears, grapes, oranges, pineapples, peaches and melons. For drinks unsweetened lemon water, or cold or hot plain water may be given. After the all fruit diet, the patient can gradually embark upon a well balanced diet, with emphasis on whole grain cereals, raw or lightly cooked vegetables and fresh fruits. The patient should avoid soft drink, candies, ice-creams, and all products made from sugar and white flour.
Yoga	• Salvasana (locust) • Bhujangasana (Cobra) • Dhanurasana (Bow)

WOMEN AND OBESITY

Some girls, who used to be slim prior to their marriage, gain weight gradually after marriage. This is due to the changed eating habits or eating rich food to, which they might not be used to previously. Perhaps a more carefree and comfortable life is also to be blamed for this. This is acceptable to them as well as to their spouses now to consider their weight gain as a sign of good health until they become pregnant. Obesity right from the first month of pregnancy has its own disadvantages. The fatty tissues in the abdomen make it difficult for the expanding uterus, as the months advance exert great pressure on the bladder and bowels, disturbing the function of these waste eliminating organs. Wrong conceptions about the needs of a pregnant woman that she should eat double the amount of food to feed her and her child to be born and she should rest and relax more to preserve her energy for the time of labour. Nothing is near the truth, because the correct way of sensible eating and mild exercises and activities till the time of delivery facilitated a normal and comfortable delivery of a healthy child.

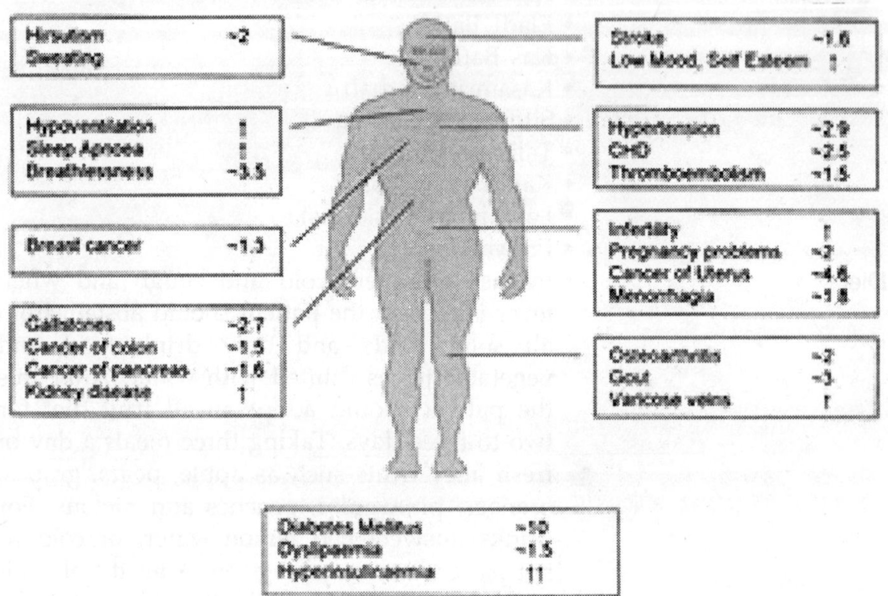

While in some cases there is reduction in weight after childbirth, in other, the young mothers keep gaining weight and remain obese for the rest of their lives. Generally two reasons can be attributed for obesity after childbirth. If normal delivery of the child is not there then this deprive the young mother of normal activities and exercises after delivery, resulting in the uterus not shrinking as it should, and gradually distention of abdomen takes place. The additional nourishment consumed undergoes poor digestion and the weight keeps increasing. Some young mothers despite normal delivery gain weight steadily because they are fed on fatty and starchy food in place of proper nutritious food under the erroneous notion that the weakness caused by labour can only be compensated by a rich diet. Sometimes young mothers, after delivery is also make rest more than it is necessary. Just as exercises is a must till almost the last stages of delivery for easy delivery, mild exercise after delivery is necessary for the contraction of the uterus to its original size. But exercise becomes more difficult if there is a weight increase. Therefore, obesity worsens the condition.

Women, who use contraceptive devices, oral contraceptives on a regular basis also tend to become obese. This is due to the effect on the hormones contained in those drugs.

Mind over body

Some women suffer from obesity for identifiable psychological reasons that manifest themselves as expressions of their underlying unhappiness and for no other reason. Such persons feel unwanted at home and outside. They develop severe complexes, become discontented with every one around and become indifferent towards anything and everything. They lose interest in every activity, which provide a pleasant diversion. In such cases, unless the underlying cause is attended to, they remain obese. Whenever they feel tense, overcome with unknown fears they seek a diversion in frequent eating. This type of eating gives them only a false sense of their tension being eased. At such times due to the absence of actual hunger, they resort to eating snacks, which please their palate. This naturally ads bulk the body.

Hormonal influence

Endocrine glands are organs, which pour internal secretion into our blood. But for these glands, the growth of our body and mind becomes defective and results in various disorders and diseases, obesity being one of them. The glands produce some chemical substances, which are called hormones. Hormone is a circulating chemical substance that is capable of acting on distant organs from its original site. The glands that function in a unique way need a mention in this chapter because a few glands and other functions are responsible for causing obesity. These are the pituitary, thyroid, adrenals, pacers and gonads.

Hormones are the agents that stirrup activity and bring about psychological changes in our behavior and bodily functions. Abnormal conditions of our health, is the direct result of an excess or deficient secretion of these hormones. Among the glands, the pituitary is the master gland that governs all other glands. It somewhat hangs from the hypothalamus, which is at the base of the brain. It monitors the activities of the other glands to produce exactly the correct amount of their respective hormones. Hypothalamus is a group of neurons that act as the centre for appetite, the stimulation of, which results in the sensation of hunger. If there is an abnormal function of this appetite centre in the hypothalamus, obesity is caused due to overeating.

Obesity also results if the hormones that the pituitary gland secretes are deficient. One notable feature of this deficiency is along with causing obesity the height of the person gets retarded particularly in the case of growing children. Girls stay short and stout and the onset of menses is delayed or absent for a very long period. In cases where this gland is overactive and secrete hormones in excess of what it should, the person grows to an abnormal size. This is known as gigantism.

The second gland that contributes obesity is the thyroid. This is situated in the neck. A deficiency in the hormones secreted by these gland results in the speedy division of cells. Such an increase in the number of cells cause obesity.

The third gland is the adrenals. These are two in number and are situated above the kidneys. The hormones that these glands, secrete, control our emotions anger, fear, etc. Excess secretion of these hormones, or when these hormones are administered in massive doses cause a severe disorder known, as Cushing's syndrome. This is also known by the name moon face. Any tumor or inflammation in this gland also causes Cushing's syndrome. The person so afflicted bloats to abnormal proportions and becomes the victim of various other disorders too, like hypertension and diabetes.

The pancreas is a very important digestive organ that secretes the digestive pancreatic juice and an essential endocrine hormone the insulin. Insulin is very essential in sugar metabolism. The stored fat from the refined carbohydrates and sugar due to the abnormal sugar metabolism result in obesity.

In some cases, if the sex hormones secreted by the ovaries in females are deficient during menopause, obesity results. Administering hormones further adds to the bulk. So is the case after hysterectomy in some women.

Overeating or Binge Eating

Addictions are of many types. All of us are addicted to something without even knowing why and how we are addicted. Generally tobacco, alcohol, drugs like opium and heroin are thought to be the things, which a person gets addicted to. But most of us are unaware of an equally serious addiction that is addiction to food. Different people are addicted to some food items. Some are addicted to carbohydrates in the form of rice or even wheat, some to spicy food, some to sweets, some to fast food and other commercial food. There are persons who get addicted even to bread and milk. Individually those foods as an addiction, to any one of these, may be harmless without visible discomfort. If abstained from, or lesser quantity of particular type of food is taken, one may feel some sort of all gone sensation in the stomach or suffer other withdrawal symptoms. But once they are introduced again, the withdrawals may disappear. As in any other addiction, the more one eats, the more the food is relished. The craving for eating keeps increasing day-by-day. Addiction to overeating is a serious problem, because it causes obesity. Overeating unwittingly begins at a very young age when it can be easily controlled or got rid of. But on being ignored or even encouraged, it reaches a stage when withdrawing or controlling it becomes extremely difficult. We often see persons overeating the type of food they are fond of addiction to isolated food items can be considered quite harmless compared to addiction to overeating. Bur if that isolated food happens to contain more calories than the isolated food happens to contain more calories than the food requires, addiction to that particular type of food will definitely be difficult to control. In case that particular food is not available, something else will be sought, which gives the satisfaction of eating the missing one. On some cases there are no such cravings for high calorie food like sweets and other processed food. A person simply eats anything that is available till his stomach is uncomfortably full. Less quantity of food makes the individual restless until her eats again after a few minutes interval.

The underlying cause for such overeating lies basically with the abnormal functions of the endocrine glands and the amount of hormones they produce. Availability of food in abundance is another reasons why addiction overeating is difficult to handle. Sometimes, competition creates greater enthusiasm to eat more, at times it happens that just for the sake of it, people over eat when they are in company. But all this leads to progressive addiction to food. When a person is engaged in some work the need to eat is not felt much as it is when he sits idle watching games, sports or even while chatting or traveling. Having nothing else to do, they indulge in eating every now and then.

Addiction to drugs, cigarettes and alcohol also cause obesity but not in every one. Sometimes, to quit the habit of smoking or drinking, some people seek substitutes happen to be food, which are high in calories. They seem to be mostly chocolates, other sweets or tasty fast food. Some psychological reasons can be attributed for such behavior. Most of the persons who decide to give up smoking or drinking have a feeling that by abstaining from these, they are depriving themselves of the pleasure they derive by indulging in them. They also feel that they should eat more of such food lest they should suffer from physical weakness. If they are advised or forced by others to quit smoking or alcohol, they almost invariably feel that they are obliging others by giving it a try. Therefore, they wish to compensate by eating what they like most, but not what could be a productive substitute.

Drugs that contain mercury and arsenic are prescribes for a variety of diseases. These if taken on a regular basis, result in obesity.

Being thin or underweight, like being overweight, is a relative term, being based on the ideal weight for a given height, built and sex. A person can be regarded, as moderately underweight if he or she weighs ten per cent below the ideal body weight and markedly so if the weight is twenty per cent below the ideal.

Symptoms

Thinness due to an inadequate calorie intake is a serious condition, especially in young people. They often feel easily fatigued; have poor physical stamina and low resistance to infections. Diseases like tuberculosis, respiratory disorders, pneumonia, circulatory diseases like heart disorders, cerebral hemorrhage, nephritis, typhoid fever, and cancer are quite common among them.

Causes

Thinness may be due to inadequate nutrition or excessive bodily activity, or both. Emotional factors or bad eating habits such as skipping meals, small meals, habitual fasting and inadequate exercise can also can cause it. Other factors include inadequate digestion and absorption of food

Height and Weight Table for Men

Weights at ages 25-59 based on lowest mortality Weight in pounds according to frame (in indoor clothing weighing 5 lbs.; shoes with 1" heels)

Height Feet Inches	*Small Frame*	*Medium Frame*	*Large Frame*
5' 2"	128-134	131-141	138-150
5' 3"	130-136	133-143	140-153
5" 4"	132-138	135-145	142-156
5' 5"	134-140	137-148	144-160
5' 6"	136-142	139-151	146-164
5' 7"	138-145	142-154	149-168
5' 8"	140-148	145-157	152-172
5' 9"	142-151	148-160	155-176
5' 10"	144-154	151-163	158-180
5' 11"	146-157	154-166	161-184
6' 0"	149-160	157-170	164-188
6' 1"	152-164	160-174	168-192
6' 2"	155-168	164-178	172-197
6' 3"	158-172	167-182	176-202
6' 4"	162-176	171-187	181-207

Height and Weight Table for Women

Weights at ages 25-59 based on lowest mortality Weight in pounds according to frame (in indoor clothing weighing 3 lbs.; shoes with 1" heels)

Height Feet Inches	*Small Frame*	*Medium Frame*	*Large Frame*
4' 10"	102-111	109-121	118-131
4' 11"	103-113	111-123	120-134
5' 0"	104-115	113-126	122-137
5' 1"	106-118	115-129	125-140
5' 2"	108-121	118-132	128-143
5' 3"	111-124	121-135	131-147
5' 4"	114-127	124-138	134-151
5' 5"	117-130	127-141	137-155
5' 6"	120-133	130-144	140-159
5' 7"	123-136	133-147	143-163
5' 8"	126-139	136-150	146-167
5' 9"	129-142	139-153	149-170
5' 10"	132-145	142-156	152-173
5' 11"	135-148	145-159	155-176
6' 0"	138-151	148-162	158-179

due to a wrong dietary pattern for a particular metabolism, metabolic disturbance such as overactive thyroid, hereditary tendencies. Disorders such as chronic dyspepsia, chronic diarrhoea, presence of intestinal worms, liver disorders, diabetes mellitus, insomnia, constipation, and sexual disorders can also lead to thinness.

Pitta body is usually thin.

Healing Options

Herbal Home Remedy	• Musk-Melon • Mango-Milk • Milk • Figs • Raisins • Good nutrient diet
Ayurvedic Suppliments	• Spirulina Plus
Diet	• Diet plays an important role in building up health for gaining weight. Under weight persons should eat frequent small meals, as they tend to feel full quickly. The number of calories it contains measures the weight building quality of food. To gain weight, the

	diet should include more calories than are used in daily activities so as to allow the excess to be stored as body fat. The allowance of 500 calories in excess of daily average needs is estimated to provide for a weight gain of half a kilogram weekly. All refined foods such as products containing white flour and sugar should be avoided as they destroy health.
Lifestyle	• Regular exercises like walking, dancing, yoga, meditation and massage are also important as they serve as relaxants, reduce stress, and induce good sleep.
Yoga	• The Shoulder Stand (Sarvang Asana) • The Plough (Hala Asana) • The Fish (Matsya Asana)

Jaundice/Hepatitis

The most common of all liver ailments, this results in an increase in the bile pigments and bilurubin in the blood, giving the skin and mucus membrane a yellow tinge. And is called 'Kamala' in Ayurveda.

Symptoms

- Extreme weaknes.
- Severe headaches.
- Constipation.
- Nausea.
- Yellow discoloration of the eyes, tongue, skin and urine.
- Dull ache in the liver region of stomach.
- Possible itching all over the body.

Root Causes

- Excessive circulation of pitta (bile pigments) in the blood. Occurs when there is any obstruction in the bile duct or impairment of the functions of the liver or excessive destruction of the red blood cells.
- Ailments as typhoid, malaria, yellow fever, tuberculosis affect the liver to some extent.
- Viral infections.

Healing Options

Herbs	• Ghritkumari (Aloe vera) • Kakmachi (Solanum nigrum) • Jaundice Berry (Berberis vultaris)

Ayurvedic Supplements	• Bhumiamla (Phyllanthus niruri) • Punarnava Mandoor • Liverol Syrup • Bhumiamla Capsule • Kumariasava
Diet	• Go for the boiled and spiceless diet. With vegetables—radish leaves, tomato, lemon . And dry fruits—dried dates with almonds and Cardemoms • Have plenty of sugarcane juice, orange juice, bitter luffa and barley water. This enhances urination, which helps eliminate excess bile pigments in the blood
Lifestyle	• Take complete rest • Avoid heat, sex and pshychic factors like anger and anxiety
Yoga	• Fish (Matsya Asana) • Shoulder Stand (Sarvang Asana) • Hidden Lotus (Baddhapadmasana)

Indigestion

Not quite a disease by itself, this condition of 'Agnimandya' in Ayurvedic terminology, it denotes a condition wherein food taken does not get digested.

Root Causes

- Aggravation of the three doshas—vata, pitta, kapha.
- Excessive intake of improper food (for more details, click diet planning).
- Psychic factors as anger, anxiety and worry.
- Fast eating habits
- Eating less of high-fiber foods.

Symptoms

- Feeling of heavy stomach
- Stomach pain
- Puking
- Vomiting
- Nausea
- Diarrhoea
- Acidity
- Burning Sensation in the chest.

Healing Options

Herbs	• Hing (Asafoetida) • Ginger (Zingiber officinale) • Lemon juice with rock salt
Ayurvedic Supplements	• Agni Bardhak Bati • Lavan Bhaskar Churna • Ajwain Ark
Diet	• Take a light fat -less diet • Have plenty of water and juices, especially lemon juice laced with a pinch of salt. • Intake of raw garlic is very beneficial
Lifestyle	• Avoid sleeping just after having a full meal. • Try to gain mental peace. • Physical exercise is a must.
Yoga	• Peacock (Mayurasan) • Shoulder Stand (Sarvangasan)

Dyspepsia

Dyspepsia is word of Greek origin meaning indigestion or difficulty indigestion. It is a common ailment and results from dietetic error.

Symptoms

Abdominal pain a feeling of undue fullness after eating, heartburn, loss of appetite, nausea or vomiting, and flatulence or gas are the usual symptoms of dyspepsia. Vomiting usually provides relief. Other symptoms are foul taste in the mouth, coated tongue, and foul breath. At times a sensation of strangling in the throat is experienced. In most cases of indigestion, the patients suffer from constipation.

Root cause

The main causes of dyspepsia are overeating, eating wrong food combinations, eating too rapidly and neglecting proper mastication and salivation of food, overeating, makes the work of the stomach, lever, kidneys and bowels harder. When the food putrefies, its poisons are absorbed into the blood and consequently the whole system is poisoned. Certain foods especially if they are not properly cooked, cause dyspepsia. Other causes are intake of fried food, rich and spicy food, excessive smoking, intake of alcohol, constipation, habit of eating and drinking together, insomnia, emotions such as jealousy, fear and anger and lack of exercise.

Healing Option

Herbs	• Lemon • Grapes • Carrot • Fenugreek

Ayurvedic Supplements	• Arogyavardhini Bati • Liverole Strong • Lashunadi Bati
Diet	• The best way to commence treatment is to adopt a light diet like soup, fruits, juices, boiled vegetables, etc. The patient may thereafter, gradually embark upon a well balanced diet consisting of fresh fruits, raw and steamed vegetables, seeds, nuts and whole grains.
Lifestyle	• The patients suffering from indigestion must always follow certain rules regarding eating, never to hurry through a meal, never to eat on a full stomach, and not to eat if appetite is lacking.
Yoga	• The Knee to Chest (Pawanmuktasan) • Vajrasana • The Lotus (Padma Asana)

Flatulence

Distension of the stomach and intestine owing to excess of wind in the system, it is called 'Adhmana' in Ayurveda.

Symptoms

- Loss of appetite
- Indigestion
- Breathlessness
- Headache
- Sleeplessness

Root Causes

- Aerophagia, or swallowing of air.
- Faulty dietary habits like eating too fast or eating too spicy food.
- Logical factors as anxiety, fear and grief.
- Hyper-salivation due to gastritis.
- Reflex from angina or chronic cholecystitis.
- Fermentation in gastro-intestinal tract due to inadequately cooked starchy foods.
- Deficiency of pachaka pitta or disorder of samana vata.

Healing Options

Herbs	• Ginger (Zingiber officinalae) • Hing (Asfoetida)
Ayurvedic Supplements	• Gaisantak Bati

	• Hingwastak Churna • Ajwain Ark
Diet	• Avoid pulses, beans, and fatty foods. • Have lots of curd and butter-milk.
Lifestyle	• Take rest after having a full meal. • Drive your worries away.
Yoga	• Peacock (Mayurasan) • Knee to Chest (Pawan Muktasan) • Leg Raises

Graying of Hair

Graying of hair is generally considered as a sign of old age. At times, graying starts even at young age. This is considered as a morbidity. In Ayurveda this is called palitya.

According to Ayurveda excessive passion, anger and phychic strain results in graying of hair. Persons suffering from chronic cold and sinusitis and those who use warm water for washing there hair are more likely to be victims of this condition.

Treatments

Bhringraja and amalaki are popularly used for the treatment of this condition. Medicated oil prepared by boiling these two drugs, viz., Mahabhringraj taila is used extremely for massaging the head. The powder of these two drugs is also used internally in a dose of one teaspoonful three times daily with milk. The oil prepared from the seeds of the Neem tree is used for inhalation twice a day for about a month. Along with this, the patient should be advised to take only milk as his diet.

Healing Options

Ayurvedic Suppliments	• Mahabhringaraj oil • Bhringarajsava • Amalaki Rasayan • Lauha Rasayan
Diet	• These therapies will be effective only when the patient observes diet restrictions. As far as possible, he should take only milk and sugar. Salt should be avoided. Sour things like yogurt are not useful. Pungent, hot and spicy food should be avoided.
Lifestyle	• The patient should not remain awake for along time at night and should be kept free from worry, anxiety and passion. If suffering from cold and sinusitis, prompt and careful treatment should be given. Hot water should never be used for washing the hair. Cold water should always be used for bathing.

Heart Disease

It is essentially a clinical syndrome of characteristic chest pain produced by increased work of the heart. It is usually relieved by rest. In most cases, it is manifested in front of the chest and mostly over the sternum. It may spread towards the left or right side of the chest. The pain radiates towards the left side very often. It may spread to the arms, neck, jaws and even the upper part of the abdomen. The left shoulder and the left arm are very often affected. The common man calls it heart disease. In Ayurveda it is known as bridroga. It is of several types depending upon the characteristic features of the pain. If the pain is acute, and of shifting nature, this is usually known as vatika bridroga. If it is associated with burning sensation, then it is called paittika bridroga. In kaphaja bridroga, the pain is usually very mild and it is associated with heaviness, nausea and cough.

Root Causes

It is caused by the obstruction to the coronary arteries. These are the blood vessels, which travel through the wall of the heart and nourish the heart muscle. Since the heart muscle spends a huge amount of energy, it needs ceaseless nourishment. It naturally demands a good supply of blood. Any impairment of these blood vessels interferes with adequate blood flow to the heart muscles. If this blood flow is significantly diminished then the heart signals its difficulties by registering pain or discomfort in the chest.

Treatment

Arjuna is the drug of choice for the treatment of this disease. This is a big tree and its bark is used as medicine. The powder or decoction of its bark is given to the patient during and even after the attack. The powder is given to the patient in a dose of 1 gm., four times a day. If the heart disease is of vatika type, it is mixed with ghee. If it is of paittika type, then milk is used. In kaphaja type of heart disease it is mixed with honey or pippali powder. For decoction usually 30 gm. of the raw powder of the bark of the drug is boiled with approximately 500 ml. of water and reduced to one-fourth. This is then filtered, honey or ghee is added to it, and given to the patient. With honey, the decoction should become cold before mixing. Ghee is mixed, when the decoction is warm, and is given to the patient as such. There are many preparations of this drug, Arjuna. Arjunarishta is commonly used by physicians. Six teaspoonfuls of this liquid drug are given to the patient twice daily after food with an equal quantity of water. Arjuna is boiled in cow's ghee, and this medicated ghee is given to the patients in a dose of 1 teaspoonful twice daily on empty stomach, mixed with a cup of warm milk. This preparation is known as Arjuna ghrita. This medicine should not be given to a person having a fat body. This is likely to add to his fat and may create more problems. Other medicines used for different types of heart diseases are Hridayarnava rasa and Prabhakara vati. These medicines are available in the form of tablets. Two tablets are given to the patient, three or four times a day, depending on the seriousness of the disease. At the time of acute attacks, Mrigamadasava is the ideal drug. It is a liquid medicine and given to the patient in a dose of ½ to 1 teaspoonful mixed with equal quantity of water. These medicines are to be used even after the attack has subsided. On exertion the patient may get the attack any time. It is, therefore, necessary for the patient to use the medicines mentioned above for about 6 months continuously.

Healing Options

Herbal Remedy	• Arjuna (Terminalia Arjuna) • Garlic (Allium sativum) • Cinnamon
Ayurvedic Supplements	• Arjunarishta
Diet	• Fried things, pulses and their preparations, and groundnut oil are prohibited. Ayurvedic physicians allow butter or ghee, and not groundnut oil. Cow's ghee, cow's milk and cow's butter are useful for the patient. Buffalo ghee and buffalo milk are not recommended. Stimulants like tea, coffee and alcoholic drinks are very harmful for such patients.
Lifestyle	• Ayurveda considers the functions of heart and mind interlinked. Disturbance in one affects the other. Therefore, patients having heart disease are advised by the Ayurvedic physicians to refrain from anxiety, worry, excessive sexual intercourse and wrathful disposition. All efforts should be made for the patient to have good sleep at night. Even rest during the day is essential. He should never be permitted to remain aware at night for long.

The patient's bowels should move regularly. If there is constipation, he is advised to take a glass of water early morning and go for a walk every day.

Rheumatism

Characterised by intense pain and inflammation of the muscles, ligaments, tendons and/or the joints, it is termed 'Amavata' in Ayurveda. Divided into chronic muscular rheumatism (affecting muscles) and chronic articular rheumatism (affecting joints), if neglected, it may even affect the heart.

Symptoms

- Fever
- Immense pain and stiffness in affected muscles in case of chronic muscular rheumatism.
- Excruciating pain and stiffness in the joints in case of chronic articular rheumatism.

Root Causes

- Accumulation in the joints of toxins (ama), formed due to improper digestion, metabolism or excreation.
- Infections from teeth, tonsils and gall bladder.
- Aggravated by exposure to cold weather.

Healing Options

Herbs	• Sallai Guggul (Boswellia sarrata) • Guggulu (Commiphora mukul) • Rasna (Vanda roxburghii) • Lohsun (Allium sativum)
Ayurvedic Supplements	• Yograj Guggul • Rashnadi Guggul • Maharashnadi Kada • Rumartho
Diet	• Avoid curd and all sour items, pulses (except moong dal), rice, meat, fish, white bread, sugar, refined cereals, fried foods, tea or coffee. • Have potato and lemon juice • Celery seeds, bitter gourd are highly beneficial.
Lifestyle	• Bowels should be cleansed daily • Soak the affected parts in hot water containing Epsom salt. Then apply Mahabishgarbh Oil. Hot water bag to the affected area is extremely beneficial. • Avoid damp place and exposure to cold weather. • Don't indulge in day-time sleeping • Limit yourself to restricted exercise
Yoga	• Plough (Hala Asana) • Bow (Dhanur Asana)
Ayurvedic massage	• Mahanaryan Taila • Mahamas Taila • Saindhavadi Taila • Rhuma Oil

Contraception is a great saviour

Women should have complete control over their sexuality and reproduction in order to take care of her own health and that of her progeny. Evidence of contraception exists in some of the earliest written records. Many contraceptive methods have been used for hundreds of years: the condom since the 16th century; cervical cap since the 1820s; the diaphragm and vaginal spermicide since the late 19th century; and intrauterine contraceptive devices (IUCDs or IUDs) since the early 20th century. According to the World Health Organization, an estimated 200 million pregnancies occur every year, 75 million of them unwanted. Unwanted pregnancies can threaten the mother's health and well-being in those who have existing health problems and in those who do not have enough family, financial, or emotional support. In places where women do not have access to safe abortion services, women may resort to unsafe procedures that can lead to death or disability. Researchers estimate that nearly 80,000 maternal deaths and hundreds of thousands of disabilities occur around the world because of unsafe abortions. The proper use of contraception can prevent the need for abortion.

Contraceptive options include the following:

- drug-free, cost-free "natural" rhythm methods and coitus interruptus
- barrier methods, which offer protection from STDs and unwanted pregnancy: condoms diaphragms, and the cervical cap, commonly used in combination with vaginal spermicides
- IUD
- hormones: oral contraceptives (the pill), injectable hormones, subdermal implants, and the emergency contraceptive pill
- sterilization (male and female)

Contraceptive Choices

The process of choosing a contraceptive is influenced by age, race, education, socio-economic status, religion, and experience with a particular contraceptive method, whichever method is chosen, proper use is critical to prevent unwanted pregnancy.

In addition to personal preference, women should consider the health risks and complications associated with the method, as well as the health risks from pregnancy, should the method fail. The risks associated with a particular method vary. Women who are considering contraception should consider the advantages and disadvantages associated with each method for women in their age group, and seek information from their doctor.

Bibliography

A Report, Series 3, No. 17 and 19. New Delhi: Office of the Registrar General. Roy Chowdhury, N.N. and K. Sikdar. 1982. 'Factors influencing maternal mortality', *Journal of Obstetrics and Gynaeology* 32, No. 4 (August): 507-10.

A utilitarian perspective, for example, supports the attribution of a privileged perspective to those most affected by particular decisions. Although classical American pragmatism is not always construed as "traditional," it clearly calls for the inclusion of non-dominant perspectives to reduce the 'fallibilism' of dominant perspectives. I develop this point in Chapter 1.

A. Gagnon J.H., 1988. Sex research and sexual conduct in the era of AIDS. *Journal of acquired Immune Deficiency Syndrome.* 1(6):593-601.

Acsadi, George T.F. and Gwendolyn Johson-Acsadu, 1990. 'Safe motherlyhood in South Asia: socio-cultural and demographic aspects of maternal health', Background Paper. Safe Motherhood, South Asia Conference, Lahore.

Agarwal, D.K. and K.N. Agarwal. 1987. 'Early childhood mortality in Bihar and Uttar Pradesh', Indian Pediatrics 24, No. 8 (August): 627-32.

Agarwal, V., S. Patil and S. Khanijo. 1982. 'Study of maternal Mortality', *Journal of Obstetrics and Gynaecology* 32, No. 5 (October): 688-92.

Ahmed, Swed, I. 1992. "Truck Drivers Are Vulnerable Group in North-East India." An abstract published in the Second International Congress on AIDS in Asia and the Pacific. Randwick, Australia: AIDS Society of Asia and the Pacific.

Ahrari, M., Kuttab, A., Khamis, S., Farahat, A.A., Darmstadt, G.L., Marsh, D.R., Levinson, F.J.: Factors associated with successful pregnancy outcomes in upper Egypt: a positive deviance inquiry. *Food Nutr Bull* 2002, 23:83-88.

AIDS Analysis, 1996, "India: 'a rapid and extensive spread of HIV'", *Incorporating AIDS and Society,* Vol. 2, No. 5, p. 11.

AIDS Control and Prevention Project of Family Health International *et al.,* 1996, The Status and Trends of the Global HIV/AIDS Pandemic, Final Report, Satellite Symposium, XI International Conference on AIDS, Vancouver.

Aim early exception to this tendency was a project developed by Bernard Gert, a philosopher at Dartmouth University. A number of projects have examined specific concepts or incorporated philosophical ethical considerations into empirical studies, and some projects have addressed legal and policy considerations. For a list of projects funded by the ELSI program, see http://nhgri.nih.gov/About_NHGBI/Der/Elsi/grant... index_html.

Airhihenbuwa Collins, O.: Health and culture : beyond the Western paradigm. Thousand Oaks, Calif., Sage Publishers 1995, xvi, 152 p.

Albeit Camus, The Rebel, trans. Anthony Bower (New York: Alfred A. Knopf, 1956), p. 22.

Albert B. Jonsen, "Casuistry and Clinical Ethics," Theoretical Medicine 7 (February 1986):65-73.

Alison Jaggar, Feminist Politics and Human Nature (Totowa, NJ: Rowman and Allanheld, 1983), p. 371.

Alkhateeb, A., Al-Alami, J., Leal, S.M., and El-Shanti, H. (1999). Fine mapping of progressive pseudorheumatoid dysplasia: A tool for heterozygote identification Genetic Testing 3, 329 333

Al-Nasser, A.N., Bamgboye, E.A., Abdullah, F.A.: Providing antenatal services in a primary healthcare system. *J Community Health,* 1994, 19:115-123.

Al-Salem, M. and Rawashdeh, N. (1993). Consanguinity in north Jordan: Prevalence and pattern, *J Biosoc Sci* 25, 553 556 [PubMed].

American Academy of Family Physicians Position Statement. September 1995.

American Academy of Pediatrics and American College of Obstetrics and Gynecology. Guidelines for perinatal care, 3rd edition. Elk Grove Village: IL: American Academy of Pediatrics. 1992.

American College of Nurse-Midwives Position Statement. Safeguarding maternal and infant health in a competitive healthcare environment. July 1995.

American College of Obstetricians and Gynecologists Committee on Obstetric Practice. Scheduled cesarean delivery and the prevention of vertical transmission of HIV infection. Committee Opinion, number 219, August 1999.

American College of Obstetricians and Gynecologists. Statement of decreasing length of hospital stay following delivery. May 23, 1995.

American Medical Association. AMANET. September, 1995.

American Society of Human Genetics. Statement on informed consent for genetic research. *Am J Hum Genet* 1996;59:471-4.

Amy Tsui *et al.*, eds., Reproductive Health in Developing Countries (Washington, DC: National Academy Press, 1997): 120.

Andrews *et al.*, p. 298.

Anirudh Krishna *et al*, 'Falling into poverty in a high-growth state: escaping poverty and becoming poor in Gujarat villages', *Economic and Political Weekly* 37(49), 6-12 December 2003.

Annas, G., Elias, S., eds. Gene Mapping: Using Law and Ethics as Guides. N.Y.: Oxford University Press, 1992.

Annas George, J. (1989), 'The Supreme Court, Privacy and Abortion' in The *New England Journal of Medicine,* Vol. 321, No. 17, pp 1200-03, October 26.

Annas, G.J. The Rights of Patients. Carbondale: Southern Illinois University Press, 1989.

Antimicrobial treatment guidelines for acute bacterial rhinosinusitis. Sinus and Allergy Health Partnership. *Otolaryngol Head Neck Surg.* 123(1 Pt 2):5-31. 2000

Anupama, H., Laxmi Reddy and R.J. Srinivasan (1989), 'Can IUCD induce uterine malignancy?', *Journal of Obstetrics and Gynaecology of India* (henceforth JOGI), Vol. 39, No. 1 (Feb.), pp. 85-87.

Appleby, L., Koren, G., Sharp, D.: Depression in pregnant and postnatal women: an evidence-based approach to treatment in primary care. Br *J Gen Pract.* 1999 Oct.; 49(447): 780-2. No abstract available.

Aras, R., N. Pai, A. Baliga, S. Jain and Naimuddin, 1989. 'Pregnancy at teenage-risk factor for lower birth weight', *Indian Pediatrics* 26, No. 8, (August): 823-25.

Aras, R., N. Pai, and A. Purandare. 1990. 'Perinatal mortality—a retrospective hospital study', *Journal of Obstetrics and Gynaecology* 40, No. 3 (June): 365-69.

Arieh Lalkin, M.D.; Ronen Loebstein, MD; Antonio Addis, PHARMD; Gideon Koren, MD, FRCPC, Therapeutic approach to hypertension during pregnancy: Extrapolation of findings from reproductive studies in animals to humans

Aristotle. The Generation of Animals transl. Peck AL. London: Heinemann, 1963.

Arora, S.K., R.C. Sharma and Lal Saran (1964), 'Pattern of sexually transmitted diseases at St. Sucheta Kripalani Hospital, N. Delhi', *Indian Journal of Sexually Transmitted Diseases* (henceforth, IJSTD, Vol. 5, No. 1.

Asano, Y., Elliott, K., Koren, G., Levin, M., Myers, M., Nathwani, D., Oxman, M.W., Schwarrrz, T.F., Whitly, R.J.: Reducing the burden of zoster associated pain-update. International Herpes Management Forum, University of Alabama. PPS Europe Ltd., 1995.

Aselton, P., Jick, H., Milunsky, A., Hunter, J.R., Stergachis, A. First-trimester drug use and congenital disorders. Obstet Gynecol. 65:451-5. 1985.

B. Weiss, E. Rao, Gupta, G. Bridging the Gap: Addressing Gender and Sexuality in HIV Prevention. International Center for Research on Women, Washington DC. (Forthcoming)

Baldo, M.H., al-Mazrou, Y.Y., Aziz, K.M., Farag, M.K., al-Shehri, S.N.: Coverage and quality of natal and postnatal care: women's perceptions, Saudi Arabia. *J Trop Pediatr* 1995, 41 Suppl 1:30-37.

Baldo, M.H., al-Mazrou, Y.Y., Farag, M.K., Aziz, K.M., Khan, M.U.: Antenatal care, attitudes, and practices., *J Trop Pediatr* 1995, 41 Suppl 1:21-29.

Bang, A.T.; Management of childhood pneumonia by traditional birth attendants, *Bull World Health Organ* 1994;72(6):897-905

Bang, R.A. *et al.* (1989), 'High prevalence of gynaecological diseases in rural Indian women', *The Lancet*, 14 Jan., pp. 85-87.

Bang, R.A. *et al.* (1989), 'High Prevalence of Gynaecological Diseases in Rural Indian Women', *The Lancet*, 14 January, 185-88.

Bang, R.A. *et al.* 1989. 'High prevalence of gynaecological diseases in rural Indian women', The Lancet, 14 January.

Bansal, M.C. and Usha Sharma. 1985.'Comparative study of septic abortions and medical termination of pregnancy', *Journal of Obstetrics and Gynaecology* 35: 705-12.

Bardhan, P.K. (1974) 'On Life and Death Questions', *Economic and Political Weekly IX*, Nos. 32-34, 1293-1304.

Barge, S., Kini, M. and Nair, S.B. (1994), Situation Analysis of MTP Facilities in Gujarat, paper prepared for the workshop on Service Delivery System in Induced Abortion between February 22-23,1994, Centre for Operations Research and Training.

Barron, S.P., Lane, H.W., Hannan, T.E., Struempler, B., Williams, J.C., Factors influencing duration of breast feeding among low-income women. *J Am Diet Assoc* 1988 Dec. 88:12 1557 61.

Bartels, D.M. *et al.* Nondirectiveness in Genetic Counseling: A survey of doctors. *Am J Med Genet* 1997;

Barton R. Burkhalter, "Assumptions and Estimates for the Application of the REDUCE Safe Motherhood Model in Uganda" (Bethesda, M.D.: University Research Corporation, unpublished analysis prepared for the SARA Project, 2000).

Baruah, M.C. *et al.* (1988), 'Clinical profit of persons seropositive for AIDS virus, *IJSTD*, Vol. 9.

Baskaran, S. (1982), 'Socio-psychological study of frequent visitors to STD clinic', *IJSTD*, Vol. 3.

Baston, H., Midwifery basics. Antenatal care: the options available. *Pract Midwife* 2002, 5:10-13.

Beauchamp and Childress, pp. 330-40.

Beauchamp, T.L., Childress, J.F., Principles of Biomedical Ethics. 3rd ed. Oxford: Oxford University Press, 1989.

Beck, K., Bodurtha, J., Human genetics and ethics education in the high school classroom. pp. 235-41 in Fujiki, N., Macer, D.R.J. eds. Intractable Neurological Disorders, Human Genome Research and Society. Christchurch: Eubios Ethics Institute, 1994.

Beck, C.T., Reynolds, M.A., Rutowski, P., Maternity blues and postpartum depression. *JOGNN* 1992; 21:287-293.

Beckwith, J., King, J., The XYY syndrome: a dangerous myth. New Scientist 14 Nov. 1974; 474-476.

Bentur, Y., Koren, G.: The three most common occupational exposures reported by pregnant women: An update, *Am J Obstet Gynecol* 165: 429-437, 1991.

Berry, L.M., Realistic Expectations of the labor coach. *J Obstet Gynecol Neonatal Nurs*, Sept/Oct 1988; 354-55.

Bertsch, T.D., Nagashima-Whalen, L., Dykeman, S., Kennell, J.H., McGrath, S.K., Labor support by first time fathers: direct observations with a comparison to experienced doulas. *J Psychosom Obstet Gyn* 1990; 11:251-60

Best Websites.

Bhalla, A.S., 1995, Uneven Development in the Third World: A Study of China and India, Basingstoke, United Kingdom.

Bhardwaj, N. *et al*. 1990. 'Socio-economic factors affecting weight gain in pregnancy', *Journal of Obstetrics and Gynaecology* 40, No. 3 (June): 327-30.

Bhargava, N.C., P.D. Ganguli and N.L. Jaisal (1981), 'An epidemiological study of gonorrhoea in males', IJSTD, Vol. 2.

Bhargava. N.C., V.K. Tewari and V.K. Pandey (1988), 'STD patients: a profile', *IJSTD*, Vol. 9.

Bhasker Rao, K., 1980. 'Maternal mortality in India-a cooperative study', *Journal of Obstetrics and Gynaccology* 30, No. 6 (December): J.C. 1988. A Study of Maternal Mortality in Anantapur District, Andhra Pradesh, India. Bangalore: Indian Institute of Management.

Bhat, M. (1987), 'Mortality in India: Levels, trends and patterns'. Unpublished Ph. D. Dissertation, University of Pennsylvania, Philadelphia, U.S.A.—(1991), 'Mortality from accidents and violence in India and China'. Research Report 91-06-1, Centre for Population Analysis and Policy, University of Minnesota, U.S.A.—(forthcoming), 'An econometric approach to the estimation of maternal mortality from incomplete data'. Paper under preparation.

Bhatia, J.C. (1988), A Study of Maternal Mortality in Anantapur District, Andhra Pradesh, India. Bangalore, Indian Institute of Management.

Bhatia, J.C. (1988), A Study of Maternal Mortality in Anantapur District, Andhra Pradesh, India. Bangalore: Indian Institute of Management.

Bhatt, R.V. and Soni, J.M. (1973), 'Criminal Abortion in Western India' in *Journal of Obstetrics and Gynaecology of India*, 23 (3).

Bhende, Asha A. 1994, "A Study of Sexuality of Adolescent Girls and Boys in Under-priviledged Groups in Bombay. *Indian Journal of Social Work*, 55(4). Bombay: Tata Institute of Social Sciences.

Bhende, Asha A., and Lata Kanitkar, 1978, Principles of Population Studies. Bombay: Himalaya Publishing House.

Bhushan Kumar *et al*. (1987), 'Pattern of sexually transmitted diseases in Chandigarh', *Indian Journal of Dermatology, Venereology and Leprology*, Vol. 53.

Blank, R.H., Redefining Human Life. Reproductive Technologies and Social Policy. Epping: Bowker Publ. 1984.

Blue Cross, Blue Shield of Minnesota: policy for postpartum stays, December, 1995

Blum, A. and P. Fargues (1990), 'Rapid estimation of maternal mortality in countries with defective data: An application to Bamako (1974-85) and other Asian countries'. Population Studies 44:155-71.

Botkin, J.R., Prenatal screening: Professional standards and the limits of parental choice. *Obstet Gynecol* 1990; 75:875-80.

Bouchard, L., Renaud, M., Kremp, O., Dallaire, L., Selective abortion: A new moral order? Consensus and debate in the medical community. *Int J Health Services* 1995; 25:65-84.

Brabin, Loretta, 'Veena Soni Raleigh and Selinah Dumella (1991), 'Pelvic inflammatory disease: a clinical syndrome with social causes', Liverpool: Liverpool School of Tropical Medicine (mimeo).

Braveman, P., *et al.* Early discharge of newborns and mothers : a critical review of the literature. *Pediatrics* 1995;96:716-725.

Breastfeeding Counselling: A Training Course", WHO/UNICEF, Geneva, 1993.

Breech Babies: What Can I Do if My Baby is Breech? (Copyright © AAFP)- This publication provides information on breech pregnancy, what it is, how a baby can be safely delivered, and what an external cephalic version is.

Briggs, G.G., Freeman, R.K., Yaffe, S.J., Drugs in Pregnancy and Lactation 6th edition,Baltimore, MD: Williams and Wilkins, 2002, p. 285.

British Medical Association (1988), Philosophy and Practice of Medical Ethics, BMA, London.

Britton, J.R., Early discharge of the term newborn: a continued dilemma. Pediatrics 1994; 94:291-295.

Bruce, J., Fundamental elements of the quality of care: a simple framework. *Stud Fam Plann* 1990, 21:61-91.

Bryanton, J., Fraser-Davey, H., Sullivan, P., Women's perceptions of nursing support during labour. *J Obstet Gynecol Neonatal Nurs,* Oct. 1994; 23(8):638-44

Buchler, pp. 9-10, 28.

Bulatao, R.A., Ross, J.A.: Rating maternal and neonatal health services in ddeveloping countries. *Bull World Health Organ* 2002, 80:721-727.

Burkhalter, "Consequences of Unsafe Motherhood in Developing Countries in 2000", Table 5.

Burns, John F., 1996 (September 22), "Denial and Taboo Blinding India to the Horror of Its AIDS Scourge." *The New York Times,* pp. 1 and 16.

Burns, John F., August 27, 1994, "India Fights Abortion of Female Fetuses." *The New York Times.*

Butt, N. *et al.* (1994): 'Histopathological changes in fallopian tubes of women using intrauterine contraceptive devices', *JOGI,* Vol. 41, No. 2 (April), pp. 223-26.

C. Dixon-Mueller, R., 1993, The sexuality connection in reproductive health. *Studies in Family Planning* 24(5):269-82.

Cairns, J.A., Shackley, P., Assessing value for money in medical screening. *J Med Screening* 1994; 1:39-44.

Campbell, I.E., Early postpartum discharge—an alternative to traditional hospital care. *Midwifery* 1992;8:132-142.

Campero, L., García, C., Díaz, C., Ortiz, O., Reynoso, S., Langer, A., "Alone, I wouldn't have known what to do": a qualitative study on social support during labor and delivery in Mexico. *Soc Sci Med,* 1998, Aug 47:3 395-403.

Cao, A., Antenatal diagnosis of beta-thalassemia in Sardinia. pp. 72-9 in Banzowski, Z., Capron, A. eds. Genetics, Ethics and Human Values: Human Genome Mapping, Genetic Screening and Therapy. Geneva: CIOMS, 1991.

Care of Mother and Baby at the Health Centre: A Practical Guide, WHO, Geneva, 1994.

Carty, E.M., Bradley, C.F., A randomized, controlled evaluation of early postpartum hospital discharge. *Birth* 1990; 17:199-204.

Casanueva, E., Lisker, R., Carnevale, A., Alonso, E., Attitudes of Mexican physicians toward induced abortion. *Int J Gynecol Obstet* 1997.

Casterline, John B. (1989), 'Maternal Age, Gravidity and Pregnancy Spacing Effect on Fetal Mortality', *Social Biology,* Vol. 36, Nos. 3-4, 186-212.

Centers for Disease Control and Prevention. Public Health Service Task Force Recommendations for use of antiretroviral drugs in pregnant HIV-1-infected women for maternal health and interventions to reduce perinatal HIV-1 transmission in the United States. February 4, 2002, http://www.hivatis.org/.

Centers for Disease Control and Prevention. Revised recommendations for HIV screening of pregnant women. *Morbidity and Mortality Weekly Report,* volume 50, RR-14, November 9, 2001.

Chadwick, R.F., What counts as success in genetic counselling? *J Med Ethics* 1993;19:43-46.

Chalmers, B., Wolman, W., Social support in labor-a selective review. *J Psychosom Obstet Gynaecol* 1993 Mar; 14(1):1-15.

Chalmers, B., Wolman, W.L., Nikodem, V.C., Gulmezoglu, A.M., Hofmeyr, G.J., Companionship in Labour; do the personality characteristics of labour supporters influence their effectiveness. *Curationis,* December 1995; 18(4):77-80

Chandrakapure and Ranganathan, 1985, 'Maternal mortality in rural Maharashtra', Paper presented at the Obstetrics and Gynaecology Conference, Aurangabad.

Charles Hartshorne and Paul Weis, eds., The Collected Papers of Charles Sanders Peirce, Vol. 2 (Cambridge: Belknap Press of Harvard University Press, 1960), #654.

Chatterjee, Meera (1990), Indian Women, Health and Productivity, Policy, Research and External Affairs Working Paper, Washington DC. World Bank.

Chatterjee, Meera, 1990, Indian Women: Their Health and Economic Productivity, World Bank Discussion Papers 109, Washington, DC.

Chatterjee, Meera, 1989, 'Socio-economic and socio-cultural influences on women's nutritional status and roles' in C. Gopalan and Suminder Kaur (eds.), Women and Nutrition in India. New Delhi: Nutrition Foundation of India.

Chaudhary, S.D. *et al.* (1988), 'Pattern of sexually transmitted diseases in Rohtak', *ISTD*, Vol. 9.

Chen, L.C. *et al.* (1974), 'Maternal mortality in rural Bangladesh'. Studies in Family Planning 5(11): 334-41.

Cheung, M.C., Goldberg, J.D., Kan, Y.W., *et al.*, Prenatal diagnosis of sickle cell anaemia and thalassaemia by analysis of fetal cells in maternal blood. *Nat Genet* 1996;14:264-8.

Chopra, A. *et al.* (1980), 'Pattern of STDs at Patiala', *IJSTD*, Vol. 11.

Chowdhry, D. Paul, 1992, Women's Welfare and Development, New Delhi: Inter India Publications.

Christopher Murray and Alan Lopez, eds., *Health Dimensions of Sex and Reproduction*, Vol. 3, Global Burden of Disease and Injury Series (Boston: Harvard University Press, 1998); and Barton, R. Burkhalter, "Consequences of Unsafe Motherhood in Asian countries in 2000: Assumptions and Estimates from the REDUCE Model" (Bethesda, M.D.: University Research Corporation, unpublished).

Clamers, B., Meyer, D., Companionship in the Perinatal Period—A Cross-Culteral Survey of Women's Experiences. *J Nurse Midwifery*, July/August 1994; 39(4):265-72

Clark, Judith F. Children's Hospital of Dartmouth. Letter for submission to the Congressional Record, September 12, 1995.

Clarke, A., Response to: What counts as success in genetic counseling? *J Med Ethics* 1993;19:47-49.

Clement, S., Candy, B., Sikorski, J., Does reducing the frequency of routine antenatal visits have long-term effects? Follow of participantes in a randomized controlled trial. *Br J Obstet Gynaecol* 1999, 106:367-370.

Committee on Fetus and Newborn. Hospital stay for healthy term newborns. *Pediatrics* 1995;96:788-790.

Conceptual bases and methodology for the evaluation of women's and providers' perception of the quality of antenatal care in the WHO Antenatal Care Randomised Controlled Trial. *Paediatr Perinat Epidemiol* 1998, 12 Suppl 2:98-115.

Conrad, P.D., *et al.* Safety of newborn discharge in less than in 36 hours in an indigent population. *AJDC* 1989;143:98-101.

Copstick, S.M., Taylor, K.E., Hayes, R., Morris, N., Partner support and the use of coping techniques in labor. *J Psychosom Res* 1986;30(4):497-503.

Czeizel, A., The Right to be born Healthy. The Ethical Problems of Human Genetics in Hungary. transl. Bokor, C.K., Bokor, G., Budapest: Academia Kiaob, 1988.

D. Heise L, 1997, Violence, sexuality and women's lives. The Gender Sexuality Reader. Lancaster RN, di Leonardo M. (eds). Routledge, New York.

Daniel Kevles, "Eugenics," in Warren T. Reich, ed., Encyclopedia of Bioethics (New York: Simon and Schuster Macmillan, 1995), p. 765.

Das Gupta, Monica, 1994, "Fertility Decline and Gender Differentials in Mortality in India," paper presented at the International Symposium on Issues Related to Sex Preference for Children in the Rapidly Changing Demographic Dynamics of Asia, Seoul.

Das Gupta, Monica, 1987, 'Selective discrimination against female children in rural Punjab, India', *Population and Development Review* 13, No. 1 (March).

Datta, K.K. *et al.* (1980), 'Morbidity Pattern among Rural Pregnant Women in Alwar, Rajasthan: A Cohort Study', *Health and Population Perspectives and Issues*, No. 3, 282-92.

Dawn, C.S. and Barn Kumar Mitra, 1990, 'Effect of food supplementation on maternal weight gain, low birth weight incidence, infant weight gain and breast feed performance', *Journal of Obstetrics and Gynaecology* 40, No. 3 (June): 313-18.

Deaven, p. 12. The project is now slated to be completed two years ahead of schedule. Nicholas Wade, "In Genome Race, Government Vows to Move Up Finish," *New York Times*, September 15, 1998, p. B10.

Denayer, L., Evers-Kieboons, G., De Boeck, K., Van den Berghe, H. (1992), Reproductive decision-making of Aunts and Uncles of a child with cystic fibrosis: Genetic risk perception and attitudes towards carrier identification and prenatal diagnosis. *Amer. J. Med. Genet.* 44: 104-111.

Department of Family Welfare (1989), Family Welfare Programme in India Year Book 1987-88, Government of India, Ministry of Health and Family Welfare, New Delhi, 178-181. Table C-12.

Department of Family Welfare, 1992, Family Welfare Programme in India. New Delhi: Government of India, Ministry of Health and Family Welfare, Department of Family Welfare.

Desai, Sonalde, 1994, Gender Inequalities and DemographicBehavior, India, New York.

DeSantis, L., Healthcare orientations of Cuban and Haitian immigrant mothers: implications for doctors. *Med Anthropol* 1989, 12:69-89.

Deva, Krishna, 1986, Khajuraho, New Delhi: Brijbasi Printers Private, Ltd.

Diallo, D., Role of iron deficiency in anemia in pregnant women in Mali, *Rev Fr Gynecol Obstet* 1995 Mar; 90(30):142-7.

Diane, B. Paul, "Eugenic Anxieties, Social Realities, and Political Choices," in Carl, F. Cranor, ed., Are Genes Us? (New Brunswick, NJ: Rutgers University Press, 1994), pp. 144, 146.

Division of Family Health, World Health Organization (1990), Measuring Reproductive Morbidity. Report of a Technical Working Group, Geneva, 30 August-1 September 1989, WHO/MCH/90.4, WHO, Geneva.

Dixon-Mueller, Ruth and Judith Wasserheit (1991), The Culture of Silence: Donna Haraway, "Situated Knowledges: The Science Question in Feminism and the Privilege of Partial Perspective," *Feminist Studies* 14 (1988): 584.

Druzin, M.L., Chervenak, F., McCullough, L.B., *et al.* Should all pregnant patients be offered prenatal diagnosis regardless of age? *Obstet Gynecol* 1993; 81:615-8.

D'Souza, Anthony A., 1979, Sex Education and Personality Development. New Delhi: Usha Publications.

Duggal, Ravi and Amin, Sucheta (1989), Cost of Healthcare : A Household Survey in an Indian District, Foundation for Research in Community Health, Bombay.

Dunn, P.M., Major ethical problems confronting perinatal care around the world. *Int J Gynaelecol Obstet* 1995 Dec., 51(3):205-10.

Durosinmi, M.A., Obebiyi, A.I., Adediran, I.A., *et al.*, Acceptability of prenatal diagnosis of sickle cell anemia (SCA) by female patients and parents of SCA patients in Nigeria. *Soc Sci Med* 1995;41:433-6.

Dutt, J. (1971), 'Psychosocial aspects of venereal diseases in teenagers', *Indian Journal of Dermatology, Venereology and Leprology*, Vol. 16.

Dutt, P.R. *et al.* (1976), 'Gandhigram' in A.R. Omran and C.C. Stanley (eds.), Family Formation Patterns and Health: An International Collaborative Study in India, Iran, Lebanon, Philippines and Turkey. *World Health Organization*, Geneva, 337-44.

E. Hong, Khuat Thu, 1998, Study on Sexuality in Vietnam: The Known and Unknown Issues. South and East Asia Regional Working Papers No. 11, Population Council, Hanoi.

E. Weisbren, B.D. Hamilton, P.J. St. James, S. Shiloh, and H.L. Levy, "Psychosocial Factors in Maternal Phenylketonuria: Women's Adherence to Medical Recommendations", *American Journal of Public Health* 85, 12(1995): 1636.

Ectopic and Molar Pregnancy (Copyright © MOD)—This fact sheet explains what ectopic and molar pregnancies are, their symptoms, how they are each diagnosed and treated, and the risk factors in future pregnancies.

Effective care in pregnancy and childbirth (Edited by: Chalmers Iain, Enkin Murray and Keirse Marc, JNC). Oxford; New York, Oxford University Press 1989, 2 v. (1516 p.).

Egnor, Margaret T., 1986, The Ideology of Love in a Tamil Family. Hobart and Smith College, unpublished. Cited by Sudhir Kakar, Intimate Relations, (1989:11).

Eidelman, A.I., Early discharge-early trouble. *J Perinatol* 1992;12:101-102.

Einarson, A., Bailey, B., Inocencion, G., Ormond, K., Koren, G., Accidental electric shock in pregnancy: A prospective cohort study, *American Journal of Obstetrics and Gynecology* 176/3 (678-681) 1997.

Einarson, A., Lyszkiewicz, D., Koren, G., The safety of dextromethorphan in pregnancy : results of a controlled study. *Chest*. 119:466-9. 2001.

El-Shanti, H., Al-Lahham, M.B., and Batieha, A. (1998), Normative standards of trunk and limb anthropometric measurements for Jordanian newborns, *Saudi Med J* 19, 702 706.

El-Shanti, H., Al-Salem, M., El-Najjar, M., *et al.* (1999). A non-sense mutation in the retinal-specific guanylate cyclase gene is the cause of Leber congenital amaurosis in a large inbred kindred from Jordan, *J Med Genet* 36, 862-865.

El-Shanti, H., Daoud, A.S., and Batieha, A. (1999). A clinical study of a large inbred kindred with pure familial spastic paraplegia Brain Dev 21, 478-482.

El-Shanti, H., Murray, J.C., Semina, E.V., Beutow, K.H., Scherpbier, T., and Al-Alami, J. (1998). The assignment of the gene responsible for progressive pseudorheumatoid Dysplasia to chromosome six and examination of COL10A1 as a candidate gene Eur, *J Hum Genet* 6, 251-256.

El-Shanti, H., Omari, H.Z., and Qubain, H.I. (1997). Progressive pseudorheumatoid dysplasia: Report of a family and review, *J Med Genet* 34, 559-563 [PubMed].

Epilepsy and Pregnancy: What You Should Know (Copyright © AAFP)—This fact sheet is for women with epilepsy who become pregnant, including the risks, the risks for the baby, how to protect you and your baby, what to expect when you are pregnant.

ESCAP (1976). Population of Sri Lanka. Country monograph series No. 4. Bangkok: United Nations.

Essential Elements of Obstetric Care at First Referral Level, WHO, 1991.

Essential elements of Obstetrics care at first referral level; 1991; WHO.

Evans, M.I., Sobiecki, M.A., Krivchenia, E.L., *et al.* Parental decisions to terminate/continue following abnormal cytogenetic prenatal diagnosis: "What" is still more important than "when." *Am J Med Genet* 1996; 61:353-5.

Evers-Kiebooms, G., Swerts, A., Van der Berghe, H., Psychological aspects of amniocentesis: anxiety feelings in three different risk groups. *Clin Genet* 1988; 33:196-206.

Evers-Kiebooms, G., Risk communication in genetic counselling and genetic risk perception. *Eur Rev Appl Psychology* 1995; 45:23-7.

F. Correa S., 1997. From reproductive health to sexual rights: achievements and future challenges. Reproductive Health Matters. 10 (November): 107-16.

Fact sheet, Population Reference Bureau, 1998.

Faden, R.R., Chwalow, A.J., Quaid, K. *et al.* Prenatal screening and pregnant women's attitudes towards abortion of defective fetuses. *Am J Publ Health* 1987; 77:288-90.

Family Planning Association of India (F.P.A.I.), 1990. Attitude and Perceptions of Educated, Urban Youth to Marriage and Sex. Bombay: S.E.C.R.T. (Sex Education Counseling Research Therapy Training) F.P.A.I.

Female Comforter During Labor Benefits Both Mother and Infant, SAN FRANCISCO (Reuters Health), Feb. 16, 2001.

FHI (Summer 1997). Better Postpartum Care Can Save Lives. Network.

Fifth Disease (Copyright © MOD)—This factsheet provides information about Fifth disease, a condition caused by parvovirus B19, signs and symptoms, and any complications during pregnancy.

Figa-Talamanca I., Maternal mortality and the problem of accessibility to obstetric care; the strategy of maternity waiting homes. *Soc Sci Med* 1996 May;42(10):1381-90.

Fleissig, A., Are women given enough information by staff during labor and delivery? Midwifery 1993 Jun; 9(2):70-5.

Fletcher, J., Situation Ethics: The New Morality. London: SCM Press, 1966.

Fletcher, J.C., Evans, M.I.: Maternal bonding in early fetal ultrasound examinations. *N Engl J Med* 1983, 308:392-393.

Fletcher, J.C., Wertz, D.C., Proposed: An international code of ethics in medical genetics. *Clin Genet* 1993; 44:37-43.

Fletcher, J.C., The morality and ethics of prenatal diagnosis. pp. 621-635 in Milunsky A. ed. Genetic Disorders of the Fetus. Diagnosis, Prevention, and Treatment. New York: Plenum Press, 1979.

Fletcher, J.C., Where in the world are we going with the new genetics? *J Cont Health Law and Policy* 1989; 5:33-50.

Fletcher, J., The Ethics of Genetic Control. Buffalo, N.Y.: Prometheus Books, 1988.

For example, while most women and men are chromosomally defined as XX and XY, respectively, some are XO, XXX, XXY, or XYY. Moreover, gender identity and sex identity (as defined by chromosomes) may be different in the same individual.

For Further Reading.

Francis, S., Collins and David Galas, "A New Five Year Plan for the U.S. Human Genome Project," *Science* 262 (October 1, 1993): 43-46.

Frequently Asked Questions—Pregnancy and Medications—This fact sheet provides information on taking medication while pregnant, the effects it might have on the baby. Also included in this publication is information on DES and the complications this might cause during pregnancy.

Friedman, R.I., 1996 (April 8), "India's Shame: Sexual Slavery and Political Corruption Are Leading to an AIDS Catastrophe." *The Nation,* pp. 11-20.

Fujiki, N., Hirayama, M., Mutoh, T., *et al.*, Japanese perspectives on ethics in medical genetics, pp. 77-91 in Fujiki, N., Bulyzhenkov, V., Bankowski, Z., eds. Medical Genetics and Society, Amsterdam: Kugler, 1991.

G. Koren, (Ed.), Third Edition: Marcel Dekker, NY 2001

Gagnon, A.J., Waghorn, K., Covell, C., A Randomized Trial of One-to-one Nurse Support of Women in Labor, *Birth,* June 1997; 24(2):71-7.

Gagnon, A.J., Waghorn, K., Supportive Care in Maternity Nurses: A Work Sampling Studin in an Intrapartum Unit. *Birth,* March 1996; 23(1): 1-6.

Ganguli, D.D. and N.C. Bhargava (1983), 'Genital infections due to chlamydia and mycoplasma: a review', *IJSTD*, Vol. 4.

Ganguli, D.D. *et al.* (1982), 'A profile of gonococcal urethritis in males', *Indian Journal of Dermatology, Venereology and Leprology,* Vol. 48, No. 3.

Ganguli, D.D. *et al.* (1985), 'Profile of gonorrhoea in males', *IJSTD*, Vol. 6.

Ganguli, D.D., J.A. Sundharam and N.C. Bhargava (1983), 'A clinico-epidemicological study of genital warts', *Indian Journal of Dermatology, Venereology and Leprology*, Vol. 49, No. 4.

Garcia, J., Bricker, L., Henderson, J., Martin, M.A., Mugford, M., Nielson, J., Roberts, T.: Women's views of pregnancy ultrasound: a systematic review. *Birth*, 2002, 29:225-250.

Garg, B.R., S. Lal and B.M.S. Bedi (1980), 'Continued endemicity of Donovanosis'. *IJSTD*, Vol. 1.

George, A., Shah, I. and Nandraj, S. (1993), Household Health Expenditures in Madhya Pradesh, Foundation for Research in Community Health, Bombay.

George, F. Cahill, "A Brief History of the Human Genome Project," in Bernard Gert, Edward, M. Berger, George, F. Cahill, Jr., K. Dassner Clouser, Charles, M. Culver, John, B. Moeschler, George, H.S. Singer. Morality and the New Genetics (Boston: Jones and Bartlett, 1996), pp. 2-3. Cahill, p. 3.

Germano, E., Bernstein, J., Home Birth and Short-Stay Delivery—Lessons in Healthcare Financing for Providers of Healthcare. *J Nurse Midwifery November*/December 1997; 42(6):489-98.

Gestational Diabetes (Copyright © American Diabetes Association)—This fact sheet explains what gestational diabetes is, how it affects the baby, and what you can do to treat it.

Gestational Diabetes: What it Means for Me and My Baby (Copyright © AAFP)—This fact sheet provides information on gestational diabetes, how it can affect you and your baby, what you can do if you have his disease, what changes you should make to your diet, and what you can do to protect you and your baby.

Gita Sen and Aditi Iyer, 'Incentives and disincentives: necessary, effective, just?', *Seminar,* 511, March 2002.

Gita Sen, 'Population: a new paradigm for old and new concerns,' in Challenge of Sustainable Development: the Indian Dynamics (eds) Ramprasad Sengupta and Anup K. Sinha, IIM Calcutta (2003); Leela Visaria and Pravin Visaria, An analysis of the long-term projections for major states of India, 1991-2101 (revised draft).

Gita Sen, Aditi Iyer and Asha George, 'Structural reforms and health equity: a comparison of NSS surveys, 1986-87 and 1995-96', *Economic and Political Weekly,* 37(14), 6-12 April 2002.

Gita Sen, Asha George and Piroska Ostlin, 'The case for gender equity in health research', *Journal of Health Management*, 4:2 (2002) and Engendering International Health: the Challenge of Equity (eds) Gita Sen, Asha George and Piroska Ostlin, The MIT Press, 2002.

Gonzalves, P., Hardin, J.J., Coordinated care early discharge of postpartum patients at Irwin Army Community Hospital. *Military Med,* 1993; 158:820-822.

Good Byron: Medicine, rationality, and experience : an anthropological perspective. The Lewis Henry Morgan lectures; 1990 Cambridge; New York, Cambridge University Press 1994, xvii, 242 p..

Gopalan, C., 1989. 'Women and nutrition in India-general consideration' in C. Gopalan and Suminder Kaur (eds.), Women and Nutrition in India. New Delhi: Nutrition Foundation of India.

Gopalan, C. and Nadamuni Naidu (1972), 'Nutrition and Fertility', *The Lancet*, 18 November, 1077-1079.

Gordis, E., Tabakoff, B., Goldman, D., *et al.*, Finding the gene(s) for alcoholism, *J Am Med Ass*, 1990; 263:2094-5.

Gordon, N.P., Walton, D., McAdam, E., Derman, J., Gallitero, G., Garrett, L., Effects of providing hospital-based doulas in health maintenance organization hospitals. *Obstet Gynecol*, 1999 Mar, 93:3 422-6.

Government of India (1966), Report of the Committee to Study the Question of Legalisation of Abortion (Shantilal Shah Committee Report), Ministry of Health and Family Planning, Government of India, New Delhi.

Government of India (1992), Family Welfare Programme in India. Year Book 1990-91, Ministry of Health and Family Welfare, Department of Family Welfare, New Delhi.

Government of India, 1995, Country Report, Fourth UN WorldConference on Women at Beijing, New Delhi.

Government of Maharashtra and UNICEF-WIO. 1991. Women and Children in Dharni: a Case Study after Fifteen Years of ICDS. Bombay: UNICEF, Western India Office.

Goyal, R.S. (1978), 'Legalisation of Abortion : A Social Perception' in Health and Population : Perspectives and issues, Vol.4, pp 302-08, October-December.

Graham, H., Oakley, A., Competing ideologies of reproduction: medical and maternal perspectives on pregnancy.

Graham, W., W. Brass and R.W. Snow, (1989). 'Estimating maternal mortality: The sisterhood method'. *Studies in Family Planning* 20(3): 125-35.

Graham, W., W. Brass, and R.W. Snow. 1989. 'Estimating maternal mortality: The sisterhood method', *Studies in Family Planning* 20, No. 3 (May/June).

Group B Strep Infection (Copyright © MOD)—This public education fact sheet provides information about the risk of GBS during pregnancy.

Group B Streptococcal Disease—Information on the causes and effects of Group B Strep infections.

Hallsdersdottir, S., Karlsdottir, S.I., Journeying through labour and delivery; preceptions of women who have given birth. *Midwifery*, June 1996; 12(2):48-61.

Haraway, pp. 581, 584.

Haring, B., Manipulation. Slough: St. Paul 1975.

Harrison, L.L., Patient education in early postpartum discharge programs. *MCN* 1990; 15:39.

Hartshorne and Weis, #654.

Hartsock, Money, Sex and Power, p. 232.

Hartsock, The Feminist Standpoint Revisited, pp. 108, 117-25, 231, 235, 238. Hartsock draws on psychoanalytic theory in developing this critique.

Hasan, I.J., Nisar, N., Womens' perceptions regarding obstetric complications and care in a poor fishing community in Karachi. *J Pak Med Assoc* 2002, 52:148-152.

Health for a change; Sue Dowling; 1983; Child Poverty Action Group.

Health Partners Position Statement: maternity lengths of stay. November, 1995.

Healthcare of women and children in developing countries; Helen M. Wallace, 1990; Third Party Publishing Company.

Heise, Lori L., 1994, Violence Against Women: The Hidden Health Burden, World Bank Discussion Papers 255, Washington, DC.

Helman Cecil: Culture, health, and illness : an introduction for health professionals. 3rd Edition Oxford; Boston, Butterworth-Heinemann 1994, viii, 446 p.

Hepburn, E.R., Genetic testing and early diagnosis and intervention: boom or burden?, *J Med Ethics* 1996; 22:105-10.

High Blood Pressure in Pregnancy—This publication contains information on high blood pressure in pregnancy. It covers the effects of high blood pressure, what pre-eclampsia is and how it is detected, and ways to prevent problems from occuring during the pregnancy.

Hind, A.S. Khattab, The Silent Endurance (Cairo: UNICEF and Population Council, 1992); and Judith A. Fortney and Jason B. Smith, The Base of the Iceberg: Prevalence and Perceptions of Maternal Morbidity in Four Asian countries (Research Triangle Park, NC: Family Health International, 1996).

HIV and Infant Feeding: Collaborative Statement by UNAIDS/UNICEF/ WHO", UNAIDS, Geneva 1997.

Hodnett, E., Nursing Support of the Laboring Woman. *J Obstet Gynecol Neonatal Nurs,* March/April 1996; 25(3):257-64.

Hodnett, E.D., Osborn, R.W., Effects of Continuous Intrapartum Professional Support on Childbirth Outcomes. *Res Nurs Health,* Oct. 1989; 12(5):289-97.

Hodnett, E.D., Caregiver support for women during childbirth (Cochrane Review). In: *The Cochrane Library,* Issue 4 2002. Oxford: Update Software.

Hofmeyer, G.J., Nikodem, V.C., Wolman, W.L., Companionship to modify the clinical birth environment: Effects on progress and perceptions of labour and breastfeeding. *Br J Obstet Gynaecol,* 1991; 98:756-64.

Holla, M., 1985. 'Vital statistics system-a major source of information on infant and child mortality', *Indian Pediatrics* 52:115-26.

Holtzman, N.A., Proceed with Caution: Predicting Genetic Risk in the Recombinant DNA Era. Baltimore: John Hopkins University Press, 1989.

Horowitz, Berny and Madhu Kishwar, 1985, "Family Life—The Unequal Deal," in Madhu Kishwar and Ruth Vanita, eds., In Search of Answers: Indian Women's Voices from Manushi, London.

Hubbard, R., Lewontin, R.C., Pitfalls of genetic testing. *New Engl J Med* 1996; 334:1192-3.

Hubbard, R., "Fetal Rights" and the new genetics. Science for the People 1984; 16(2):7-9.

Human Genome Organization Ethics Committee. Statement on the Principled Conduct of Genetics Research, March 1996.

Hundley, V.A., Milne, J.M., Glazener, C.M., Mollison, J., Satisfaction and the three C's: continuity, choice and control. Women's views from a randomized controlled trial of midwifery-led care. *Br J Obstet Gynaecol* 1997 Nov; 104(11):1273-80.

Hurst Jane (1991). 'Abortion in Good Faith : The History of Abortion in the Catholic Church : The Untold Story' in *Conscience,* Vol. XII, No. 2, March-April 1991.

Hurvitz, J.R., Suwairi, W.M., Van Hul, W., *et al.* (1999). Mutations in the CCN gene family member WISP3 cause progressive pseudorheumatoid dysplasia, *Nat Genet* 23, 94 98.

Hyppolito, S.B., Alternative model for low risk obstetric care in Third World rural and peri-urban areas, *Int J Gynaecol Obstet,* 1992, Jun; 38 Suppl:S63-66.

ICMR (1989), Illegal Abortions in Rural Areas, Indian Council for Medical Research, New Delhi.

ICMR (1991), Evaluation of Quality of Family Welfare Services at Primary Health Center Level, Indian Council for Medical Research, New Delhi.

India Registrar General, 1992, Final Population Totals, Series 1, Paper-2 of 1992, New Delhi, 1995, SRS Based Abridged Life Tables 1988-92, Occasional Paper No. 4 of 1995, New Delhi, 1996a, Fertility and Mortality Indicators 1993, New Delhi, 1996b, *Sample Registration Bulletin,* Vol. 30, No. 1, New Delhi.

India, Ministry of Health and Family Welfare (1981). The Report of the Working Group on Health for All By 2000 A.D. New Delhi: National Institute of Health and Family Welfare (reprinted 1983).

India: Issues in Women's Health, The World Bank, January 25th, 1996.

India's Progress Towards Reproductive Health Goals: ICPD + 5. India Country Paper, Ministry of Health and Family Welfare (MOHFW), February 1999.

Indian Council of Medical Research (1982) Report of the ICMR Working Group, *American Journal of Clinical Nutrition,* 35: 1442.

Indian Council of Medical Research (1991), 'HIV infection: current status and future research plans, *MMR Bulletin,* Vol. 21, No. 12 (December), pp. 125-44.

Inequalities between men and women in nutrition and family welfare services: an in-depth enquiry in an Indian village, Social Action 38 (October-December).

Information kit, World Health Day 1998, WHO.

Integrating maternal and child health services with primary healthcare; 1990; WHO.

International Institute for Population Studies and ORC Macro (2000). 21.National Family Health Survey (NFHS 2), 1998-99: India. Mumbai: IIPS.. Intervention and Current Best Practices; Promoting Quality Maternal and Newborn Care.

International Institute for Population Sciences, 1995, India National Family Health Survey, 1992-93, Bombay.

International Institute of Population Sciences, Bombay and Department of Sociology, Marathwada University, Aurangabad (1985) Baseline Survey of Fertility, Mortality, and Related Factors in Maharashtra, July.

International Institute of Population Sciences, Bombay, and Population Research Centre, M.S. University, Baroda (1985) Baseline Survey on Fertility, Mortality and Related Factors in Rural Gujarat, December.

International Women's Health Coalition.

Is Mother/Infant HIV Transmission Preventable? (Copyright © University of California)-This fact sheet from the Center for AIDS Prevention Studies includes statistical information on breastfeeding and perinatal HIV transmission.

It may of course be argued that the fetus or potential child is more drastically affected by Julia's decision than she is. Among those who are autonomous, however. Julia is clearly the one most affected. 'Whether the impact on the fetus is morally compelling depends on the moral status attributed to it, an issue that appears irresolvable by philosophical or public consensus.

Ito, S., Koren, G., Estimation of fetal risk from aerosolized pentamidine in pregnant healthcare workers. *Chest* 106: 1460-1462, 1994.

Ito, S., Koren, G., Exposure of pregnant women to ribavirin-contaminated air: risk assessment and recommendations, *J Ped Infect Dis* 12: 2-5, 1993.

Iyenger, L., 1975, 'Influence of the diet on the outcome of pregnancy in Indian women', in Proceeding of the 9th International Congress of Nutrition, Mexico, 1972, Vol. 2, Karger, *Nutrition*, pp. 48-53.

J. Dobbing, "Maternal Nutrition in Pregnancy and Later Achievement of Offspring,' Early Human Development 12 (1985): 1-8; W.B. Hanley, Linsao, W. Davidson, and C.A.F. Moes, "Maturation within Early Treatment of Phmenylketonmiria," *Pediatric Research* 4 (1970): 318-27.

Jacob Marv *et al.* (1989), 'Epidemiology and clinical profile of genital herpes', *Indian Journal of Medical Research*, Vol. 89.

Jacobson Jodi (1990), The Global Politics of Abortion, World Watch Institute, World Watch Paper No. 97, Washington DC.

Jacobson, Jodi L. (1991), Women's Reproductive Health, The Silent Emergency, Washington, D.C., Worldwatch Institute Paper 102 (June).

Jaffrey, Zia, 1996. The Invisibles: A Tale of the Eunuchs of India. New York: Pantheon Books.

Jain, M.L. and Dinesh Agarwal, 1986. 'Utilization of maternal services in an I.C.D.S. block', *Journal of Obstetrics and Gynaecology* 36, No. 5, October 842-44.

Jain, S., *et al.* (1989), 'Clinicobacteriological evaluation of pelvic inflammatory disease amongst women in state protective and aftercare homes', *IJSTD*, Vol. 2.

Jambai, A., Maternal health, war, and religious tradition: authoritative knowledge in Pujehun, Sierra Leone. *Med Anthropol Q*, 1996 Jun; 10(2):270-86

Jamison, D., W.H. Mosley, A.R. Measham, J.L. Bobadilla, 1993. Disease Control Priorities in Developing Countries. New York: Oxford University Press.

Jansson, P., Early postpartum discharge. *Am J Nursing* 1985; 85:547-550.

Jayasingh, P. *et al.* (1984), 'Effect of V.D. on knowledge and attitude to sex', *IJSTD*, Vol. 5, No. 1.

Jayasingh, R., T.B.B.S.V. Ramanaiah and S.G. Fernandes (1985a), 'Pattern of sexually transmitted diseases in Madurai, India', *Genitourinary Medicine*, Vol. 61.

Jejeebhoy, Shireen and Saumya Rama Rao (1992), 'Unsafe motherhood: a review of reproductive health in India', Paper presented at seminar on Future of Health and Development in India, N. Delhi (January), published in the present volume.

Jejeebhoy, Shireen J. and Saumya Rama Rao, 1995, "Unsafe Motherhood: A Review of Reproductive Health," in Monica Das Gupta,

Jesani Amar and Anantharam Saraswathy (1990), Private Sector and Privatisation in the Healthcare Services, Foundation for Research in Community Health, Bombay.

Jeyapaul, K. *et al.* (1985), 'Reasons for promiscuity', IJSTD, Vol. 6, No. 2.

Jeyasingh, P., T.B.B.S.V. Ramanaiah and Baiasubramaniam (1985b), 'Teenagers with STDs', *IJSTD*, Vol. 6.

John J. McDermott, ed., The Writings of William James New York: Modern Library, 1968), pp. 629-45, 136-52.

John Ladd, "The Ethics of Participation," in J. Roland Pennock and John W. Chapman, Participation in Politics Nomos 16 (New York: Lieber-Atherton, 1975), p. 101. Ladd imputes this viev to Kurt Baler in The Moral Point of View (New York: Random House, 1965), p. 107.

Johnson, Cate *et al.*, 1996, "Domestic Violence in India," unpublished report to USAID/INDIA.

Johnson, F. Catherine, 1996,"Violence Against Women in India:The Law as Protector?," paper presented at the Association of Women in Development International Conference, Washington, DC.

Joint WHO/UNICEF/UNFPA Policy Statement on Traditional Birth Attendants", WHO, Geneva, 1992.

Journal Reproductive Health Matters, 2002, 10(19), pp. 190-192. The entire issue was devoted to sex-selection and sex-selective abortion.

Justus Buchler, ed., Philosophical Writings of Peirce (New York: Dover Publications, 1955), pp. 4, 38, 42-59, 160, 288, 356.

Kaiya, H., Macer, D., Japanese muscular dystrophy families are more accepting of fetal diagnosis than patients. *Eubios J Asian Int Bioethics* 1996;6:103-4.

Kakar, Sudhir, and K. Chowdhary, 1970. Conflict and Choice: Indian Youth in a Changing Society. Bombay: Somaiya Publications.

Kakar, Sudhir, 1989, Intimate Relations: Exploring Indian Sexuality. Chicago: University of Chicago Press. New Delhi: Penguin Books India (P) Ltd.

Kamalajayaram, V. and T. Parameswari, 1988, 'A study of septic abortion cases in the last 6 years', *Journal of Obstetrics and Gynaecology* 38, No. 4 (August): 389-92.

Kanitkar, Tara and R.K. Six-ha. 1989, 'Antenatal care services in five states of India', in S.N. Singh, M.K. Premi, P.S. Bhatia and Ashish Bose, *Population Transition in India,* Vol. 2, pp. 201-11, Delhi: B.R. Publishing Corporation.

Kannan, K.P. *et al.* (1991), HeaLth Status in Rural Kerala: A Study of the Linkages Between Socio-economic Status and Health Status. Integrated Rural Technology Centre of the Kerala Sastra Sahitya Parishad, February.

Kannappan, N.N. *et al.* (1984), 'Level of knowledge about STD among college students', *IJSTD*, Vol. 5.

Kapil, U., 1990, 'Promotion of safe motherhood in India', *Indian Pediatrics* 27, No. 3 (March): 232-38.

Kapur, Promilla, 1973, Love, Marriage, and Sex. Delhi: Vikas Publishing House.

Kapur, T.R. (1982), 'Pattern of sexually transmitted diseases in India', *Indian Journal of Dermatology, Venereology and Leprology,* Vol. 48.

Karkal Malini (1970), A Bibliography of Abortion Studies in India, International Institute of Population Studies, Bombay.

Karkal Malini (1991), 'Abortion Laws and the Abortion Situation in India' in *Issues in Reproductive and Genetic Engineering*, Vol. 4, No. 3, pp. 223-30.

Katherine Montgomery Hunter, "Narrative," in Warren Reich, ed., The Encyclopedia of Bioethics (New York: Macmillan, 1995).

Keenan, P., Benefits of massage therapy and use of a doula during labor and childbirth. *Altern Ther Health Med* 2000 Jan.; 6:66-74.

Kelkar, Govind, 1992, Violence Against Women: Perspectives and Strategies in India, *Indian Institute of Advanced Study,* Occasional Papers 30, New Delhi.

Kenen, R.H., The at-risk health status and technology: a diagnostic invitation and the 'gift' of knowing. *Soc Sci Med* 1996; 42:1545-53.

Kennell, J., Klaus, M., McGrath, S., Robertson, S., Hinkley, C., Continuous emotional support during labor in a US hospital. A randomized controlled trial. *JAMA,* 1991, May 1, 265:17; 2197-2201.

Khan, M.E. and C.V.S. Prasad, 1983, Under-utilization of Health Services in Rural India: A Comparative Study of Bihar, Gujarat and Kerala. Baroda: Operations Research Group.

Khan, M.E. and Singh, Ratanjeet (1987), Woman and her role in the family decision-making process: a case study of Uttar Pradesh, India', *Journal of Family Welfare*, Vol. 33, No. 4 (June).

Khan, M.E., Richard Anker, S.K. Ghosh Dastidar and Sashi Bairathi, 1988.

Khan, M.E., S.K. Ghosh Dastidar and R. Singh, 1986. 'Nutrition and health practices among rural women—a case study of Uttar Pradesh, India', *Journal of Family Welfare* 33, No. 1 (September).

Khattak, S., K-Moghtader, G., McMartin, K., Barrera, M., Kennedy, D., Koren, G., Pregnancy outcome following gestational exposure to organic solvents: a prospective controlled study. *JAMA* 1999, Sep 15; 282(11):1033.

Khattak, S., K-Moghtader, G., McMartin, K., Barrera, M., Kennedy, D., Koren, G., Pregnancy outcome following gestational exposure to organic solvents: a prospective controlled study *JAMA* 1999, Mar 24-31; 281(12):1106-9.

Khoury, S.A. and Massad, D. (1992), Consanguineous marriage in *Jordan Am J Med Genet* 43, 769 775 [PubMed]

Klaus, M.H., Kennell, J.H., *et al.*, Effects of social support during parturition on maternal and infant morbidity. *Br Med J* 1986; 193:585-87.

Klaus, M.H., Kennell, J.H., The doula: an essential ingredient of childbirth rediscovered. *Acta Paediatr* 1997, Oct. 86:10 1034-6.

Klein, Susan, A Book for Midwives, The Hesperian Foundation, 1995.

Kleinman Arthur: Patients and healers in the context of culture : an exploration of the borderland between anthropology, medicine, and psychiatry. Comparative studies of health systems and medical care; No. 3, Berkeley, University of California Press 1980, xvi, 427 p.

Knipe, D.M., 1991, Hinduism. New York/San Francisco/London: Harper/ Collins.

Koenig, M.A. *et al.* (1988), 'Maternal mortality in Matlab, Bangladesh. 1976-85', *Studies in Family Planning* 19(2):69-80.

Kogi-Makau, W., Role of traditional birth attendants in the dissemination of advice on nutrition (letter) World Health Forum 1992; 13(2-3):197-9

Konar, Hiralal (1992), 'Changing trends in septic abortion', *JOGI*, Vol. 42, No. 3 (June).

Koren, G., Chang, N., Gonen, R., Klein, J., Weiner, L.H., Demshar, H.P., Pizzolato, S., Shime, J., Lead exposure in mothers and their newborn babies in greater Toronto, 1989. *Can Med Assoc J* 142: 1241-1244, 1990.

Koren, G., Khattak, S., Pregnancy outcome following gestational exposure to organic solvents: Author's response. *Teratology*, 1999 Dec.; 60(6):330-1.

Koren, G., Matsui, D., Bailey, B., DEET-based insect repellents: safety implications for children and pregnant and lactating women, *CMAJ* Aug. 5, 2003; 169(3).

Koren, G., Sharav, T., Pastuszak, A., *et al.*, A multicenter prospective study of reproductive outcome following carbon monoxide poisoning in *Pregnancy Reproduct Toxicol* 5: 397-403, 1991.

Koren, G., Chickenpox during pregnancy; small but real risk. *Can Fam Physicians* 41: 1477-1478, 1995.

Koren, G., Lead risk during pregnancy, *Can J Fam Physicians* 42: 414-415, 1996.

Koren, G., The risks of pregnancy in epilepsy. In: Neurology Specialist Program, 1990. *Medifacts*, Ottawa, Ontario.

Krishnaji, N. (1987), 'Poverty and Sex Ratio-Some Data and Speculations', *Economic and Political Weekly*, XXII, 892-97.

Krishnaraj Maithreyi (1991), Women and Science: Selected Essays, Himalaya Publishing House, Bombay.

Kristen, I. McMartin, M.S.C., Gideon Koren, M.D., FRCPC, Exposure to organic solvents: Does it adversely affect pregnancy?

Kumar, Harish, S. Aneja, V.K. Prasad, S.K. Arora and D.N. Mullick. 1988, 'Tetanus neonatorum: clinico-epidemiological profile', *Indian Pediatrics* 25, No. 11 (November): 1054-57.

Kumar, Vijay and Inderjit Walia. 1983.'Beliefs and practices of birth attendants during antenatal period in a rural area', *Journal of Obstetrics and Gynaecology* 33, No. 4 (August): 460-65.

Kunhilakshmi, T.V., K. Vijayalakshmi and C.N. Sowmini (1980), 'STDs among the inmates of vigilance home, Madras', IJSTD, Vol. 1.

Kuppermann, M., Gates, E., Washington, E., Racial-ethnic differences in prenatal diagnostic test use and outcomes: Preferences, socio-economics, or patient knowledge?, *Obstet Gynecol* 1996; 87:675-82.

Kurt Bayertz, GenEthics, trans. Sarah L. Kirkhy (New York: Cambridge University Press, 1994), p. 23.

Kwast, B.E., Building a community-based maternity program. *Int J Gynaecol Obstet* 1995 Jun; 48 Suppl:S67-82.

Kwast-B-E, Reduction of Maternal and perinatal mortality in rural and per-urban settings; European *Journal of Obstetrics, Gynecology and Reproductive Biology;* 1996 Oct., 69(1), pp. 47-53.

Ladd, pp. 102, 103.

Langer, A., Campero, L., Garcia, C., Reynoso, S., Effects of psychosocial support during labour and childbirth on breastfeeding, medical interventions, and mothers' well-being in a Mexican public hospital: a randomised clinical trial. *Br J Obstet Gynaecol*, 1998 Oct., 105:10 1056-63.

Langer, A., Villar, J., Romero, M., Nigenda, G., Piaggio, G., Kuchaisit, C., Rojas, G., Al-Osimi, M., Miguel Belizan, J., Farnot, U., Al-Mazrou, Y., Carroli, G., Ba'aqeel, H., Lumbiganon, P., Pinol, A., Bergsjo, P., Bakketeig, L., Garcia, J., Berendes, H., Are women and providers satisfied with antenatal care? Views on a standard and a simplified, evidence-based model of care in four developing countries. *BMC Womens Health*, 2002, 2:7.

Larry, L. Deaven, "Mapping and Sequencing the Human Genome.' in Carl F. Cramor, ed., Are Genes Us? (New Brunswick, NJ: Rutgers University Press, 1994), p. 13.

Laslo-Baker, D. *et al.*, Child neurodevelopmental outcome and maternal occupational exposure to solvents. *Arch Pediatr Adolesc Med.* 2004 Oct., 158(10):956 61.

Leg Cramps (Copyright © Smart Moms, Healthy Babies)—This publications provides information on leg cramps and how to avoid getting them during your last trimest of pregnancy.

Leslie, Joanne, 1991, 'Women's nutrition: the key to improving health in Asian countries?' Health Policy and Planning 6, No.J. A., K.K. Deshmukh and K.S. Iyer, 1986. 'Maternal mortality due to sepsis', *Journal of Obstetrics and Gynaecology* 36, No. 3 (June): 411-13.

Levy, M., Koren, G., Maternal and fetal safety of Hepatitis B vaccine in pregnancy. *Am J Perinatol* 8: 227-231, 1991.

Licu, T.A., Watson, S.E., Washington, A.E., The cost-effectiveness of prenatal carrier screening for cystic fibrosis. *Obstet Gynecol* 1994, 84:903-12.

Life Saving Skills Manual for Midwives", *American College of Nurse-Midwives*, 3rd Edition, Washington, DC, 1997.

Lincoln, C. Chen and T.N. Krishnan, eds., Women's Health in India: Risk and Vulnerability, Bombay.

Linda, J. Nicholson, ed., Feminism/Postmodernism (New York: Routledge, 1990), is an excellent collection of articles on postmodern feminism.

Lippman, A., Prenatal genetic testing and screening: Constructing needs and reinforcing inequities. *Amer J Law Med* 1991; XVII:15-50.

Listeriosis and Food Safety Tips—This brochure provides information about the risks associated with listeriosis for pregnant women, newborns, older adults and people with weakened immune systems.

Lori, B. Andrews, Jane, E. Fullarton, Neil, A. Holtzman, and Arno, G. Motulsky, eds., Assessing Genetic Risks (Washington, DC: National Academy Press, 1994).

Lozoff, B., Jordan, B., Malone, S., Childbirth in cross-cultural perspective. *Marriage Fam Rev* 1988; 35-60.

Luthra, Usha *et al.* (1992), 'Reproductive :act infections in India: need for comprehensive reproductive health policy and programs' in A. Germain *et al.*, Reproductive Tract Infections, New York: Plenum Press.

Macer, D., Niimura, Y., Umeno, T., Wakai, K., Bioethical attitudes of Japanese university doctors, and members of Japan Association of Bioethics, *Eubios J Asian Int Bioethics* 1996; 6:33-48.

Macer, D., Perception of risks and benefits of *in vitro* fertilization, genetic engineering and biotechnology. *Soc Sci Med* 1994; 38:23-33.

Macer, D.R.J., Asada, Y., Tsuzuki, M., Akiyama, S., Macer, N.Y., Bioethics in high schools in Australia, New Zealand and Japan. Christchurch: Eubios Ethics Institute, 1996.

Macer, D.R.J., *et al.*, International perceptions and approval of gene therapy *Hum Gene Therapy* 1995; 6:791-803.

Macer, D.R.J., Attitudes to Genetic Engineering: Japanese and International Comparisons. Christchurch: Eubios Ethics Institute, 1992.

Macer, D.R.J., Bioethics for the People by the People. Christchurch: Eubios Ethics Institute, 1994.

Macer, D.R.J., Bioethics: Descriptive or prescriptive? *Eubios J Asian Int Bioethics* 1995; 5:144-6.

Macer, D.R.J., Shaping Genes: Ethics, Law and Science of Using Genetic Technology in Medicine and Agriculture. Christchurch: Eubios Ethics Institute, 1990.

Macer, D.R.J., The "far east" of biological ethics. *Nature* 1992; 359:770.

Macer, D. No to "genethics", *Nature* 1993; 365:102.

Mackey, M.C., Lock, S.E., Women's Expectations of the Labor and Delivery Nurse. *J Obstet Gynecol Neonatal Nurs,* Nov./Dec0 1989; 18(6):505-12.

MacKinney, Lorren C. (1952), 'Medical Ethics and Etiquettes in Early Middle Ages : The Persistence of Hippocratic Ideals', *Bulletin of the History of Medicine,* Vol.XXVI No.1, January-February 1952.

Mahadevan, K., N.S. Murthy, P.R. Reddy, P.J. Reddy, V. Gowri, and S. Sivaraju, 1985, Infant and Childhood Mortality in India. Delhi: Mittal Publications.

Majeed, H.A., Rawashdeh, M., El-Shanti, H., Qubain, H., Khuri-Bulos, N., and Shahin, H.M. (1999), Familial Mediterranean fever in children: the expanded clinical profile Q, *J Med* 92, 309-318.

Majumdar, N., and T.N. Madan, 1956, Social Anthropology. Bombay: Himalaya Publishing House.

Mane, P., and S.A. Maitra, 1992, AIDS Prevention: The Socio-Cultural Context in India. Bombay: Tata Institute of Social Sciences.

Manning-Orenstein, G., A birth intervention: the therapeutic effects of Doula support versus Lamaze preparation on first-time mothers' working models of caregiving. *Altern Ther Health Med,* 1998 Jul, 4:4 73-81.

March of Dimes Genetic testing and gene therapy. National Survey Findings, Sept. 1992.

Mari Bhat, P.N., K. Navaneetham and S. Irudaya Rajan, 1992, 'Maternal mortality in India: estimates from an econometric model', Population Research Centre, Dharwad: Working Paper 24 (January).

Maria, C. Lugones and Elizabeth, V. Spelman, "Have We Got a Theory for You! Feminist Theory, Cultural Imperialism, and the Demand for 'The Woman's Voice Women's Studies' International Forum 6 (1983): 573-81, and Elizabeth, V. Spelman, Inessential Woman: Problems of Exclusion in Feminist Thought (Boston: Beacon Press, 1988).

Marquisa Lavelle Moerman, "Growth of the Birth Canal in Adolescent Girls," *American Journal of Obstetrics and Gynecology* 143, No. 5 (1982): 528-32; and Justin, C. Konje and Oladapo, A. Ladipo, "Nutrition and Obstructed Labor," *American Journal of Clinical Nutrition* 72, No. 1 (2001): 291S-97S.

Marteau, T.M., Towards informed decisions about prenatal testing: A review. *Prenatal Diagnosis* 1995; 15:1215-26.

Martinez-Frias, M.L., Rodriguez-Pinilla, E., Epidemiologic analysis of prenatal exposure to cough medicines containing dextromethorphan: no evidence of human teratogenicity. *Teratology*, 63:38-41, 2001

Maternal Personality, Evolution and the Sex Ratio: Do Mothers Control the Sex of the Infant? by Valerie J. Grant (1998, Routledge).

Maternal-Fetal Toxicology: A Clinician's Guide

Mathai, Rachel *et al.* (1990), 'HIV seropositivity among patients with sexually transmitted diseases in Vellore', *Indian Journal of Medical Research*, Vol. 91 (July).

Mathai, Saramma T., 1989, 'Women and the health system' in C. Gopalan and Suminder Kaur (eds.), Women and Nutrition in India. New Delhi: Nutrition Foundation of India.

Mathur, V. and P. Rohatgi, 1981, 'Maternal mortality in septic abortion', *Journal of Obstetrics and Gynaccology* 31, No. 2 (April): 272-75.

May, K.., Is it time to fire the coach? Childbirth Educator Winter 1988-89; 30-5.

Mbizvo, M.T., Reproductive and sexual health; *Central African Journal of Medicine*; 1996 March, 42(3), pp. 80-5.

McCourt, C., Page, L., Hewison, J., Vail, A., Evaluation of One-toOne Midwifery: Women's Responses to Care. *Birth*, June 1998; 25(2):73-80.

McKay, S., Smith, S.Y., "What are they talking about? Is something wrong?" Information sharing during the second stage of labor. *Birth*, 1993, Sep., 20(3):142-7.

McMartin, K.I., Chu, M., Kopecky, E., Einarson, T.R., Koren, G., Pregnancy outcome following maternal organic solvent exposure: a meta-analysis of epidemiologic studies, *Am J Ind Med.* 1998 Sep.; 34(3):288-92.

McMartin, K.I., Koren, G., Proactive approach for the evaluation of fetal safety in chemical industries.Teratology, 1999 Sep.; 60(3):130-6.

McNiven, P., Hodnett, E., O'Brien-Pallas, L.L., Supporting Women in Labor: A working Sampling Study of the Activities of Labor and Delivery Nurses. *Birth*, March 1992; 19(1):3-9.

Medica Medical Policy for Vaginal Delivery: discharge criteria. September, 1994.

Meerar Sahib, K.P. *et al.* (1990), 'Pattern of genital ulcers in and around Mangalore', *JISTE*, Vol. 11.

Mehta, A., 1983, 'Strategies for reduction of perinatal mortality in India', *Journal of Obstetrics and Gynaecology* 33, No. 6 (December): 721-33.

Mehta, A. and K. Jayant, 1981, 'Perinatal mortality survey in India (1977-79) Part I, identification of health intervention needs', *Journal of Obstetrics and Gynaecology* 32, No. 2 (April):183-215.

Mehta, S., M.E. Khan, R.B. Gupta, M.M. Gandotra and O.S. Ojha, 1983, Role of Health Service Delivery on Acceptance of Family Planning. New Delhi: ICMR, mimeo.

Mennie, M.E., Compton, M.E., Gilfillan, A., *et al.*, Prenatal screening for cystic fibrosis: psychological effects on carriers and their partners. *J Med Genet* 1993; 30:543-8.

Miller, S.R., Schwartz, R.H., Attitudes toward genetic testing of Amish, Mennonite, and Hutterite Families with Cystic Fibrosis. *Am J Pub Health* 1992; 82:236-42.

Milunsky, A., Commercialization of clinical genetic laboratory services: In whose best interest? *Obstet Gynecol* 1993; 81:627-9.

Milunsky, A., Heredity and Your Family's Health. Baltimore: John Hopkins University Press, 1992.

Ministry of Health and Family Welfare, Central Bureau of Health Intelligence, Directorate General of Health Services, 1987. Health Information of India. New Delhi: Government of India Press.

Ministry of Health and Family Welfare. 1989. Family,' Welfare Programme in India: Yearbook 1987-88. New Delhi: Ministry of Health and Family Welfare.

Ministry of Health and Family Welfare. 1990. Family Welfare Programme in India: Yearbook 1988-89. New Delhi: Ministry of Health and Family Welfare.

Ministry of Welfare, Department of Women and Child Development. 1991. 15 Years of ICDS, an Overview. New Delhi: Government of India.

Minnesota Department of Health, Statute 144.125. Tests of infants for inborn involved in newborn metabolic screening program, 1994.

Minnesota Health Statistics 1994. January 1996.

Minnesota Hospital and Healthcare Partnership: distribution of length of stay by discharge. October 1995.

Minnesota Medical Association Resolution. November, 1995.

Minnesota Nurses Association Resolution. November, 1995.

Miscarriage (Copyright © MOD)—This fact sheet explains some of the reasons why a miscarriage can occur, the tests that can be done following a miscarriage, how to prevent future miscarriages, and the recovery time you should expect before becoming pregnant again.

Mishra, D., Gurmohan Singh and D. Sharma (1988), 'Unsuspected gonococcal infection, candidiasis and trichomonmiasis in females', *IJSTD*, Vol. 9.

Mitra, I. and B.N. Khara, 1983, 'Maternal Mortality (a review of the current status in a teaching institution)', *Journal of Obstetrics and Gynaecology* 33, No. 2 (April): 209-13.

MNH (2001), Best Practices: Preventing Postpartum Hemorrhage. Baltimore: Maternal and Neonatal Health.

MNH (2001), Birth Preparedness and Complication Readiness: A Matrix of Shared Responsibility. Baltimore: Maternal and Neonatal Health.

Mondal Aftab Uddin, (1991), 'Induced abortions in rural society and need for people's awareness', *JOGI*, Vol. 41, No. 4 (August).

Morgan, D., Krueger, R., When to Use Focus Groups and Why?

Morning Sickness (Copyright © AAFP)—This publication discusses morning sickness, how long it will last, and how to help relieve morning sickness.

Mother and Baby Package", WHO, Geneva, 1994.

Motulsky, A.G., Societal problems in human and medical genetics. *Genome* 1989; 31:870-5.

Munthe, C., The moral roots of prenatal diagnosis. Ethical aspects of the early introduction and presentation of prenatal diagnosis in Sweden. Gothenburg: Centre for Research Ethics, *Studies in Research Ethics* No. 7, 1996.

Murray and Lopez, eds., Health Dimensions of Sex and Reproduction: 280.

Murray and Lopez, eds., Health Dimensions of Sex and Reproduction: 170-74.

Murray and Lopez, eds., Health Dimensions of Sex and Reproduction: 252-55.

Murray and Lopez, eds., Health Dimensions of Sex and Reproduction: 219-39.

Murray and Lopez, Health Dimensions of Sex and Reproduction; Burkhalter, "Consequences of Unsafe Motherhood in Asian countries in 2000"; and A. Prual *et al.*, "Severe Maternal Morbidity From Direct Obstetric Causes in West Africa: Incidence and Case Fatality Rates," *Bulletin of the World Health Organization* 78, No. 5 (Geneva: WHO, 2000): 593.

Murthy, G.V., Anil Goswami and Saroja Narayanan. 1990. 'Utilization patterns.of antenatal services in an urban slum', *Journal of Obstetrics and Gynaecology* 40, No. 1 (February), 42-46.

Murthy, G.V.S. *et al.* (1987), 'A Study of Pregnancy Wastage in a Rural Area of Haryana', Health and Population: Perspectives and Issues, No. 10, 26-34.

Murugan, S. *et al.* (1986), 'Pattern of late syphilis: a decade study', *IJSTD*, Vol. 7.

Nafisa Beebi, 1987. 'Five year study of maternal mortality at the Institute of Obstetrics and Gynaecology, Madras (1981-85)', *Journal of Obstetrics and Gynaecology* 37, No. 6: 820-22.

Nagel could respond to this criticism by claiming that tIme timings that matter roost to individual persons matter to all of them (p. 11). My rejoinder to this response is that morality asks more, and sometimes less or other than merely dealing with what matters most to everyone.

Nair, P.S., Muralidhar Vemuri, and Fanjdar Ram. 1989. Indian Youth. New Delhi: Mittal Publications.

Nancy, C.M., Hartsock, Money, Sex, and Power (Boston: Northeastern University Press, 1985), and The Feminist Standpoint Revisited and Other Essays (Boulder, CO: Westview Press, 1998), pp. 105-32.

Nandraj, Sunil (1994), 'Beyond the Law and the Lord : Quality of Private Healthcare' in *Economic and Political Weekly*, Vol. XXIX No. 27, pp. 1680-85, July 2.

Narayan, S., 1988, Social Anthropology. Delhi: Gian Publishing House.

National Council of Applied Economics Research (1992a). Household Survey of Medical Care, NCAER, New Delhi.

National Council of Applied Economics Research (1992b) Rural Household Healthcare Needs and Availability. NCAER, New Delhi.

National Crime Records Bureau, 1995, Crime in India-1994, New Delhi.

National Family Health Survey 2: India. International Institute for Population Sciences, 1999-2000.

National Institute of Health and Family Welfare (1985), Levels of Fertility, Mortality, Family Welfare, and Utilization of Health and Family Welfare Services—A Baseline Report of Eight Project Districts Madhya Pradesh, October.

National Nutrition Monitoring bureau (1980) Consolidated Report for 1975-79. National Institute of Nutrition, Hyderabad.

National Research Council, The Consequences of Maternal Morbidity and Maternal Mortality: Report of a Workshop (Washington, DC: National Academy Press, 2000): 6, 17.

National Sample Survey Organization (1980), 28th Round Survey on Morbidity (1973-74), Sarvekshana, July-October.

National Women's Hospital Annual Report. 1996 Inhouse Publication.National Childbirth Trust, 1993.

Nausea and Vomiting (Copyright © Smart Moms, Healthy Babies)-This fact sheet explains why morning sickness occurs, and provides some tips on how you can relieve your nausea and vomiting.

Nelkin, D.A., Tancred, L., Dangerous Diagnostics: The Social Power of Biological Information. New York: Basic Books, 1989.

Nelson, L.J., Milliken, N., Compelled medical treatment of pregnant women. *J Am Med Ass* 1988; 259:1060-6.

New trends in Maternal and Child Health, Moscow 1974, Regional office for Europe, World Health Organization.

Nigam Franesh and Mukhija, R.D. (1986), 'Pattern of sexually transmitted at Gorakhpur', *IJSTD*, Vol. 7.

Nitwe, M.T., S.V. Desai and V.R. Walvekar (1989), 'Teenage pregnancy: a health hazard', *JOGI*, Vol. 39, No. 3 (June).

Nolan, M., Supporting women in labour: the doula's role. *Mod Midwife* 1995 Mar 5:3 12-5.

Norr, N.F., Nacion, K., Outcomes of postpartum early discharge, 1960-86. A comparative review. *Birth* 1987; 14:135-141.

Note that I have identified equality as an ethical rather than psychological or empirical norm. Paradoxically, equality deserves to be supported, and is in fact supported, as an ethical norm by people who are psychologically attracted to inequality and pursue it in their empirical affairs. Most of us tend to promote the advantaged side of inequality in our own behalf.

Nulman, I., Laslo, D., Koren, G., Treatment of epilepsy in pregnancy Drugs. 1999 Apr.; 57(4):535-44. Review.

Obstetrics Care; Kathryn M. Andolsek; 1990; published by Lea and Febiger

O'Cathain, A., Thomas, K., Walters, S.J., Nicholl, J., Kirkham, M., Women's perceptions of informed choice in maternity care. *Midwifery* 2002, 18:136-144.

Of course, patterns emerge in treatment and ethical dilemmas and in ways of addressing them effectively; these patterns are useful and necessary but inadequate to the particularities of each situation. Laura Purdy (personal communication, August 3, 1998) believes that partiality and universalizability are compatible so long as the partiality practiced is judged permissible for everyone in that situation. As suggested above, however (n. 11), no one is ever in precisely the same situation as any other.

Pachauri, S. and A. Jamshedji, 1983, 'Risks of teenage pregnancy', *Journal of Obstetrics and Gynaecology* 33, No. 3 (June): 477-82.

Panat, S.P. and S.S. Mehendale, 1987, 'Maternal Mortality-review of 6 years', *Journal of Obstetrics and Gynaecology* 37, No. 3 (June): 527-29.

Parasuraman, R., *et al.* 1992, "STD and AIDS in Homosexuals." Abstracts of the Second International Congress on AIDS in Asia and the Pacific. Rand Wick, Australia: AIDS Society of Asia and the Pacific, p. 200.

Parvovirus B19 Infection and Pregnancy—This fact sheet provides information about parvovirus B19 infection and pregnancy. It describes illnesses caused by this infection (including Fifth Disease) the signs and symptoms, the affects it has during pregnancy, results of blood tests, and treatment.

Pastuszak, A., Levy, M., Shick Boschetto, B., Zuber, C., Feldkamp, M., Gladstone, J., BarLevy, F., Jackson, E., Meschino, W., Koren, G., Outcome after maternal varicella infection in the first 20 weeks of pregnancy. *N Engl J Med* 330; 901-905, 1994.

Pastuszak, A.L. *et al.*, Outcome after maternal varicella infection in the first 20 weeks of pregnancy. *N Engl J Med*. 1994, Mar 31; 330(13):901-5.

Pastuszak, A.L., Koren, G., Varicella infection in pregnancy. *N Engl J Med* 331: 482, 1994.

Paul, B.K., Maternal Mortality in Africa: 1980-87, *Soc Sci Med* 1993, Sep.; 37(6); 745-52.

Pavitharn, K. (1988), 'Effects of sexually transmitted diseases on the foetus and neonate', *Indian Journal of Dermatology Venerology and Leprology*, Vol. 54.

Pawar, M.S., 1991, "Prostitution and the Girl Child." *Indian Journal of Social Work*, 52(1).

Petchesky Rosalind Pollack (1986), Abortion and Women's Choice : The State, Sexuality and Reproductive Freedom, Verso, London.

Phillips, F.S. and Ghouse, N. (1976), 'Septic Abortion—Three Year Study, 1971-73. Hazards of Septic Abortion as compared to Medical Termination of Pregnancy at Government Earkine Hospital, Madurai' in *Journal of Obstetrics and Gynaecology of India*, 26 (5).

Pittard, W.B. and Geddes, K.M., Newborn hospitalization: a closer look. *J Pediatrics* 1988; 112:257-261.

Planning Commission, Government of India, 1985, 'Steering Group Report Part III. Rural and Urban Health Services in the Seventh Plan', *Indian Journal of Pediatrics*, 52: 217-22.

Post, M., Preventing Maternal Mortality through Emergency Obstetric Care; SARA Issues Papers, April 1997.

Pradeep Kumar *et al.* (1990), 'Trichomoniasis and candidiasis in consorts of females with vaginal discharge', *IJSTD*, Vol. II.

Prasad, Shally, 1996, "Instituting Measures to Address Violence Against Women in India," paper presented at the Association of Women in Development International Conference, Washington, DC.

Pre-eclampsia (Copyright © AAFP)—This handout provides information on the symptoms of pre-eclampsia, possible treatments and the risks to the women and her pregnancy.

Pregnancy: What to Expect When It's Past Your Due Date (Copyright © AAFP)-This fact sheet provides information on overdue pregnancy, how the due date is determined, and why your doctor may decide to induce labor, and if so, how labor is medically induced.

Prendiville, W.J., Elbourne, D., McDonald, S., Active versus expectant management of the third stage of labour. In: Neilson, J.P., Crowther, C.A., Hoidnett, E.D., Hofmeyer, G.J., Keirse, MJNC (eds). Pregnancy and Childbirth Module of the Cochrane Database of Systematic Reviews, (updated 3 June 1997). Available in the Cochrane Library (database on disk and CDROM). The Cochrane Collaboration, Issue 3. Oxford: Update Software; 1997. Updated quarterly.

Presidents' Commission for the study of ethical problems in Medicine, and Biomedical and Behavioural Research. Screening and Counseling for Genetic Conditions: the ethical, social and legal implications of genetic screening, counseling and education programs. Washington D.C.: U.S.G.P.O., 1983.

Prolonged use of a nasograstric tube for feeding involves risks of dislodgement and aspiration into tlme esophagus.

Raichowdhuri, G., Veena Ganju and Rupali Dewan, 1990, 'Review of maternal mortality over nine year period at Safdarjang Hospital, New Delhi', *Journal of Obstetrics and Gynaecology* 40, No. 1 (February): 84-88.

Raina Jay (1992), 'New Rules for Nursing Homes Soon' in *Hindustan Times*, New Delhi, January 15.

Rama Krishnaiah, Y. *et al.* (1989), 'Clinical profile of STD clinic patients seropositive for HIV antibodies', *IJSTD*, Vol. 10.

Ramachandran, Prema, 1989, 'Nutrition in pregnancy' in C. Gopalan and Summinder Kaur (eds.), Women and Nutrition in India. New Delhi: Nutrition Foundation of India.

Ramachandran, Prema. 1989a, 'Lactation-nutrition-fertility interaction' in C. Gopalan and Suminder Kaur (eds.), Women and Nutrition in India. New Delhi: Nutrition Foundation of India.

Ramachandran, Prema, 1992, "Women's Vulnerability." *Seminar*, 396:21-25.

Ramalingaswami, V., 1985, The state of life: Report of the National Seminar on reducing incidence of low birth weight babies in India. New Delhi: National Institute of Public Cooperation and Child Development.

Ramanath, T.B.B.S.V. *et al.* (1981a), 'Level of Knowledge about STD, *IJSTD*, Vol. 2.

Ramanath, T.B.B.S.V. *et al.* (1981b), 'Pshchosocial factors and attitudes of patients towards STDs', *IJSTD*, Vol. 2.

Ramasuren, R. (1992), 'Sexual behaviour and conditions of healthcare potential risks in HIV transmission to India' in T. Dyson (ed.), Sexual Behaviour and Networking, Anthropological and Socio-culture Studies on the Transmission of HIV, Liegs Derouaux Ordins.

Ramsey, P., Fabricated Man: The Ethics of Genetic Control. New Haven: Yale University Press, 1970.

Rao, V.N. and Pense, G.A. (1975), 'Analysis of Acceptors of MTPs in Maharashtra' in *The Journal of Family Welfare*, No.XXII, pp.64-73.

Rao, Vijaycmdra and Francis, Bloch, 1993, "Wife-beating, Its Causes and Its Implications for Nutrition Allocations to Children: An Economic and Anthropological Case-Study of a Rural South-Indian Community," University of Michigan, Population Studies Center, Research Report No. 93-298, Ann Arbor.

Raphael, D., Support and variation, the needs of the breast-feeding woman. *Acta Paediatr Jpn*, 1989 Aug, 31:4 369-72.

Reddy, G., D. Narayana, P. Eswar, and A.K. Sreedharan, 1983, "A Report on Urban (Madras) College Students' Attitudes Towards Sex." *Antiseptic*, September, pp. 1-5.

Registrar General and Census Commissioner India. 1991. Provisional Population Totals (Rural-Urban Distribution), (New Delhi), paper number 2 of 1991.

Registrar General of India (1979), Survey Report on Levels, Trends and Differentials in Fertility. India, Ministry of Home Affairs New Delhi.

Registrar General, 1987, Survey of causes of death (Rural): annual report 2984 and 2986.

Registrar-General of India (1988), Fertility in India-An Analysis of 1981 Census Data. Census of India, 1981, Occasional Paper No. 13 of 1988, Demography Division, Ministry of Home Affairs, New Delhi.

Registrar-General of India (1989), Sample Registration System, 1988, New Delhi, Ministry of Home Affairs, Government of India.

Reid, M., Garcia, J., Women's view of care during pregnancy and childbirth.

Report 5 of the Council on Scientific Affairs (A-95). Impact of 24-hour postpartum stay on infant and maternal health.

Report on confidential enquiries into maternal deaths in the United Kingdom 1991-1993, HMSO, 1996.

Reproductive tract infections among women in the third world. New York:

Researchers Identify Risk Factors for Pre-eclampsia in Hypertensive Women-Information about the risks of hypertension before and during pregnancy.

Revel, M., Genetic Counseling. pp. 9-38 in Proceedings of the Third Session of the International Bioethics Committee, Paris: UNESCO, 1996.

Richard, A. McCormick, "Blastomere Separation," Hastings Center Report 24,2, (March-April 1.994): 14-46.

Riggs, J.W., Blanco, J.D., Post partum complications in management of labour and delivery. Ed. Creasy, R.K., Ch. 10:223-255. Blackwell, 1996.

Robertson, J.A., Procreative liberty and the control of conception, pregnancy, and childbirth. *Virginia Law Review* 1983; 69:405-64.

Romito, P., Zaleteo, C. Social history of a research project: a study on early postpartum discharge. *Soc Sci Med* 1992; 34:227-235.

Rona, R.J., Beech, R., Mandalia, S., *et al.*, The influence of genetic counseling in the era of DNA testing on knowledge, reproductive intentions and psychological well-being. *Clin Genet* 46; 1994:198-204.

Rosemarie Tong, Feminist Thought (Boulder, CO: Westview Press, 1998), p. 7.

Rosenzweig, M. and T.P. Schultz (1982), 'Market Opportunities, Genetic Endowment and Intra-Family Research Distribution—Survival in Rural India', *American Economic Review*, 72, 803-15.

Ross, Susan Rae (1998), Promoting Quality Maternal and Newborn Care: A Reference Manual for Program Managers, CARE.

Rovet, J., Cole, S., Nulman, I., Scolnik, D., Altmann, D., Koren, G., The effects of maternal epilepsy on children's neurodevelopment, *Child Neuropsychol* 1: 1-8, 1995.

Roy Choudhary, S. and O.N. Jayaswal, 1989, 'Infant and early childhood mortality in urban slums under ICDS scheme—a prospective study', *Indian Pediatrics* 26, No. 6 (June): 544-49.

Royston, Eric and Sue Armstrong (eds.), 1989, Preventing Maternal Deaths. Geneva: World Health Organization.

S.K. Khanna, 1997, Traditions and Reproductive Technology in an Urbanizing North Indian Village, *Soc. Sci. Med.*, 44, 171-180.

S.S. Sheth and A.N. Malpani, Inappropriate use of new technology: Impact on women's health, *International Journal of Gynecology and Obstetrics*, 58 (1997) 159-165; V. Hingorani and G. Shroff, Natural sex selection for safe motherhood and as a solution for population control, *International Journal of Gynecology and Obstetrics*, 56 (1995) S169-S171.

S.S. Wadley, 1993, Family composition strategies in rural north India. *Soc. Sci. Med.* 37, 1367-1376.

Sadik, Nafis, 1980, 'Family planning: improving the health of women', Draper Fund Report: 9 (October)

Safe Motherhood Factsheet, Family Care International and the Safe Motherhood Interagency Group, October 1997.

Safe Vitamin A Dosage During Pregnancy and Lactation: Recommendations and a Report of a Consultation", WHO and The Micronutrient Initiative, Geneva, 1998.

Sai, Fred T. and Janet Nassim, 1989, 'The need for a reproductive health approach International *Journal of Gynaecology and Obstetrics, Supplement* 3:103-13.

Samasuhban, R., Nigel Cook and B. Singh (1990), 'Educationa, Approach to Leprosy Contact: A Study of Knowledge, Attitudes and Practices in Two Poor Localities in Bombay', Bombay, Centre for Social and Technological Studies.

Sandra Harding, The Science Question in Feminism (Ithaca, NY: Cornell University Press, 1986), p. 195.

Sangeeta Krishna, 2002, Death Wish for Daughters: Son Preference and Daughter Aversion in Bihari Folk Songs, Manushi, v. 131.

Sanyal, M.K., T.N. Mukherjee and A.K. Chatterjee (1989), 'MTP: a four years study in rural medical college of West Bengal', *JOGI,* Vol. 39, No. 1 (February).

Sanyal, Ratna *et al.* (1991), 'Study on septic abortion in a rural medical college', *JOGI,* Vol. 41, No. 4 (August).

Sara Ruddick, Maternal Thinking: Toward a Politics of Peace (New York: Ballantine Books, 1989).

Saramma Thomas Mathai (1989), 'Women and the Health System' in C. Gopalan and Suminder Kaur (eds.) Women and Nutrition in India Nutrition Foundation of India Special Publication series no. 5, Hyderabad.

Sarbajna, Shankar (1991), 'Intrauterine device as a means of contraception in our population', *JOGI,* Vol. 41, No. 4 (August).

Savara, M. (1992), 'Sexuality', *Seminar,* 396 (August).

Savara, Mira, and C.R. Shridhar, 1992, "Sexual Behaviour of Urban Educated Indian Women. Results of a Survey." *Journal of Family Welfare,* 38(1):30-43.

Schachter, J. *et al.* (1975), 'Chlamydial infection in women with cervical dysphasia', *American Journal of Obstetrics and Gynaecology,* Vol. 123.

Schatz, M., Zeiger, R.S., Harden, K., Hoffman, C.C., Chilingar, L., Petitti, D., The safety of asthma and allergy medications during pregnancy. *J Allergy Clin Immunol,* 1997, 100:301-6.

Schwartz, R.M., Short stay hospitalization for mother and newborns: concerns and issues. submitted to Maternal and Child Health Bureau. Providence: RI: The National Perinatal Information Center. November 1994. *Science* 248 (May 20, 1990): 1023.

Scot, Hilda (1974), Does Socialism Liberate Women, Beacon, Boston, pp.190 as quoted by Petchesky Rosalind Pollack in 'Abortion and Women's Choice: The State, Sexuality and Reproductive Freedom, Verso, London.

Scott, K.D., Berkowitz, G., Klaus, M., A comparison of intermittent and continuous support during labor: a meta-analysis. *Am J Obstet Gynecol,* 1999 May, 180:5 1054-9.

Scott, K.D., Klaus, P.H., Klaus, M.H., The obstetrical and postpartum benefits of continuous support during childbirth. *J Womens Health Gend Based Med* 1999, Dec.; 8:1257-64.

Seal, K., Maternity mayhem. Maternity 1995. See Carol Gilligan, "Moral Orientation and Moral Development," in Eva Feder Kittay and Diana, T. Meyer, eds., Women and Moral Theory (Totowa, NJ: Rowman and Littlefield, 1987), pp.19-33.

Seibold, C., Miller, M., Hall, J., Midwives and women in partnership: the ideal and the real, *Aust J Adv Nurs* 1999, 17:21-27.

Seller, M.J., Genetic counseling, pp. 961-970 in Gillon, R., ed. Principles of Healthcare Ethics. London: John Wiley and Sons Ltd, 1994.

Sen Gupta, Amit and A.G. Gode, 1988, 'A comparative study of maternal mortality and morbidity in a teaching hospital of Northern India'. *Journal of Obstetrics and Gynaecology* 38, No. 2: 177-81.

Sen, Iyer and George (2002); *ibid.*

SFI, Safe Motherhood Resource Guide. Available on the web.

Sharma, N. and P. Bali, 1989, 'Care of the newborn by traditional birth attendants', *Indian Padiatrics* 26, No. 7 (July): 649-53.

Shaw, G.M., Todoroff, K., Velie, E.M., Lammer, E.J., Maternal illness, including fever, and medication use as risk factors for neural tube defects. *Teratology* 57:1-7, 1998.

Shearer, B., Birth Assistant: new ally for the parents-to-be. *Childbirth Educator Spring*, 1989; 26-31.

Shortness of Breath During Pregnancy (Copyright © Smart Moms, Healthy Babies)—This fact sheet explains the shortness of breath you may experience during your third trimester, as the baby's weight presses on your diaphragm and digestive organs.

Sibley, L., Obstetric First Aid in the community-partners in safe motherhood. *J Nurse Midwifery*, 1997, Mar.-Apr.; 42(2):117-21

Siddappa, K.,V., Jagannath Kumar and A.K. Bajaj (1990), 'Pattern of STDs at Davangere', *IJSTD*, Vol. 11.

Simkin, P., Just Another Day in a Woman's Life? Women's Long-term Perceptions of Their First Birth Experience. Part I, *Birth*, Dec. 1991; 18:4, Part II, *Birth*, June 1992; 19:2.

Simone de Beauvoir, "The Second Sex," in Mary Briody Mahowald, ed., Philosophy of Woman (Indianapolis: Hackett, 1992), p. 82.

Singer, E., Public attitudes toward genetic testing. *Pop Res and Policy Rev*, 1991; 10:235-55.

Singh, K.G., M.K. Joshi and A.K. Bajaj (1990), 'Pattern of STDs in Allahabad', *IJSTD*, Vol. 11.

Singh, Meharban and V.K. Paul, 1988, 'Strategies to reduce perinatal and neonatal mortality', *Indian Pediatrics* 25, No. 6 (June): 499-509.

Singh, Meharban, 1986, 'Hospital based data on perinatal and neonatal mortality in India', *Indian Pediatrics* 23, No. 8 (August): 579-84.

Singh, Surinder, Jagjeet Singh, Sushila Mittal, R.K.D. Goel, Tejbir Singh and S.K. Oberoi, 1988, 'A study of antenatal services in rural area of district Bathinda of Punjab', *Journal of Obstetrics and Gynaecology* 38, No. 1 (February): 22-26.

Situation Analysis on the Reproductive health of women in Pakistan.; 1995; College of Physicians and Surgeons , Pakistan.

Snow, V., Mottur-Pilson, C., Hickner, J.M. Principles of appropriate antibiotic use for acute sinusitis in adults. *Ann Intern Med.* 20;134:495-7, 2001.

Some authors have questioned the ternm "maternal-fetal conflict" on grounds that tlme disagreements to which the term refers generally occur between clinicians and pregnant women. Typically, both want what is best for the fetus but they have different views on bow to pursue that goal. Ellen, J. Stein, 'Maternal-Fetal Conflict: Reformulating the Equation," in Andrew Grubb, ed., Challenges in Medical Care (Chichester: John Wiley and Sons, 1992), pp. 91-92.

Some of the material developed here is drawn from my article on Treatment of Myopia: Feminist Standpoint Theory and Bioethics," in Susan, W. Wolf, ed., Feminism and Bioethics (New York: Oxford University Press, 1996), pp. 95-111.

Sosa, R., Kennell, J., Klaus, M., Robertson, S., Urrutia, J., The effect of a supportive companion on perinatal problems, length of labor, and mother-infant bonding interaction. *N Engl J Med,* Sept. 11, 1980; 303(11):597-600.

Successful Focus Groups. Advancing the State of the Arte (Edited by: Morgan, D.). Sage Focus Edition 1993, 3-19.

Sundari, T.K. (1993), 'Can Health Education Improve Pregnancy Outcome? Report of a Grassroots Action-Education Campaign'. *Journal of Family Welfare,* March.

Super, M., Pembrey, M., Morrison, P.J. *et al.,* Non-directive genetic counseling. *Lancet* 1991; 338:1266-8.

Suresh Mohammed, 'The Ugandan response to HIV/Aids: some lessons for India', *The National Medical Journal of India* 16(5), 2003.

Susan Sherwin, No Langer Patient (Philadelphia: Temple University Press, 1991), p. 75.

Suzuki, D., Knudtson, P., Genethics: The Clash Between the New Genetics and Human Values Boston:Harvard University Press, 1989.

Swelling and Varicose Veins, During Pregnancy (Copyright © Smart Moms, Healthy Babies)—During your second and third trimesters, you may experience swelling in your legs and ankles, or varicose veins. These symptoms are normal during pregnancy, and this fact sheet provides tips to relieve your discomfort.

T. Mikkelsen B., Training in the management of critical obstetrics problems; *European Journal of Obstetrics,* Gynecology and Reproductive Biology; 1996 March, 65(1), pp. 149-51.

Tata Institute of Social Sciences, October 1994, *Indian Journal of Social Work,* Bombay, 55(4).

Taylor, K., Copstick, S., Psychological care in labour. *Nurs Mirror,* July 24, 1985; 161(4):42-3.

Teebi, A.S., (1994), Autosomal recessive disorders among Arabs: An overview from *Kuwait, J Med Genet* 31, 224-233 [PubMed].

Teich, A.H. and Frankel, M.S., eds., The Genome, Ethics and the Law: Issues in Genetic Testing. Washington: AAAS, 1992.

Thankappan, K.R. and V. Ramankutty (1990), 'Immunization Coverage in Kerala and the Role of the Integrated Child Development Scheme Programme', *Health Policy and Planning*, Vol. 5, No. 3, 267-73.

Thayaparan B; Prevention and control of tetanus in childhood. *Curr Opin Pediatr*, 1998 Feb.; 10(1):4-8.

The "if" in this statement is intended to allow for tIme possibility that the interests of one party are never precisely the same as those of another.

The democratic justification for participation may be construed as a deontological argument, e.g., one based on the inalienable right of persons to participate in the development of social policies that affect them. Admittedly, utilitarian arguments may be invoked to curtail as well as to demand participation by non-dominant groups. The utilitarian rationale for their participation gives priority to the greatest number of subjects to whom utility is to he applied; this is a democratic interpretation of utilitarianism. The utilitarian rationale opposing their participations gives priority to the best consequences (greatest happiness), wInch may be achieved undemocratically by allowing the exclusion of specific groups or individuals.

The European Group of Advisors on Ethical Issues Related to Biotechnology. Ethical aspects of prenatal diagnosis. Brussels: European Commission, Feb. 1996.

The potential of the traditional birth Attendant" WHO offset publication, No 95, World Health Organisation, Geneva, 1986.

The QED defines genetics as "that branch of biology which is concerned with the study of natural development when not complicated by human interference" and as the scientific study of heredity and variation." Heredity is defined property of organic beings, in virtue of which offspring inherit the nature and characteristics of parents and ancestors generally." *The Oxford English Dictionary*, 2nd ed. (Oxford: Clarendon Press, 1989), Vol. 6, p. 440, and Vol. 7, p. 163.

The Working Group on Antiretroviral Therapy and Medical Management of HIV-Infected Children. Guidelines for the use of antiretroviral agents in pediatric HIV infection. December 13, 2001

The World Bank, 1996, Improving Women's Health in India, Washington, DC.

Thomas, Nagel, Equality and Partiality (New York: Oxford University Press, 1991), pp. 10-20.

Thorpe, K., Harker, L., Pike, A., Marlow, N., Women's views of ultrasonography. A comparison of women's experiences of antenatal ultrasound screening with cerebral ultrasound of their newborn infant. *Soc Sci Med* 1993, 36:311-315.

Thurston, N.E., *et al.*, Evaluation of an early postpartum discharge program. *Canadian J Pub Health* 1985; 76:384-387.

Till, C., Koren, G., Rovet, J.F., Prenatal exposure to organic solvents and child neurobehavioral performance. *Neurotoxicol Teratol* 2001; 23: 235-45

Till, C., Westall, C.A., Rovet, J.F., Koren, G., Effects of maternal occupational exposure to organic solvents on offspring visual functioning: a prospective controlled study. *Teratology* 2001; 64: 134-41.

Tinker, Anne, Patricia Daly, Cynthia Green, Helen Saxenian, Rama Lakshminarayanan, and Kirrin Gill, 1994, Women's Health and Nutrition: Making a Difference. World Bank Discussion Paper 256. Washington, D.C.: World Bank

Tom, L., Beauchamp and James Childress, The Principles of Biomedical Ethics (New York: Oxford University Press, 1979, 1983, 1989, 1994).

Toxoplasmosis and Pregnancy (Copyright © AAFP)-Toxoplasmosis is an infection that occurs during pregnancy and can affect the unborn child. This fact sheet explains prevention of toxoplasmosis, and treatment methods.

Trakroo, P.L. and S.D. Kapoor (1990), A Study to Identify Problems and Patterns of Acceptability and Utilization of Healthcare Services by Scheduled Caste Population in Rural India. National Institute of Health and Family Welfare, New Delhi.

Treatment of PKU means dietary restriction that avoids the onset or exacerbation of symptoms.

Trigg, M.E., Geier, M.R., On the relationship between academic and private genetic services. *Am J Hum Genet* 1992; 51:890-1.

Tsui *et al.*, eds., Reproductive Health in Developing Countries: 122-23.

U.S. Bureau of the Census, International Programs Center, 1995, HIV/AIDS in Asia, Research Note No. 18, Washington, DC.

U.S. Congress, Office of Technology Assessment. Cystic fibrosis and DNA tests: Implications of carrier screening. Washington D.C.: U.S.G.P.O., 1992.

U.S. Congress, Office of Technology Assessment. New Developments in Biotechnology, 2: Public Perceptions of Biotechnology-Background Paper. Washington D.C.: U.S.G.P.O., 1987.

Uma Narayan, 1997, Dislocating cultures: Identities, traditions and third world feminism, Routledge.

UNESCO International Bioethics Committee, Universal Declaration on the Human Genome and Human Rights. Paris: UNESCO 1997.

UNICEF website; www.unicef.org

UNICEF Women-friendly health services; The Women and Maternal Health Project inBangladesh. Bangladesh

United Nations Children's Fund(UNICEF), 1995, The Progress of Indian States, New Delhi.

Urinary Tract Infections During Pregnancy (Copyright © AAFP)-This publication contains information on Urinary Tract infections (UTI), how it can affect your baby, how it can be treated, and what to do to prevent them from reoccurring.

V. Fauveau; Maternal tetanus; International Journal of Gyn and Obs, 1993, 40; 3-12.

Vehvilainen-Julkunen, K., Liukkonen A. Father's experiences of childbirth. *Midwifery,* March 1998; 14(1):10-7.

Verp, M.S., Heckerling, P.S., Use of decision analysis to evaluate patients' choices of diagnostic prenatal test. *Am J Med Genet* 1995; 58:337-44.

Victor, A., MeKusick, *Mendeltan Inheritance in Man,* 11th ed., Vol. 1 (Baltimore: Johns Hopkins University Press, 1994), p. xvii.

Vijay Kumar, B.R. Garg and M.C. Baruah (1990), 'A clinical study of genital ulcers', *IJSTD,* Vol. 11.

Villar, J., Ba'aqeel, H., Piaggio, G., Lumbiganon, P., Miguel Belizan, J., Farnot, U., Al-Mazrou, Y., Carroli, G., Pinol, A., Donner, A., Langer, A., Nigenda, G., Mugford, M., Fox-Rushby, J., Hutton, G., Bergsjo, P., Bakketeig, L., Berendes, H., Garcia, J., WHO antenatal care randomised trial for the evaluation of a new model of routine antenatal care. *Lancet,* 2001, 357:1551-1564.

Visaria, P. 1971. The Sex Ratio of the Population of India. Monograph No. 10, *Census of India,* Volume 1, New Delhi: Manager of Publications.

von Dadelszen, P., Ornstein, M.P., Bull, S.B., Logan, A.G., Koren, G., Magee, L.A., Fall in mean arterial pressure and fetal growth restriction in pregnancy hypertension: a meta-analysis. *Lancet,* 2000 Jan. 8; 355(9198):87-92.

W.B. Hanley, J.T.R. Clarke, and W. Schoonheyt, "Maternal Phenylketonuria (PKU)—A Review," *Clinical Biochemistry* 20 (June 1987): 149-56.

W.B. Hanley, R. Koch, H.L. Levy, R. Matalon, B. Rouse, C. Azen, and F. de la Cruz, "The North American Maternal Phsenylketonuria Collaborative Study, Develop-mental Assessment of the Offspring: Preliminary Report," *European Journal of Pediatrics* 155, Suppl. 1 (July 1996): 5169-72; R. Koch, C. Azen, E.C. Friedman, K. Fishier, C. Baumann-Frischsling, and T. Lin, *European Journal of Pediatrics* 155, Suppl. 1 (July 1996): S90-92; and R. Koch, H. Ley, W. Hanley, R. Matalong, B. Rouse, F. Trefx, and F. de ha Crux, "Outcome Implications of the International Maternal Phenylketonuria Collaborative Study (MPKUCS)," *European Journal of Pediatrics* 155, Suppl. 1 (July 1996): S162-64.

Waisbren, S.E., Shiloh, S., St. James, P., Levy, H.L., Psychosocial factors in maternal phenylketonuria: Prevention of unplanned pregnancies. *Am J Public Health,* 1991; 81:299-304.

Waldenstrom, U., Axelsson, O., Nilsson, S., Eklund, G., Fall, O., Lindeberg, S., Sjodin, Y., Effects of routine one-stage ultrasound screening in pregnancy: a randomised controlled trial. *Lancet* 1988, 2:585-588.

Waldenström, U., Borg, I.M., Olsson, B., Sköld, M., Wall, S., The Childbirth Experience: A Study of 295 New Mothers. *Birth,* September 1996; 23(3):144-53.

Waldenstrom, U., Early discharge as voluntary and involuntary alternatives to a longer postpartum stay in hospital-effects on mother's experiences and breast-feeding. *Midwifery,* 1989; 5:189-196.

Walia, I. (1988), 'Health Services and the Rural Pregnant, *The Nursing Journal of India,* September.

Wang, D., Mao, X., Qian, S., Clinical observation on Doula delivery. *Chung Hua Fu Chan Ko Tsa Chih,* 1997, Nov. 32:11 659-61.

Warren, M.A., Gendercide: The Implications of Sex Selection. Totowa, N.J.: Rowman and Allanheld, 1985.

Wasserheit, J.N. and Holmes, K.K. (1992), 'Reproductive tract infections: challenges for international health policy, programs and research' in A. Germain *et al.,* Reproductive Tract Injections, N. York: Plenum Press.

Watson, E.K., Marchant, J., Bush, A., Williamson, B., Attitudes towards prenatal diagnosis and carrier screening for cystic fibrosis among the parents of patients in a paediatric cystic fibrosis clinic. *J Med Genet.,* 1992; 29:490-1.

Watts, Alan, 1974, Erotic Spirituality: The Vision of Konarak. New York: Collier Books.

Weinrich, James D., 1987, Sexual Landscapes: Why We An What We Are, Why We Love Whom We Love. New York: Scribners.

Welkenhuysen, M., Evers-Kiebooms, G., Decruyenaere, M., Van den Berghe, H., Unrealistic optimism and genetic risk. *Psychology and Health,* 1996; 11:479-492.

Welkenhuysen, M. *et al.,* Adolescents' attitude towards carrier testing for cystic fibrosis and its relative stability over time. *Eur J Hum Genet* 1996; 4:52-62.

Well, S.I. [?], *Am J Perinatol,* September 1993.

Wertz, D.C., Fletcher, J.C., Berg, K., Guidelines on Ethical Issues in Medical Genetics and the Provision of Genetics Services. Geneva: World Health Organization, 1995, rev 1996 (Document: WHO/HDP/GL/ ETH/95.1).

Wertz, D.C., Fletcher, J.C. eds., Ethics and human genetics: A cross cultural perspective. Heidelberg: Springer-Verlag, 1989.

Wertz, D.C., Fletcher, J.C., Fatal Knowledge? Prenatal diagnosis and sex selection. Hastings Center Report, 1989; 19(3): 21-27.

Wertz, D.C., Rosenfield, J.M., Janes, S.R., Erbe, R.W., Attitudes toward abortion among parents of children with cystic fibrosis. *Am J Pub Health* 1991; 81:992-6.

White Ribbon Alliance India (2000), Safe Motherhood at Home: Realities, Perspectives and Challenges-A Report. New Delhi: WRAI.

WHO (1998), Postpartum Care of the Mother and Newborn: A Practical Guide, WHO, Geneva.

WHO (2000), Improving Access to Quality Care in Family Planning: Medical Eligibility Criteria for Contraceptive Use. Geneva: WHO Reproductive Health and Research.

Williams, Walter, 1986, The Spirit and the Flesh: Sexual Diversity in American Indian Culture. Boston: Beacon Press.

Wolman, W.L., Chalmers, B., Hofmeyr, G.J., Nikodem, V.C., Postpartum depression and companionship in the clinical birth environment: A randomized, controlled study. *Am J Obstet Gynecol,* May 1993; 168(5):1388-93.

Women and Children in Healthcare: An Unequal Majority (New York Oxford University Press, 1993), pp. 3-19.

Women, health, and reproduction (Edited by: Roberts Helen). London; Boston, Routledge and Kegan Paul 1981, xii, 196 p..

World Bank, 1993, World Development Report 1993: Investing in Health. New York: Oxford University Press.

World Bank, 1994, A New Agenda for Women's Health and Nutrition. Washington, D.C.: The World Bank.

World Bank, 1994, Population and Development: Implications for The World Bank. Washington, D.C.: The World Bank.

World Bank, 1994, World Bank HIV/AIDS Activities. Population, Health, and Nutrition Department. Washington, D.C.: The World Bank.

World Bank, 1995, Investing in People: The World Bank in Action. Washington, D.C.: The World Bank.

World Bank, 1995, Working with NGOs. Operations Policy Department. Washington, D.C.: The World Bank.

World Bank, 1996, Improving Women's Health in India. Washington, D.C.: The World Bank.

World Health Organization (1981), Non-gonococcal Urethritis and Other Sexually Transmitted Diseases of Public Health importance, Technical Report Series Geneva: WHO.

World Health Organization, 1996, "Revised 1990 Estimates of Maternal Mortality: A New Approach by WHO and UNICEF," WHO/FRH/MSM/96.11, Geneva.

www.commitnit.com/st2001/sld-3263.html, Safer Motherhood 2000: Towards A Framework for Behavior Change to reduce maternal death

www.who.int/reproductive-health/publication/MSM_98_3/MSM_98_3_chapter12.en.html

www.who.int/rht/document/reduction-of- maternal-mortality 02-Nov-00

Yanover, M.J.; Jones, D.; Miller, M.D.; Perinatal care of low-risk mothers and infants. *N. Engl. J. Med.* 1976; 294:702-705.

Zechmeister, I., Foetal images: the power of visual technology in antenatal care and the implications for women's reproductive freedom. *Healthcare Anal* 2001, 9:387-400.

Zhang, J., Bernasko, J.W., Leybovich, E., Fahs, M., Hatch, M.C., Continuous labor support from labor attendant for primiparous women: a meta-analysis. *Obstet Gynecol,* 1996 Oct., 88:4 Pt 2 739-44

Zimmerli, W.C., Who has the right to know the genetic constitution of a particular person?, pp. 93-110 in Human Genetic Information: Science, Law and Ethics, Ciba Foundation Symposium 149. Amsterdam: Elsevier North Holland, 1990.

Index

Abnormal Fetal Prevention, 260
Abortion, 85
    Causes, 97
    Scenario, 89
After Birth Supervision, 27
After Childbirth;
    Mother Needs Critical Care, 23
Ageing Polpulation, 209
AMA (American Medical Association), 86
Aneschesia and Pain Relief, 9
Antisperm Antibodies, 140
Appropriate Antenatal Care, 24
Assisted Hospital Birth, 61
Azoospermia, 138

B.B.T. (Basal Body Temperature), 143
Birth Injuries, 261
Bleeding in the Brain, 76
Breast Cancer, 182
Breastfeeding;
    Counteracting Common Myths, 64

Caesarean Delivery, 1
Cancer Control, 197
Care of Newborn, 50
Cervical Cancer, 187
Caesarean Section;
    Complications, 14, 18
    Reasons, 17
Childbirth Complications, 260
Childbirth;
    First Stage Management, 4
    Second Stage Management, 5
    Risks Involved, 12
Chlamydia, 121
CHW (Community Health Workers), 27
Clinical Data, 25
CNM (Certified Nurse Midwife), 62
Colorectal Cancer, 203
Complications;
    Detection and Management, 24
Coping Skills, 78
Counseling for Breastfeeding, 48

Dealing with HIV, 59
Delivery Care, 26
Domestic Violence, 280
Dowry Mania, 108
DPP (Diabetes Prevention Program), 206
DUB (Dysfunctional Uterine Bleeding), 190
Dwindling Public Health Expenditure, 90

Emergency Childbirth Situation, 67
Emergency Contraception, 101
Endometrial Biopsy, 145
Endometriosis;
    Management, 150

Family Welfare Services, 273
Female Infertility, 148
    Interventions, 148
Fertility;
    How to Resore?, 146
Fertility is a Team Work, 131
Fetal Distress, 10
Fillingim, Rager B., 167

Gamete Intrafallopian Transfer, 148
Gestational Diabetes, 206
Global Maternity Coverage, 220
Gonorrhoea, 121

Health and Diseases in Women;
    Ayurvedic Point of View, 312
Health Education, 25
    Effectiveness, 211
Health Partners, 258
Herpes, 122
Hormonal Assessment, 144
Hormonal Defects, 137
Hormone Therapy, 147
HPV Infection, 185
Hypertension, 41

IDD (Iodine Deficiency Disorder), 25
India;
    Women's Health, 275
Inevitable Abortion, 97
Invision on the Uterus, 8

Induced Abortion, 92
Infant and Maternal Mortality, 195
Infertile Couple, 135
Infertility, 120
  Exclusive Male Factors, 134
Integrating Services, 28
Intracy to Plasmic Sperm Injection, 148

Johnson, John M., 166

Laboratory Measures, 36
Labour;
  First Stage, 43
  Second Stage, 44
  Third Stage, 44
LAM (Lactational Amenorrhea Method), 49
Legal Abortions, 100
Leong, N.K.Y., 264

Major Maternal Problems, 31
Male;
  Physical Examination, 139
Male Responsibility, 272
Mal-presentations, 10
Maternal Discharge;
  Guidelines, 242
Maternal Health;
  Interventions to Improve, 34
Maternal Medical Conditions, 11
Maternal Morbidity, 23
  Causes, 30
  Global, 23
Maternal Nutrition, 25
Maternity Care, 220
Menstrual Regulation, 115
Menstruation, 130
Missed Abortion, 98
MMA (Minnesota Medical Association), 237
MNA (Minnesota Nurses Association), 237
MTP (Medical Termination of Pregnancy), 87

National Diabetes, 206
Newborn;
  Care, 232
New Parents;
  Help, 72
NFHS (National Family Health Survey), 286
Normal Body Changes, 54
Normal Childbirth, 1
Normal Labour;
  Stages, 43

Obsteric Emergency, 47
Optional Feeding Practices, 64
Oral Contraceptives, 169, 186
Ovarian Cancer, 203, 205
Ovaries, 130

Patient Education, 39
Physical Examination, 37
Politics Abortion, 87
Poor Nutrition, 186
Post-Delivery Care, 223
Postpartum Best Practices, 46
Postpartum Care, 236
PPD (Postpartum Depression), 53
PPH (Postpartum Hemorrhage), 47
  Risk, 58
  Management, 58
Pregnancy;
  Screening for Syphilis, 72
  Nutrition, 170
  Related Deaths, 95, 217
  Induced Hypertension, 33
Premature Delivery, 260
Premature for Births, 73
Premature Labour, 41
Premature Rupture of Membranes, 41
Prematurity Risk Factors, 38
Premenstrual Syndrome, 193
Previous Cesarean Section, 40
Primary Diabetic Prevention, 61
Prolonged Labour, 32
Prostate Cancer, 203, 205
Promote Family Planning, 34

Recurrent Abortion, 94
Recurrent Trauma, 99
Reproductive Health, 278
Reproductive Health Services;
  Components, 269
Retained Placenta, 48
Risk for Fetus, 13
Risks for;
  Baby, 18
  Mother, 12, 18

Safe Motherhood Indicators, 29
Safe Motherhood Services, 66
Secondary Infertility, 152
Selective Abortions, 103
Semen Examination, 138
Septic Abortion, 98
Shah, Shantilal, 87
Skin Cancer, 203, 205
SPA (Sperm Penetration Assay), 139
Spermatogeness, 135
Sperm Retrieval, 148
Sperm Washing, 148

Spontaneous Abortion Prognosis, 111
Support for Breastfeeding, 63
Systocia, 10

Test of Fertilization Potential, 140
Threatened Abortion, 97
Toe Twisting, 183
Tooth Decay, 215
Treatment for PCOs, 150
Tubal Patency, 145

Unassisted Childbirth, 63
Unexplained Infertility, 126
Unsafe Abortions, 94
Uterine Atony, 56
Uterine Massage, 59

Vaginal Birth after a Cesarean, 19
Vaginal Bleeding, 41
VBAC;
  Benefits, 20
  Risks, 20

What is Infertility?, 154
What is Intimacy?, 142
WHO (World Health Organisation), 31, 285
Why Emergency Oral Contraception?, 102
Women and Obesity, 323
Women and Welfare Benefits, 303
Women's Prime of Life;
  Diseases and Medical Conditions, 164
World Bank Project, 173